Nonalcoholic Fatty Liver Disease

Guest Editor

ARUN J. SANYAL, MBBS, MD

CLINICS IN LIVER DISEASE

www.liver.theclinics.com

Consulting Editor
NORMAN GITLIN, MD

August 2012 • Volume 16 • Number 3

SAUNDERS an imprint of ELSEVIER, Inc.

W.B. SAUNDERS COMPANY

A Division of Elsevier Inc.

1600 John F. Kennedy Boulevard, Suite 1800 • Philadelphia, PA 19103-2899

http://www.theclinics.com

CLINICS IN LIVER DISEASE Volume 16, Number 3
August 2012 ISSN 1089-3261, ISBN-13: 978-1-4557-4916-4

Editor: Kerry Holland

Clinics in Liver Disease (ISSN 1089-3261) is published quarterly by Elsevier Inc., 360 Park Avenue South, New York, NY 10010-1710. Months of issue are February, May, August, and November. Business and Editorial Offices: 1600 John F. Kennedy Blvd., Ste. 1800, Philadelphia, PA 19103-2899. Customer Service Office: 3251 Riverport Lane, Maryland Heights, MO 63043. Periodicals postage paid at New York, NY and additional mailing offices. Subscription prices are $271.00 per year (U.S. individuals), $134.00 per year (U.S. student/resident), $365.00 per year (U.S. institutions), $360.00 per year (foreign individuals), $185.00 per year (foreign student/resident), $440.00 per year (foreign instituitions), $313.00 per year (Canadian individuals), $185.00 per year (Canadian student/resident), and $440.00 per year (Canadian institutions). Foreign air speed delivery is included in all *Clinics* subscription prices. All prices are subject to change without notice. **POSTMASTER:** Send address changes to *Clinics in Liver Disease*, Elsevier Health Sciences Division, Subscription Customer Service, 3251 Riverport Lane, Maryland Heights, MO 63043. **Customer Service: Telephone: 1-800-654-2452 (U.S. and Canada); 314-447-8871 (outside U.S. and Canada). Fax: 314-447-8029. E-mail: journalscustomer service-usa@elsevier.com (for print support); journalsonlinesupport-usa@elsevier.com (for online support).**

Reprints. For copies of 100 or more of articles in this publication, please contact the Commercial Reprints Department, Elsevier Inc., 360 Park Avenue South, New York, NY 10010-1710. Tel.: 212-633-3812; Fax: 212-462-1935; E-mail: reprints@elsevier.com.

Clinics in Liver Disease is covered in *MEDLINE/PubMed (Index Medicus)*, Science Citation Index Expanded, Journal Citation Reports/Science Edition, and Current Contents/Clinical Medicine.

Printed and bound by CPI Group (UK) Ltd, Croydon, CR0 4YY
Transferred to Digital Print 2012

Contributors

GUEST EDITOR

ARUN J. SANYAL, MBBS, MD, FACP
Charles Caravati Professor of Medicine, Chairman, Division of Gastroenterology, Hepatology and Nutrition, VCU Medical Center, Richmond, Virginia

AUTHORS

PAUL ANGULO, MD
Professor of Medicine, Section Chief of Hepatology, Division of Digestive Diseases & Nutrition, Department of Medicine, University of Kentucky Medical Center, Lexington, Kentucky

BRITTANY N. BOHINC, MD
Fellow Physician, Department of Endocrinology, Diabetes, and Metabolism, Duke University Hospital, Durham, North Carolina

ANNA MAE DIEHL, MD
Florence McAlister Professor of Medicine, Chief, Division of Gastroenterology, Duke Liver Center, Duke University, Durham, North Carolina

MICHAEL FUCHS, MD, PhD, FEBG, AGAF
Associate Professor of Medicine, Division of Gastroenterology, Hepatology and Nutrition, Virginia Commonwealth University School of Medicine, Richmond, Virginia

JACOB GEORGE, MD, PhD
Professor, Storr Liver Unit, Westmead Millennium Institute; Department of Gastroenterology and Hepatology, University of Sydney, Westmead Hospital, Westmead, New South Wales, Australia

GARFIELD A. GRANDISON, MD
Clinical Fellow, Division of Digestive Diseases & Nutrition, Department of Medicine, University of Kentucky Medical Center, Lexington, Kentucky

EVELYN HSU, MD
Assistant Professor of Pediatrics, Division of Pediatric Gastroenterology and Hepatology, Seattle Children's Hospital, Seattle, Washington

SOLEDAD LARRAIN, MD
Visiting Physician Investigator, Division of Gastroenterology and Hepatology, Department of Medicine, Northwestern University Feinberg School of Medicine, Chicago, Illinois

JAMES L. LEVENSON, MD
Professor, Department of Psychiatry, Virginia Commonwealth University, Richmond, Virginia

SUZANNE E. MAHADY, MD
Storr Liver Unit, Westmead Millennium Institute, Department of Gastroenterology and Hepatology, University of Sydney, Westmead Hospital, Westmead; Sydney School of Public Health, University of Sydney, Camperdown, New South Wales, Australia

SCOTT C. MATHERLY, MD
Transplant Hepatology Fellow, Division of Gastroenterology, Hepatology and Nutrition, Department of Internal Medicine, Virginia Commonwealth University Medical Center, Richmond, Virginia

ARTHUR J. MCCULLOUGH, MD
Department of Gastroenterology and Hepatology, Cleveland Clinic Lerner College of Medicine at Case Western Reserve University, Cleveland Clinic, Cleveland, Ohio

KAREN MURRAY, MD
Professor of Pediatrics, Division Chair, Division of Pediatric Gastroenterology and Hepatology, Seattle Children's Hospital, Seattle, Washington

TOMMY PACANA, MD
Division of Gastroenterology, Hepatology and Nutrition, Virginia Commonwealth University School of Medicine, Richmond, Virginia

MANGESH R. PAGADALA, MD
Department of Gastroenterology and Hepatology, Cleveland Clinic, Cleveland, Ohio

CARLOS J. PIROLA, PhD, FAHA
Department of Molecular Genetics and Biology of Complex Diseases, Institute of Medical Research A Lanari-IDIM, University of Buenos Aires-National-Council of Scientific and Technological Research (CONICET), Ciudad Autónoma de Buenos Aires, Argentina

PUNEET PURI, MBBS, MD
Assistant Professor of Medicine, Division of Gastroenterology, Hepatology and Nutrition, Department of Internal Medicine, Virginia Commonwealth University Medical Center, Richmond, Virginia

MARY E. RINELLA, MD
Associate Professor of Medicine, Division of Gastroenterology and Hepatology, Department of Medicine, Northwestern University Feinberg School of Medicine, Chicago, Illinois

SILVIA SOOKOIAN, MD, PhD
Department of Clinical and Molecular Hepatology, Institute of Medical Research A Lanari-IDIM, University of Buenos Aires-National Council of Scientific and Technological Research (CONICET), Ciudad Autónoma de Buenos Aires, Argentina

KAREN E. STEWART, PhD
Assistant Professor, Department of Psychiatry, Virginia Commonwealth University, Richmond, Virginia

Contents

Preface   ix

Arun J. Sanyal

**The Genetic Epidemiology of Nonalcoholic Fatty Liver Disease: Toward a
Personalized Medicine**   467

Silvia Sookoian and Carlos J. Pirola

> The understanding of the genetic bases of complex diseases such as non-
> alcoholic fatty liver disease opens new opportunities and challenges. This
> article explores new tools designed toward moving genomic data into clin-
> ical medicine, providing putative answers to more practical questions.

**The Relevance of Liver Histology to Predicting Clinically Meaningful Outcomes in
Nonalcoholic Steatohepatitis**   487

Mangesh R. Pagadala and Arthur J. McCullough

> Nonalcoholic fatty liver disease (NAFLD) has emerged as the most preva-
> lent chronic liver disease. Nonalcoholic steatohepatitis (NASH), the more
> severe form of NAFLD, has an increased risk for progression to cirrhosis.
> The available data suggest increased morbidity and mortality among those
> patients with advanced histologic severity such as NASH and fibrosis.
> Despite the lack of a universally accepted histologic definition of NAFLD
> and inconsistency among pathologists regarding histologic findings es-
> sential to the diagnosis of NASH, a few studies have identified specific his-
> tologic findings (particularly fibrosis regardless of stage) that are able to
> predict NAFLD-related mortality as being most important.

Mechanisms of Simple Hepatic Steatosis: Not So Simple After All   505

Scott C. Matherly and Puneet Puri

> Nonalcoholic fatty liver disease is becoming an epidemic. Fat is typically
> stored in adipose tissue in the form of triglycerides (TGs). The deposition
> of TGs in the liver is the result of an imbalance between the amount of en-
> ergy taken in and the amount used. This balance is maintained by a com-
> plex interplay between the dietary intake of nutrients, the hormonal
> response to the nutrients, and their effect on both the liver and adipose tis-
> sue. Disruption of this system is what leads to the development of steato-
> sis and is the focus of this article.

A Myriad of Pathways to NASH   525

Soledad Larrain and Mary E. Rinella

> Nonalcoholic steatohepatitis (NASH) is defined histopathologically by
> the presence of macrovesicular steatosis, cellular ballooning, and inflam-
> mation. NASH represents a complex multifactorial disease that typically
> occurs within the context of the metabolic syndrome. NASH lacks homo-
> geneity, and other forms of NASH can present atypically. Less than 50% of

patients with NASH respond to pharmacologic treatment, which speaks to this heterogeneity. The authors discuss drugs, disease entities, and nutritional states that can cause or exacerbate underlying NASH indirectly through worsening insulin resistance or directly by interfering with lipid metabolism, promoting oxidative injury, or activating inflammatory pathways.

Mechanisms of Disease Progression in NASH: New Paradigms   549

Brittany N. Bohinc and Anna Mae Diehl

The incidence of nonalcoholic fatty liver disease is increasing at an astonishing rate in the US population. Although only a small proportion of these patients develop steatohepatitis (NASH), those who do have a greater likelihood of developing end-stage liver disease and complications. Research on liver fibrosis and NASH progression shows that hedgehog (Hh) is reactivated after liver injury to assist in liver repair and regeneration. When the process of tissue repair and regeneration is prolonged or when Hh ligand and related genes are aberrantly regulated and excessive, tissue repair goes awry and NASH progresses to cirrhosis and hepatocellular carcinoma.

Can Nash Be Diagnosed, Graded, and Staged Noninvasively?   567

Garfield A. Grandison and Paul Angulo

Nonalcoholic bland steatosis and nonalcoholic steatohepatitis (NASH) are stages in the spectrum of nonalcoholic fatty liver disease (NAFLD). NASH may progress to end-stage liver disease. Liver biopsy distinguishes between patients with NASH and no NASH and can stage fibrosis. Markers of hepatocyte apoptosis hold promise as noninvasive tests for NASH diagnosis. Several scoring systems that combine routine clinical and laboratory variables and some proprietary panels can assist in predicting fibrosis severity. Noninvasive imaging modalities are reasonably accurate available tools to determine severity of fibrosis in NAFLD, but none of them yet can replace liver biopsy.

Is Nonalcoholic Fatty Liver Disease in Children the Same Disease as in Adults?   587

Evelyn Hsu and Karen Murray

Nonalcoholic fatty liver disease (NAFLD) is the leading cause of chronic liver disease in children, and can present in toddlerhood. There is a differential distribution of NAFLD in children based on race and gender. The gold standard for diagnosis and classification of pediatric NAFLD is liver biopsy although ongoing studies aim to identify and define noninvasive investigations for pediatric NAFLD. Treatments that have been shown to be successful in adult NAFLD, such as insulin sensitizers and Vitamin E, have not been proven to be as definitively successful in children with NAFLD.

The Cardiovascular Link to Nonalcoholic Fatty Liver Disease: A Critical Analysis   599

Tommy Pacana and Michael Fuchs

Nonalcoholic fatty liver disease (NAFLD) is the most common chronic liver disease in Western countries and can progress from simple steatosis to nonalcoholic steatohepatitis and finally to liver cirrhosis. NAFLD is considered to be the hepatic manifestation of the metabolic syndrome because both share common features, which implicates a role of NAFLD in the development and progression of cardiovascular disease (CVD). The diagnosis of NAFLD deserves special attention in clinical practice for cardiovascular risk screening and surveillance strategies to allow for early targeted intervention in selected individuals at risk of future cardiovascular events.

Psychological and Psychiatric Aspects of Treatment of Obesity and Nonalcoholic Fatty Liver Disease

615

Karen E. Stewart and James L. Levenson

Chronic illnesses incur a tremendous cost to American lives in dollars and quality of life. Outcomes in these illnesses are often affected by psychological, behavioral, and pharmacologic issues related to mental illness and psychological symptoms. This article focuses on psychological and psychiatric issues related to the treatment of obesity and nonalcoholic fatty liver disease (NAFLD), including available weight-loss interventions, the complex relationship between psychiatric disorders and obesity, and special considerations regarding use of psychiatric drugs in patients with or at risk for NAFLD and obesity. Recommendations for collaborative care of individuals with comorbid NAFLD and psychological disorders/symptoms are discussed.

Management of Nonalcoholic Steatohepatitis: An Evidence-Based Approach

631

Suzanne E. Mahady and Jacob George

Nonalcoholic fatty liver disease (NAFLD) and its progressive form, nonalcoholic steatohepatitis (NASH), are an increasingly common cause of chronic liver disease in the developed world, with NASH projected to be the leading cause of liver transplantation in the United States by 2020. This review of NASH management addresses current data from the perspective of levels of evidence for therapeutic options in NASH, including lifestyle modification, drug therapies, and bariatric surgery. In particular, behavioral therapies to assist patients in adopting lifestyle changes are highlighted and a research agenda for future NASH management is presented.

Index **647**

CLINICS IN LIVER DISEASE

FORTHCOMING ISSUES

November 2012
Alcoholic Liver Disease
David Bernstein, MD, *Guest Editor*

February 2013
Novel and Combination Therapies for HCV
Paul J. Pockros, MD, *Guest Editor*

May 2013
Cholestatic Liver Diseases
Cynthia Levy, MD, *Guest Editor*

RECENT ISSUES

May 2012
Approach to Consultations for Patients with Liver Disease
Steven L. Flamm, MD, *Guest Editor*

February 2012
Hepatic Encephalopathy: An Update
Kevin D. Mullen, MD, FRCPI and
Ravi K. Prakash, MBBS, MD, MRCP (UK),
Guest Editors

November 2011
Liver Transplant: Reaching the Half Century
Cynthia Levy, MD, and Paul Martin, MD,
Guest Editors

RELATED INTEREST

Neurologic Clinics, February 2010, (Vol. 28, No. 1)
Neurology and Systemic Disease
Alireza Minagar, *Guest Editor*

NOW AVAILABLE FOR YOUR iPhone and iPad

Preface

Advances and Evolving Concepts in Nonalcoholic Fatty Liver Disease

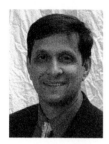

Arun J. Sanyal, MBBS, MD
Guest Editor

The field of nonalcoholic steatohepatitis (NASH) continues to evolve rapidly. This issue of *Clinics in Liver Disease* captures many of the advances and evolving concepts that will be relevant for clinicians who take care of patients with nonalcoholic fatty liver disease. In an era where personalized medicine is not just a concept but a reality in many areas, such as the use of IL-28 gene status to determine therapeutic strategies for hepatitis C, there has been remarkable advances in the understanding of the genetic predisposition to NASH and activation of disease pathways relevant to disease progression. These are comprehensively reviewed by Dr Sookian. There is considerable sampling variability with liver biopsies and there are intra- and interobserver variability in assessment of liver histology that confound evaluation of the role of liver biopsies in defining prognosis in NASH. The controversies associated with this subject are thoughtfully reviewed by Dr McCullough. The limitations of liver biopsies and their interpretation are driving research to developing noninvasive biomarkers that can identify those with disease and its progression versus regression. The current state of the art is summarized lucidly by Dr Angulo. It is also now appreciated that the liver has a limited repertoire for expressing a disease phenotype and that steatosis and liver injury can result from a multitude of molecular pathways. Clinical scenarios that can cause NASH but are not classically related to obesity-related NASH and their associated pathophysiology are reviewed by Dr Rinella. Advances in the understanding of classical steatosis and disease progression are also reviewed with a view toward providing translational insights into how this knowledge can be used to prevent or treat the disease in the future. The critical role of behavioral factors that drive eating and exercise behaviors and the impact of drugs used to treat such conditions are often underplayed in the clinical literature. A very practical and clinically relevant analysis

Clin Liver Dis 16 (2012) ix–x
doi:10.1016/j.cld.2012.06.001
1089-3261/12/$ – see front matter © 2012 Elsevier Inc. All rights reserved.

of these conditions is provided to help clinicians manage patients in their practice along with a state-of-the-art review of best practices in the management of NASH. We believe that this compilation of reviews will bring practicing clinicians in both academic and community settings up to date with the major advances in the field and will enhance their clinical practice.

Arun J. Sanyal, MBBS, MD
Charles Caravati Professor of Medicine
Chairman, Division of Gastroenterology, Hepatology and Nutrition
VCU Medical Center, West Hospital, 14th Floor
West Wing, PO Box 980341
Richmond, VA 23298, USA

E-mail address:
asanyal@mcvh-vcu.edu

The Genetic Epidemiology of Nonalcoholic Fatty Liver Disease
Toward a Personalized Medicine

Silvia Sookoian, MD, PhD[a,*], Carlos J. Pirola, PhD[b,*]

KEYWORDS

- Nonalcoholic fatty liver disease • Nonalcoholic steatohepatitis • Adiponutrin
- PNPLA3 • Epigenetics • Systems biology • Genetics • Drug targets

KEY POINTS

- Nonalcoholic fatty liver disease (NAFLD) is a complex disorder that develops from the interplay of a myriad of genetic and environmental factors.
- Until some years ago, the most helpful strategy in the search for genes underlying complex diseases such as NAFLD was to look at candidate genes.
- The knowledge of the genetic bases of NAFLD has tremendously benefited from recent advances in genotyping technology and information generated by genome-wide association studies.
- Now, systems biology offers the opportunity to get more insight in its pathophysiology and opens new avenues for novel treatments.

INTRODUCTION

This review, very far from the collected and summarized information about the current knowledge of the genetic epidemiology of nonalcoholic fatty liver disease (NAFLD), attempts to build new integrated ways to understand the genetic architecture of the

Funding: This study was partially supported by grants PICT 2008-1521 and PICT 2010-0441 (Agencia Nacional de Promoción Científica y Tecnológica), and UBACYT CM04 (Universidad de Buenos Aires). S.S. and C.J.P. belong to Consejo Nacional de Investigaciones Científicas (CONICET).
Disclosures: None.
[a] Department of Clinical and Molecular Hepatology, Institute of Medical Research A Lanari-IDIM, University of Buenos Aires–National Council of Scientific and Technological Research (CONICET), Combatientes de Malvinas 3150 Ciudad Autónoma de Buenos Aires-1427, Argentina; [b] Department of Molecular Genetics and Biology of Complex Diseases, Institute of Medical Research A Lanari-IDIM, University of Buenos Aires–National-Council of Scientific and Technological Research (CONICET), Combatientes de Malvinas 3150 Ciudad Autónoma de Buenos Aires-1427, Argentina
* Corresponding authors. Instituto de Investigaciones Médicas A. Lanari-IDM CONICET, Combatiente de Malvinas 3150, Buenos Aires (1427), Argentina.
E-mail addresses: sookoian.silvia@lanari.fmed.uba.ar; pirola.carlos@lanari.fmed.uba.ar

Clin Liver Dis 16 (2012) 467–485
doi:10.1016/j.cld.2012.05.011
1089-3261/12/$ – see front matter © 2012 Elsevier Inc. All rights reserved.

disease. Hence, based on current knowledge about a disease-associated *PNPLA3* gene variant, the authors postulate new paradigms of NAFLD pathogenesis. Also proposed is a systems biology approach in the search of joining effects of genetic variants from multiple pathways. Based on the information of previously reported loci associated with the genetic risk of NAFLD, candidate genes from the entire genome are prioritized to show putative unexplored genes as potential modifiers of the biology of the disease. An important question is whether it is possible to rapidly translate the knowledge about genetic susceptibility of NAFLD into more individualized decision making and personalized medicine. If so, can the diagnostic and therapeutic strategies be improved? This article attempts to answer whether disease-associated gene variants can help select therapeutic targets. Therefore, an effort is made to translate the current findings of NAFLD-associated gene-risk variants into therapeutic target identification. Finally, the article further explores DNA sequence variation to introduce relevant knowledge about the role of epigenetics in NAFLD.

Nonalcoholic fatty liver disease (NAFLD) is a complex disorder that develops from the interplay of a myriad of genetic and environmental factors. This concept clearly characterizes the nature of the disease as highly heterogeneous and influenced by multiple critical pathways. The challenge, as well the prospect of the genomic era, lies in the ability to integrate all the information about the genetic components of a disease to better understand its pathogenesis as well as its treatment strategies.

Until some years ago, the most helpful strategy in the search for genes underlying complex diseases such as NAFLD was to look at candidate genes. The candidate genes for NAFLD were then selected based either on their known or presumed function or on their biological plausibility in the disease pathophysiology; a recent comprehensive review summarizes the major findings on candidate-gene association studies in NAFLD.[1] Most candidate-gene association studies showed a small effect on the susceptibility of developing fatty liver, and a few of them demonstrated an effect on disease progression.[2–5]

The knowledge of the genetic bases of NAFLD has tremendously benefited from recent advances in genotyping technology and information generated by genome-wide association studies (GWAS). In fact, the first GWAS on NAFLD[6] has not only expanded our knowledge about the genetic component of the disease but has also contributed to the understanding about the role of genes on the histologic severity.[7] In this particular GWAS, differing from the most common genome scans, Romeo and colleagues[6] specifically surveyed nonsynonymous sequence variations along the entire genome. As a result, the missense rs738409 C/G single-nucleotide polymorphism (SNP) implying an amino acid change from isoleucine (I) to methionine (M) at the position 148 (I148M) of the protein encoding by the patatin-like phospholipase domain–containing 3 gene (*PNPLA3*), also known as adiponutrin, was strongly associated with increased hepatic fat content measured by ^{1}H magnetic resonance spectroscopy. After further replication in several populations around the world, including adults and children, the G allele in the forward strand was significantly and unequivocally associated with increased risk of hepatic triglyceride accumulation and fatty liver disease, as shown in a recent meta-analysis.[7] In fact, carriers of the GG homozygous genotype show 73% higher lipid fat content than do carriers of the CC genotype. Surprisingly, even though ethnic differences in the susceptibility to NAFLD are evident,[8] the effect of the *PNPLA3* variant transcends racial or ethnic boundaries, as Asian and Caucasians have an almost identical effect (odds ratio [OR] 3.26 vs 3.11). A significantly higher effect was demonstrated in females, however, than in males, a sexual dimorphism discussed later.[7] In conclusion, the risk effect of the rs738409 on developing fatty liver is perhaps one of the strongest ever reported for a common variant modifying the genetic susceptibility for complex diseases (explaining 5.3% of the total variance), and seems to follow an additive model, at least for liver fatty accumulation.[7]

Moreover, the rs738409 is nowadays the most replicated gene variant in the study of the genetic component of disease severity as, after pooling liver biopsies of 2124 NAFLD patients, nonalcoholic steatohepatitis (NASH) was more frequently observed in GG than in CC homozygous carriers (OR 3.488, 95% confidence interval [CI] 1.859–6.545; data from 2124 patients).[7] Even more surprising is that a large body of literature about replication studies of *PNPLA3* and NAFLD is constantly generated, with more articles published annually than the entire evidence accumulated until now about candidate-gene association studies for this disease. Thus, the enthusiasm about newly discovered loci has vanished and the newly discovered rs738409 SNP far more widely covered than the previously proposed candidate genes.

Although no doubts exist about the impact of the rs738409 on the natural history of NAFLD, several important questions still remain unanswered and some other questions could be resolved, based on the current knowledge about the impact of the *PNPLA3* variant on NAFLD; this review introduces some ideas on this matter.

PNPLA3 AND NAFLD: FROM GENES TO DISEASE PATHOGENESIS. *PNPLA3* AND THE LIVER "FAT REMODELING" HYPOTHESIS

Considering that NAFLD is a polygenic and multifactorial disease that results from complex interactions among multiple genetic factors in addition to a collection of environmental exposures, it makes probably no sense to attribute to *PNPLA3* the whole burden of the genetic risk of the disease. Thus, the first question to arise after the findings of the NAFLD GWAS is how a single variant in a single gene is able to cause, by itself, such a strong impact on the biology of the disease. Certainly SNPs that alter the coding sequence and result in a nonsynonymous change have more chance of leading to a pronounced effect in the protein function that markedly affects the disease or trait of interest. That would be case for the rs738409, which involves a coding variant that encodes the amino acid substitution I148M; this change in the amino acid sequence seems to cause a loss of protein function, altering the hydrolysis of glycerolipids, more popularly known as fatty acid triesters of glycerol or triacylglycerols (TAG).[9]

One may wonder whether the disruption of the hydrolysis of glycerolipids is so important in the context of NAFLD. Previous evidence showed that defects or perturbations in the hydrolysis of glycerolipids (both neutral and phospholipids) are associated with the cluster of metabolic disorders, characteristics of the metabolic syndrome, including type 2 diabetes, obesity, and NAFLD.[10]

The hydrolysis of TAG to diacylglycerol (DAG) is primarily achieved by the enzyme PNPLA2 and putatively by PNPLA3.[11] In fact, there is a group of genes (PNPLA1 to PNPLA9) that encode for proteins (enzymes) containing a patatin-like domain with broad lipid acyl-hydrolase activity and with specificities for diverse substrates such as triacylglycerols, phospholipids, and retinol esters.[12] In this regard the strong effect of the rs738409 variant is surprising, considering that the PNPLA3 protein shares domains with several family members and is coexpressed with PTGES (prostaglandin E synthase). In silico function prediction of the *PNPLA3* gene[13] shows that only PNPLA2, PNPLA3, PNPLA8, and PLA2G6 have carboxylesterase and lipase activities ($P<4.8$ and 9.4×10^{-5}) and PNPLA3, PNPLA8, and PLA2G6 have phospholipase A2 activity ($P<1.6 \times 10^{-4}$), indicating that the release of arachidonic acid and its product, prostaglandin E_2, may have a role in the pathogenesis of NAFLD. Supporting this observation, Puri and colleagues[14] recently showed that NASH is associated with increased levels of the proinflammatory product 15-hydroxyeicosatetraenoic acid (HETE) and 11-HETE, a nonenzymatic oxidation product of arachidonic acid.

In addition, neutral lipid, triglyceride, or glycerolipid catabolic processes are shared by only PNPLA2 and PNPLA3 ($P<.05$). Although these aspects deserve further investigation, the functional redundancy explained previously can also explain the paradoxic results observed in mice with global targeted deletion of *Pnpla3*, which do not reproduce the biological effect reported in humans.[15,16]

The hallmark feature of NAFLD is the abnormal accumulation of TAG and DAG in the hepatocytes. The evidence showed that stored hepatic TAG are largely hydrolyzed to DAG and then reesterified before being secreted as very-low-density lipoprotein TAG.[17] In this process, there is a critical step of remodeling of DAGs, which are reesterified to TAG before being secreted. Overall, these data may support the hypothesis proposed by Jenkins and colleagues[18] suggesting that PNPLA3 might stimulate triacylglycerol/fatty acid cycling (fatty acid reesterification). Taking into account this evidence, it is reasonable to speculate that PNPLA3 plays a role in hepatic lipid partitioning while also bearing in mind that DAG is a potent activator of protein kinases C (PKCs) with potential metabolic effects per se, as activation of some conventional and novel PKCs in response to increased levels of DAG have been shown to counteract insulin signaling.[19] Hence, in this scenario and considering the strong impact of rs738409 on the natural history of NAFLD, the contribution of the knowledge of the disease-associated genes, at least but not last, leads one to advice about changing the paradigm of the NAFLD pathogenesis and starting to revise the "2-hit hypothesis" to explain the molecular events triggering the disease. Supporting this notion, recent evidence clearly showed that changes in lipid partitioning in the liver are associated with an increase in liver cell apoptosis,[20] a common finding in patients and rodent models of NAFLD.[21,22]

PNPLA3 AND GENE BY SEX INTERACTION: DOES THE RS738409 VARIANT EXPLAIN SEXUAL DIMORPHISM OF NAFLD?

As a final comment, the findings about the rs738409 brought new answers to poorly explored questions, for instance, the role of sexual dimorphism in the pathogenesis of NAFLD. As already mentioned, meta-regression analysis of pooled data from all the published evidence showed a negative association between the effect of rs738409 on liver fat content and the proportion of male individuals in the studied populations.[7] Despite the explanation of this gene by sex interaction still being unknown, one may speculate that the effect of *PNPLA3* and, putatively, the rs738409 risk variant may be modulated by sex hormones. This explanation is in agreement with previous evidence that PNPLA3 levels are strongly influenced by metabolic status and hormones, such as insulin.[23] Reinforcing the previous concept about the role of PNPLA3 on lipid remodeling, sexual hormones, such as estrogen, modulate lipogenic genes, including *SREBP-1c*, and participate in adiposity and fuel partitioning.[24]

NAFLD AND GENETIC SUSCEPTIBILITY: SYSTEMS BIOLOGY APPROACHES AND THE SEARCH OF JOINING EFFECTS OF GENETIC VARIANTS FROM MULTIPLE PATHWAYS

As summarized earlier, several SNPs in different genes or loci have been proposed as potential modifiers (albeit modest) of the genetic risk of NAFLD, even though the mechanism behind the association between the associated gene variant and the disease may be unknown. Instead of understanding the effect of each reported variant independently, one should consider integration of the current knowledge about the genetic influence of NAFLD into common pathways of the disease, and ask whether common regulatory pathways or common physiologic processes link the pathophysiology of NAFLD with the metabolic syndrome.

To answer these questions, the authors used systems biology approaches to integrate genomic, molecular, and physiologic data to decipher putative pathways that connect all the available information about genes suspected to play a role in the susceptibility of NAFLD. This approach is designed to analyze and integrate genomic, transcriptomic, and/or proteomic data to inferred from genetic signals–related pathways of disease. Furthermore, systems biology introduces a new concept for revealing the pathogenesis of human disorders, and suggests that the presence of common physiologic processes and molecular networks influences the risk of a disease.

Based on this hypothesis, different systems biology approaches were proposed, such as gene-enrichment analysis and the use of a protein-protein interaction network.

For this purpose, the authors built a candidate gene list using as template the published evidence about the genetic component of NAFLD from all the candidate-gene association studies, including *PNPLA3* (the input gene list is given in **Table 1**). The list includes 58 reported loci with variants associated with either fatty liver or NASH, as mentioned previously.[1]

Functional enrichment analysis of the gene list was performed by the bioinformatic resource ToppGene Suite (http://toppgene.cchmc.org) and ToppCluster (http://toppcluster.cchmc.org/), based on Transcriptome, Proteome, Regulome (TFBS and miRNA), Ontologies (GO, Pathway), Phenotype (human disease and mouse phenotype), Pharmacome (Drug-Gene associations), literature cocitation, and other features. The analysis showed that the 58 reported loci could be integrated into several common functional pathways, of which the highly ranked are shown in **Fig. 1**. The predicted pathways are mainly enriched with mechanisms of cellular control of lipid and lipoprotein metabolism. Thus, the associated genes strongly suggest the role of lipotoxicity in the pathogenesis of NAFLD. Moreover, as shown in **Table 2**, highly predicted biological processes were observed, most of them related to the regulation of lipid homeostasis and the cellular lipid metabolic process, and whereby *PNPLA3* was jointly included with other related genes.

Gene-enrichment analysis also detected common physiologic processes that potentially link the pathophysiology of NAFLD with the metabolic syndrome; for example, 3 pathways were predicted that are involved in cardiovascular system regulation (see **Table 2**).

In addition, a functional association analysis was performed that included protein and genetic interactions, pathways, coexpression, colocalization, and protein domain similarity, using the bioinformatic resource GenMANIA.[13] Several genes are regarded as direct "neighbors" of the *PNPLA3* considering coexpression or colocalization, physical interactions, belonging to the same pathways, or having shared protein domains (**Fig. 2**). Most of them are not obvious *PNPLA3*-related genes, but then again, some interesting associations with prostaglandin-endoperoxide synthases (ie, *PTGS2*) emerged that may explain the beneficial effect of indomethacin on the liver fat accumulation observed in an experimental rodent model of NAFLD.[25]

GENE PRIORITIZATION BASED ON PREVIOUS REPORTED LOCI SHOWS NUCLEAR RECEPTORS AND HYPOXIA AS MOLECULAR MEDIATORS OF NAFLD PATHOGENESIS

As already mentioned, the enthusiasm about the discovery of novel loci associated with NAFLD is nowadays vanishing, and this could have a negative impact on our ability

Table 1
Candidate gene list based on the published evidence about the genetic component of NAFLD

Gene Symbol	Ensembl ID	Gene Name Description
PEMT	ENSG00000133027	Phosphatidylethanolamine N-methyltransferase
MTTP	ENSG00000138823	Microsomal triglyceride transfer protein large subunit precursor
APOC3	ENSG00000110245	Apolipoprotein C-III precursor (Apo-CIII)
NR1I2	ENSG00000144852	Orphan nuclear receptor PXR (pregnane X receptor)
FABP2	ENSG00000145384	Fatty acid-binding protein, intestinal
DGAT1	ENSG00000185000	Diacylglycerol O-acyltransferase 1
DGAT2	ENSG00000062282	Diacylglycerol O-acyltransferase 2
ACSL4	ENSG00000068366	Long-chain-fatty-acid–CoA ligase 4
ADRB3	ENSG00000188778	β3-Adrenergic receptor (β3 adrenoceptor)
ADRB2	ENSG00000169252	β2-Adrenergic receptor (β2 adrenoceptor)
LIPC	ENSG00000166035	Hepatic triacylglycerol lipase precursor
APOE	ENSG00000130203	Apolipoprotein E precursor (Apo-E)
CLOCK	ENSG00000134852	Circadian locomotor output cycles protein kaput
ENPP1	ENSG00000197594	Ectonucleotide pyrophosphatase/phosphodiesterase 1
IRS1	ENSG00000169047	Insulin receptor substrate 1
ADIPOQ	ENSG00000181092	Adiponectin precursor
ADIPOR1	ENSG00000159346	Adiponectin receptor protein 1
ADIPOR2	ENSG00000006831	Adiponectin receptor protein 2
PPARA	ENSG00000186951	Peroxisome proliferator-activated receptor α
PPARG	ENSG00000132170	Peroxisome proliferator-activated receptor γ
PPARGC1A	ENSG00000109819	Peroxisome proliferator-activated receptor γ coactivator 1α
TCF7L2	ENSG00000148737	Transcription factor 7-like 2
GCKR	ENSG00000084734	Glucokinase regulatory protein
MC4R	ENSG00000166603	Melanocortin receptor 4
SPINK1	ENSG00000164266	Pancreatic secretory trypsin inhibitor precursor
LEPR	ENSG00000116678	Leptin receptor precursor
TNF	ENSG00000204490	Tumor necrosis factor precursor (TNF-α)
TNFSF10	ENSG00000121858	Tumor necrosis factor ligand superfamily member 10
IL6	ENSG00000136244	Interleukin-6 precursor
CD14	ENSG00000170458	Monocyte differentiation antigen CD14 precursor
GCLC	ENSG00000001084	Glutamate–cysteine ligase catalytic subunit
SOD2	ENSG00000112096	Superoxide dismutase [Mn], mitochondrial precursor
HFE	ENSG00000010704	Hereditary hemochromatosis protein precursor (HLA-H)
UGT1A1	ENSG00000167165	UDP-glucuronosyltransferase 1–8 precursor
UCP1	ENSG00000109424	Mitochondrial brown fat uncoupling protein 1
PTGS2	ENSG00000073756	Prostaglandin G/H synthase 2 precursor
ABCB11	ENSG00000073734	Bile salt export pump (ATP-binding cassette subfamily B member 11)
MIF	ENSG00000099964	Macrophage migration inhibitory factor
CYP2E1	ENSG00000130649	Cytochrome P450 2E1
SERPINA1	ENSG00000197249	α1-Antitrypsin precursor

(continued on next page)

Table 1
(continued)

Gene Symbol	Ensembl ID	Gene Name Description
MTHFR	ENSG00000177000	Methylene tetrahydrofolate reductase
IL1B	ENSG00000125538	Interleukin-1β precursor
TLR4	ENSG00000136869	Toll-like receptor 4 precursor
CFTR	ENSG00000001626	Cystic fibrosis transmembrane conductance regulator
STAT3	ENSG00000168610	Signal transducer and activator of transcription 3
AGTR1	ENSG00000144891	Type-1 angiotensin II receptor
KLF6	ENSG00000067082	Krueppel-like factor 6
PNPLA3	ENSG00000100344	Adiponutrin (iPLA2-ε) (calcium-independent phospholipase A2ε) (Patatin-like phospholipase domain-containing protein 3)
FDFT1	ENSG00000079459	Squalene synthetase
COL13A1	ENSG00000197467	α1 type XIII collagen isoform 1
PDGFA	ENSG00000197461	Platelet-derived growth factor A chain precursor
LTBP3	ENSG00000168056	Latent-transforming growth factor β–binding protein 3 precursor
EFCAB4B	ENSG00000130038	EF-hand calcium binding domain 4B
NCAN	ENSG00000130287	Neurocan core protein precursor
LYPLAL1	ENSG00000143353	Lysophospholipase-like protein 1
GCKR	ENSG00000084734	Glucokinase (hexokinase 4) regulator 1
PPP1R3B	ENSG00000173281	Protein phosphatase 1, regulatory (inhibitor) subunit 3B

to better understand the disease pathogenesis. Hence, the already known associated disease loci might serve as a template to look further for gene variants involved in the disease susceptibility. This approach benefits from examining previously proposed candidate gene loci in a more systematic manner. For this reason, the authors performed a comprehensive analysis of candidate regions generated by the freely accessible ENDEAVOUR software available at http://homes.esat.kuleuven.be/~bioiuser/endeavor/endeavor.php, which specifically focused on the previous loci reported to be associated with NAFLD susceptibility (see **Table 1**).

ENDEAVOUR is a software application for the computational prioritization of candidate genes underlying biological processes or diseases, based on their similarity to known genes involved in a disease as previously described.[26] The hypothesis of prioritization by ENDEAVOUR is that candidate test genes are ranked based on their similarity with a set of known training genes. This attractive methodology allows performance of gene prioritization based on the biological plausibility of a gene-disease association and on the knowledge of the protein function. In addition, this strategy allows expansion of the selection of putative candidate genes and prediction of new targets, as the authors have reported previously for other components of the metabolic syndrome.[27] Surprisingly, a prioritized list of candidate genes, along with the rankings per data source, showed interesting loci never previously explored that could be tested for gene-associated risk variants (**Fig. 3**). For instance, the results of gene prioritization ranked very highly 2 nuclear receptors, the *NR1H4* or farnesoid X nuclear receptor, a ligand-activated transcription factor that functions as a receptor for bile acids such as chenodeoxycholic acid, lithocholic acid, and deoxycholic acid, and the *RXRA* or retinoid X receptor, a nuclear receptor that mediates the biological

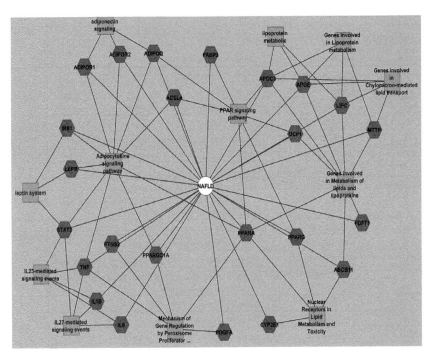

Fig. 1. Functional enrichment analysis of loci previously associated with NAFLD: predicted disease pathways. Disease pathways were obtained by the Toppcluster tool, and the analysis was based on combined data from the following resources: BioCyc, GenMAPP, KEGG pathway, MSigDB: C2.cp—BioCarta, MSigDB: C2.cp—Reactome, 430MSigDB: C2.cp— Sigma-Aldrich, MSigDB: C2.cp—Signaling Gateway, MSigDB: C2.cp—Signaling Transduction KE, MSigDB: C2.cp—SuperArray, NCI-Nature Curated, PantherDB, Pathway Ontology, SMPDB. List of pathway IDs in the figure: Adipocytokine signaling pathway, hsa04920; Adiponectin signaling, PW:0000563; PPAR signaling pathway, hsa03320; Nuclear receptors in lipid metabolism and toxicity, BIOCARTA NUCLEAR RS PATHWAY; Genes involved in chylomicron-mediated lipid transport, REACTOME CHYLOMICRON-MEDIATED LIPID TRANSPORT; Genes involved in the metabolism of lipids and lipoproteins, REACTOME METABOLISM OF LIPIDS AND LIPOPROTEINS; IL27-mediated signaling events, il27pathway; Genes involved in lipoprotein metabolism, REACTOME LIPOPROTEIN METABOLISM; Mechanism of gene regulation by peroxisome proliferators via PPARα, BIOCARTA PPARA PATHWAY; Leptin system, PW:0000363; Lipoprotein metabolic, PW:0000482; IL23-mediated signaling events, il23pathway.

effects of retinoids by their involvement in retinoic acid-mediated gene activation. This information is a reminder of the important role the bile acids might have in the regulation of lipid homeostasis,[28] and suggests that these candidate genes may be attractive pharmacologic targets. It should be emphasized that bile acids may act through the elevation of incretins,[29] and this family of substances has been proved to be effective in improving NAFLD.[30]

Moreover, the data mining also identified *HIF1A* (hypoxia-inducible factor 1, α subunit), a transcription factor involved in the regulation of cellular response to hypoxia. Hypoxia is a pathogenic disease pathway largely ignored in NAFLD, but is now recognized as a putative mediator of initial metabolic changes in the liver[21,22] and in the progression of inflammation and liver damage.[31,32] Other examples that are worth noting are *HNF4A*, a type 2 diabetes–associated gene,[33] members of the

Table 2
Functional enrichment analysis of NAFLD candidate genes associated loci: predicted biological process

Gene Ontology (GO) ID	GO: Biological Process	Gene List
GO:0030730	Sequestering of triglyceride	ENPP1 IL1B PPARA PPARG TNF
GO:0006641	Triglyceride metabolic process	ACSL4 APOC3 APOE DGAT1 DGAT2 LIPC MTTP **PNPLA3**
GO:0008610	Lipid biosynthetic process	ABCB11 ACSL4 APOC3 APOE CFTR DGAT1 DGAT2 FDFT1 LIPC MIF PDGFA PEMT **PNPLA3** PTGS2 TNF
GO:0045834	Positive regulation of lipid metabolic process	ADIPOQ AGTR1 APOE IL1B IRS1 PPARA PPARG PPARGC1A PTGS2 TNF
GO:0009891	Positive regulation of biosynthetic process	ADRB2 APOE CLOCK IL1B IL6 IRS1 KLF6 MC4R NR1I2 PDGFA PPARA PPARG PPARGC1A PTGS2 SOD2 STAT3 TCF7L2 TLR4 TNF
GO:0006869Ii	Lipid transport	ACSL4 ADIPOQ APOC3 APOE CFTR FABP2 IL1B LIPC MTTP PPARA PPARG
GO:0045598	Regulation of fat cell differentiation	ADIPOQ ENPP1 IL6 PPARG PTGS2 SOD2 TNF
GO:0009893	Positive regulation of metabolic process	ADIPOQ ADRB2 ADRB3 AGTR1 APOE CLOCK GCKR GCLC IL1B IL6 IRS1 KLF6 MC4R MIF NR1I2 PDGFA PEMT PPARA PPARG PPARGC1A PTGS2 SOD2 STAT3 TCF7L2 TLR4 TNF
GO:0044255	Cellular lipid metabolic process	ACSL4 ADIPOQ ADIPOR1 ADIPOR2 AGTR1 APOC3 APOE CYP2E1 DGAT1 DGAT2 FABP2 FDFT1 IRS1 LIPC MIF MTTP PDGFA PEMT **PNPLA3** PPARA PPARG PPARGC1A PTGS2 UCP1 UGT1A1
GO:0050727	Regulation of inflammatory response	ADIPOQ ADRB2 AGTR1 APOE IL1B IL6 MIF PPARG PTGS2 TLR4 TNF
Common physiologic processes link the pathophysiology of NAFLD with metabolic syndrome		
GO:0008217	Regulation of blood pressure	DIPOQ ADRB2 ADRB3 AGTR1 MIF PPARA PPARG PTGS2 SOD2
GO:0003013	Circulatory system process	ADIPOQ ADRB2 ADRB3 AGTR1 APOE CFTR GCLC MIF MTHFR PPARA PPARG PTGS2 SOD2
GO:0008015	Blood circulation	ADIPOQ ADRB2 ADRB3 AGTR1 APOE CFTR GCLC MIF MTHFR PPARA PPARG PTGS2 SOD2

uncoupling protein family (ie, *UCP3*), which may play an important role in burning fat, STAT proteins, serpins such as angiotensinogen (*AGT*), and other proinflammatory substances. In fact, the participation of the renin-angiotensin system in the pathophysiology of NAFLD was anticipated by the protection against NAFLD previously reported for losartan, an angiotensin-2 type 1 receptor (AT1R) blocker.[34] Details about the whole set of the top 100 prioritized genes are shown in **Fig. 3**.

Once more, an important topic to highlight is that despite the 2-hit hypothesis still being the leading theory guiding current research on NAFLD, biological evidence

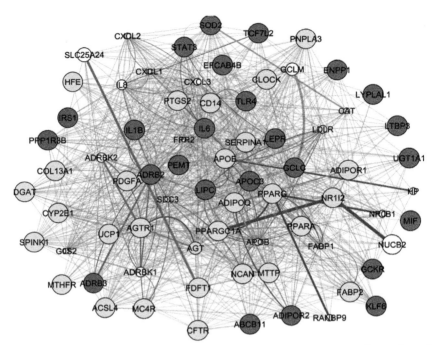

Fig. 2. Functional association analysis of protein and genetic interactions focused on the *PNPLA3* gene. Pathways, coexpression, colocalization, and protein domain similarity were analyzed by the bioinformatic resource GenMANIA. Yellow nodes (genes) are considered to be direct "neighbors" of the *PNPLA3*. The remaining gray circles are the listed genes in **Table 1**. In addition, 20 new predicted genes are incorporated (*white circles*) in the network. Edges interconnecting nodes mean: coexpression, violet (weight: 70.2%); colocalization, brown-bordeaux (11.9%); physical interactions, deep blue (11.1%); pathways, light blue-turquoise (3.4%); shared protein domains, green (0.2%).

strongly suggests that there are other impaired metabolic scenarios that play a key role in the development and progression of NAFLD, for instance, hepatocellular hypoxia, which may lead to the generation of reactive oxygen species, mitochondrial changes, and inflammation along with the associated insulin resistance state.[21]

GENETIC ARCHITECTURE OF NAFLD. CAN GENES FROM DISEASE-ASSOCIATED VARIANTS HELP US TO SELECT THERAPEUTIC TARGETS? TRANSLATING FINDINGS OF NAFLD-RISK GENE VARIANTS INTO THERAPEUTIC TARGET IDENTIFICATION

The tremendous progress on the knowledge of the human genome variation and the explosion of studies exploring the genetic component of a disease offer the unique opportunity to translate this information into the design and identification of promising therapeutic targets. Thus the authors used the available information about gene variants associated with NAFLD risk to address this challenge, and some interesting findings were observed. For example, a remarkable observation concerns drug prediction from functional enrichment analysis. After using the candidate gene list (see **Table 1**) it was found that rosiglitazone, troglitazone, and vitamin E were not only highly predicted, but clustered more than 20 genes out of the 58 reported loci (**Table 3**). Therefore, one might infer that the use of these drugs is strongly supported not only by the

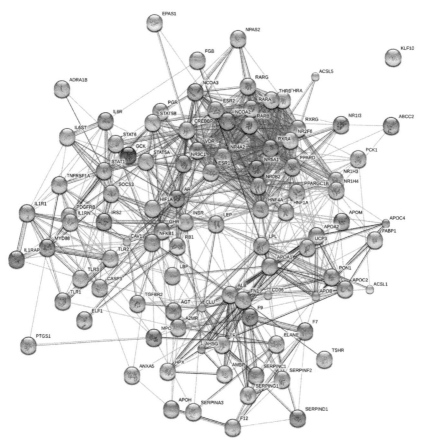

Fig. 3. Best candidates of the whole human genome prioritization for the evaluation of the genetic component of NAFLD. Prioritization was built by the bioinformatic tool ENDEAVOUR, and the figure shows results of the cluster analysis of the first 100 prioritized candidate genes from the whole human genome (23,712 genes) with a significant association with the training set. Analysis was performed using the STRING resource (Search Tool for the Retrieval of Interacting Genes/Proteins), which is a database of known and predicted protein interactions. The interactions include direct (physical) and indirect (functional) associations.

clinical phenotype but also by the associated disease gene variants analyzed in an integrative manner. This concept promptly redirects one to the straightforward question: can variations in key genes that encode proteins of disease-associated pathways influence the treatment response? The answer to this question is critical introducing personalized medicine, and some ideas are outlined as follows.

The Web resource STITCH (Search Tool for Interactions of Chemicals; http://stitch.embl.de/), which explores known and predicted interactions of chemicals and proteins, was used to look for interactions of vitamin E. Through this resource, chemicals or drugs are linked to other chemicals and proteins by evidence derived from experiments, databases, and the literature. These associations create a network that can be used to predict and further explore putative mechanisms or putative genes involved in the compound action, among other things. The results of interactions of

Table 3
Functional enrichment analysis of NAFLD candidate genes associated loci: predicted drug

Database ID	Predicted Drug	Gene List
CID000077999	Rosiglitazone	*ABCB11 ACSL4 ADIPOQ ADIPOR1 ADIPOR2 AGTR1 APOC3 APOE CFTR DGAT2 GCKR IL1B IL6 IRS1 MTTP NR1I2* **PNPLA3** *PPARA PPARG* <u>*PPARGC1A*</u> *PTGS2 SERPINA1 SPINK1 TNF UCP1*
CID000005591	Troglitazone	*ABCB11 ACSL4 ADIPOQ ADIPOR1 ADIPOR2 APOE CYP2E1 ENPP1 IL1B IL6 IRS1 LIPC NR1I2* **PNPLA3** *PPARA PPARG* <u>*PPARGC1A*</u> *PTGS2 SOD2 STAT3 TNF TNFSF10 UCP1 UGT1A1*
CID000004829	Pioglitazone	*ABCB11 ACSL4 ADIPOQ ADIPOR1 ADIPOR2 AGTR1 APOC3 APOE CYP2E1 IL6 IRS1 LIPC MTTP PPARA PPARG PTGS2 SOD2 STAT3 TCF7L2 TNF TNFSF10 UCP1*
CID000004091	Metformin	*ADIPOQ ADIPOR2 AGTR1 ENPP1 IL6 IRS1 LIPC PPARA PPARG PPARGC1A PTGS2 TCF7L2 TNF*
CID000005056	Resveratrol	*ADIPOQ APOC3 APOE CYP2E1 GCLC IL1B IL6 KLF6 NR1I2 PPARA PPARG* <u>*PPARGC1A*</u> *PTGS2 SOD2 STAT3 TNF TNFSF10 UGT1A1*
CID000002116	Vitamin E	*APOC3 APOE CYP2E1 GCLC HFE IL1B IL6 LIPC MTTP NR1I2* **PNPLA3** *PPARG PTGS2 SOD2 TNF*
D003474	Curcumin	*ADIPOQ CD14 CFTR CYP2E1 GCLC IL1B IL6 KLF6 MIF NR1I2 PPARG PTGS2 SOD2 STAT3 TCF7L2 TLR4 TNF TNFSF10 UGT1A1*
CID000001106	Stearoyl-coenzyme A	*ADIPOQ ADIPOR2 DGAT2 FDFT1 GCKR LEPR MC4R* **PNPLA3** *PPARA PPARG PTGS2 STAT3*
D011794	Quercetin	*APOE CFTR CYP2E1 GCLC IL1B IL6 MIF NR1I2* **PNPLA3** *PPARA PPARG* <u>*PPARGC1A*</u> *PTGS2 SOD2 STAT3 TCF7L2 TNF TNFSF10 UGT1A1*
CID000000778	Homocysteine	*ADIPOQ APOC3 APOE GCLC IL6 MIF MTHFR PEMT* **PNPLA3** *PPARA PPARG SOD2 TNF*
CID000000965	Oleic acid	*ACSL4 ADIPOR1 ADIPOR2 APOC3 APOE DGAT1 DGAT2 FABP2 LIPC MTTP* **PNPLA3** *PPARA PPARG PPARGC1A PTGS2 SOD2 UCP1*
CID000000303	Bile acid	*ABCB11 APOC3 APOE CYP2E1 ENPP1 FDFT1 LIPC MTTP NR1I2 PPARA PPARG PPARGC1A PTGS2 UGT1A1*
D007213	Indomethacin	*AGTR1 CYP2E1 GCLC IL1B IL6 PPARA PPARG PTGS2 SERPINA1 SOD2 TCF7L2 TLR4 TNF UGT1A1*
Compounds Associated with Drug-Induced Fatty Liver		
CID000003285	Estrogen	*ABCB11 ADIPOQ ADRB2 ADRB3 AGTR1 APOC3 APOE CFTR CYP2E1 IL1B IL6 IRS1 LIPC NR1I2 PEMT PPARA PPARG PPARGC1A PTGS2 SERPINA1 SOD2 STAT3 TNF UGT1A1*
D011374	Progesterone	*ADIPOQ ADIPOR2 ADRB2 ADRB3 CFTR CYP2E1 ENPP1 FDFT1 IL1B IL6 IRS1 NR1I2 PDGFA PPARG* <u>*PPARGC1A*</u> *PTGS2 SOD2 TLR4 TNF TNFSF10 UGT1A1*
CID000003003	Dexamethasone	*ABCB11 ADIPOQ ADIPOR2 ADRB2 ADRB3 AGTR1 APOC3 APOE CD14 CYP2E1 ENPP1 GCLC IL1B IL6 IRS1 MC4R MIF NR1I2* **PNPLA3** *PPARA PPARG* <u>*PPARGC1A*</u> *PTGS2 SERPINA1 SOD2 STAT3 TCF7L2 TNF TNFSF10 UGT1A1*

Prediction of related drugs was performed based on annotations from the following resources: CTD (Comparative Toxicogenomics Database), CTD Marker, CTD Therapeutic, Drug Bank, and STITCH (Search Tool for Interactions of Chemicals).

vitamin E are shown in **Fig. 4**. Vitamin E shows a chemical-protein interaction with CYP4F2 (cytochrome P450, family 4, subfamily F, polypeptide 2) which, in liver microsomes, is involved in a nicotinamide adenine dinucleotide phosphate–dependent electron transport pathway. Moreover, CYP4F2 oxidizes a variety of structurally unrelated compounds, including steroids, fatty acids, and xenobiotics, and starts the process of inactivating and degrading leukotriene B$_4$, a potent mediator of inflammation. In addition, vitamin E also shows chemical-protein interactions with PLA2G1B (phospholipase A$_2$), group IB (pancreas) that catalyzes the calcium-dependent hydrolysis of the 2-acyl groups in 3-*sn*-phosphoglycerides releasing arachidonic acid, whose importance was aforementioned; APOB (apolipoprotein B), a major protein constituent of chylomicrons; PRKCA (protein kinase C, α), a calcium-activated, phospholipid-dependent, serine- and threonine-specific enzyme; ALOX5 (arachidonate 5-lipoxygenase Z), which catalyzes the first step in leukotriene biosynthesis; SOD2 (superoxide dismutase 2, mitochondrial); and GSR (glutathione reductase), which maintains high levels of reduced glutathione in the cytosol (see **Fig. 4**).

Perhaps this information could be used as a prognostic and predictive tool to guide therapeutic decisions. Looking at genetic variants of *CYP4F2*, perhaps one may better predict patients' treatment response and distinguish between responders and nonresponders to therapy. However, this is an open question that needs to be answered in future research and future clinical trials.

In addition, the authors inquired as to which of the highly predicted drugs or chemical components incorporated *PNPLA3* in the functional analysis (see **Table 3**). *PNPLA3* was found to be associated with some of the already proven pharmacologic agents, with reasonable efficacy on improving fatty liver, such as rosiglitazone and vitamin E,[35] but also with some other compounds that have never been tested in

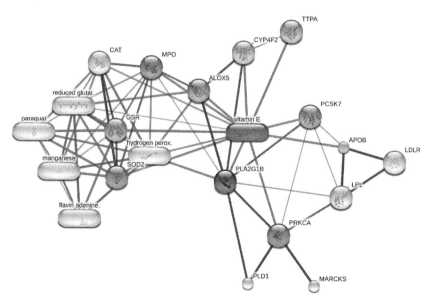

Fig. 4. In silico prediction of interactions between drugs and target proteins: Network around Vitamin E. Network prediction was performed by the STITCH resource. Protein-protein interactions are shown in blue, chemical-protein interactions in green, and interactions between chemicals in red. Chemicals are represented as pill-shaped nodes, whereas proteins are shown as spheres.

humans such as quercetin, a flavonoid widely distributed in nature. Despite this information, more thorough research is needed because some evidence in previous experimental works showed that flavonoids operating on the redox state can improve diet-induced fatty liver,[36] and quercetin decreases de novo fatty acid and TAG synthesis in rat hepatocytes.[37] Some other compounds, such as homocysteine and oleic acid, were also highly predicted in association with *PNPLA3* (see **Table 3**).

Not surprisingly, compounds that are well known to be associated with drug-induced fatty liver, such as corticosteroids and sexual hormones, were also highly predicted in association with a great majority of the target genes, including *PNPLA3* (see **Table 3**), suggesting that the pathogenesis of abnormal liver triglyceride accumulation involves common disease pathways.

In addition, the coactivator *PPARGC1A*, with its transcriptional activity modulated by epigenetic factors, and which seems to participate in the pathogenesis of insulin resistance and NAFLD,[38] was highly predicted by most of the drug compounds (see **Table 3**).

Finally, the transcription factor *STAT3*, previously reported as being involved in the genetic susceptibility of NAFLD progression and severity,[2] was also predicted for several compounds, including resveratrol, a well-known compound explored in animals but scarcely in humans, with beneficial effects on the various aspects of body homeostasis.[39]

GENES AND NAFLD: MODERN MEDICINE AND FUTURE CHALLENGES

The understanding of the genetic risk of complex diseases opens new opportunities and challenges and more practical questions. For example, can we rapidly translate the knowledge about NAFLD genetic susceptibility into more individualized decision making and personalized medicine? If so, can we improve the diagnostic and therapeutic strategies?

The ideal situation would be the design of tools based on the patient's genetic profile that would allow improved diagnosis and tailored treatment without invasive procedures and with minimal adverse events. Perhaps the clearest attempt to combine genetic data and clinical features was performed by Kotronen and coworkers.[40] Their study evaluated the performance of predicting NAFLD by combining routine clinical and laboratory data and the rs738409 genotypes. Surprisingly, however, the addition of the rs738409 patient's information into the disease modeling to create a score only improved the accuracy of the prediction by less than 1%.

An interesting and attractive use of the genetic data as mentioned previously is the idea to replace invasive procedures such as liver biopsy by risk alleles. Unfortunately, in this regard the incorporation of genetic information is not yet very promising, as traditional and noncanonical risk factors, when combined properly, have a good predictive power.[41] Hence, we would have to rely on genetic variants with stronger risk effects to observe better results in terms of disease prediction, in comparison with the current serologic biomarkers or even the more simple algorithms.[42]

Assuming that both environmental and genetic influences are likely involved in the NAFLD treatment response to a given drug, can we expect that all patients will equally respond to the therapy? Certainly we cannot. In this framework, gene variants with a proven effect on the biology and natural history of the disease, such as rs738409, could be included in future tailored therapeutic regimens to better predict, for instance, drug response. In this context, one may speculate that carriers of the G allele of the rs738409 variant might show less improvement in histologic outcomes compared with homozygous for the C allele. Thus, it would be interesting to stratify the treatment response and, in particular, adjust drug doses to the patient genotype. Conversely, as already proved for a myriad of drug targets, namely, angiotensin I–converting enzyme (peptidyl-dipeptidase A or ACE) or AT1R, carriers of the G allele of the rs738409 variant might show a better response for a drug designed for binding to the PNPLA3 protein. In fact, in vitro assays using recombinant PNPLA3 showed that the wild-type enzyme hydrolyzes emulsified triglycerides, and the 148M substitution abolishes this activity.[43] Structural protein modeling also predicted that this substitution may restrict access of substrate to the catalytic serine at residue 47 by enhancing the distance between the proximal Asp^{166} and Cys^{47}, as shown in **Fig. 5**. More studies using crystallographic analysis should be done to confirm these assumptions and test putatively active drugs.

THE POTENTIAL ADVANCE GENERATED BY NEXT-GENERATION SEQUENCING TECHNIQUES

Great promise has been raised by the emergence of high-throughput next-generation sequencing technologies, initially applied, but not restricted, to the discovery of rare variants causing Mendelian diseases not only in the exome but also in the

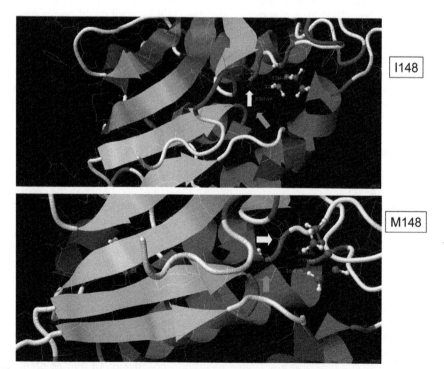

Fig. 5. The use of genetic information to optimize drug therapy: Structure protein modeling of *PNPLA3* rs738409. Structural protein prediction shows that the I148M substitution may restrict access of substrate to the catalytic serine at residue 47 by enhancing the distance between the proximal Asp^{166} and Cys^{47}. Green arrows show Ser^{47} and white arrows show Asp^{166}. Prediction was built using the SWISS-MODEL resource at http://swissmodel.expasy.org/, and visualization of chemical structure in 3D was prepared in Jmol at http://www.jmol.org/.

whole genome, as the techniques have become more available and cheaper. In fact, the 1000 Genome Project (http://browser.1000genomes.org) will contribute powerful information to the better understanding of human genetic variation. In addition, exome sequencing is being adapted to explore the contribution of rare variants (present in <1% of the population) to the "missing" heritability of complex diseases. It is commonly stated that association studies "discover disease genes," a misinterpretation that is taken too often. The fact is that associated markers map to block linked SNPs that may extend more than 100 kb and may contain several genes, and there is no guarantee of the functional involvement of the variant in the genetic effect. Fine mapping to the functional variant requires the identification of all candidate polymorphisms, obtaining the sequence of the entire region for the discovery of all the variants to explain the association in a large number of cases and controls. Moreover, as discussed recently,[44] next-generation sequencing is faced with problems in the selection of the best design to obtain good statistical power, the method of filtering neutral variants, and subsequent identification of true disease-associated polymorphisms and the development of efficient bioinformatics algorithms for the management of this huge amount of information.

Haplotype analysis of *PNPLA3* shows that the rs738409 is in moderate linkage disequilibrium (LD) ($r^2 = 0.65$) with the other variants, including the rs6006460 and rs2294918. Thus, this scenario precludes any imputation across the *PNPLA3* locus centered on the rs738409, and suggests that the I148M variant might be the causal variant in the susceptibility of fatty liver. Nevertheless, annotation of nearby SNPs in LD (proxies) with the rs738409 based on HapMap data and nearby loci shows other loci, such as SAMM50, which is a component of the sorting and assembly machinery (SAM) complex of the outer mitochondrial membrane. Of interest is that a nonsynonymous SNP (rs3761472) in *SAMM50* was associated with elevated liver enzymes,[45] suggesting that SAMM50 could be a good candidate for follow-up studies.

BEYOND DNA SEQUENCE VARIATION: THE ROLE OF EPIGENETICS IN NAFLD

Other genetic factors beyond DNA sequence variation play a critical role in the etiology of NAFLD and could potentially explain the interaction between the disease, the environmental influences, and other phenotypes. Among these factors, epigenetic modifications are the best candidates.

Epigenetics is important in understanding the pathophysiology of NAFLD because, in addition to biological plausibility, epigenetic modifications regulate chromosome organization and gene transcription by definition and are, in turn, highly controlled by environmental stimuli, including nutritional status; are highly dynamic; and can occur de novo but are potentially transmitted to the next generation.

In this context, the authors hypothesize that NAFLD is intimately associated with the status of insulin resistance and that both conditions are strongly linked by local epigenetic modifications occurring in the liver tissue before or after fat transformation. The authors observed that methylation levels of the promoter of the transcriptional coactivator, peroxisome proliferator-activated receptor γ coactivator 1α (*PPARGC1A*), in the liver tissue of patients with NAFLD correlate with HOMA-IR (homeostasis model assessment–estimated insulin resistance) and plasma fasting insulin levels.[38] Accordingly, it was also observed that liver abundance of *PPARGC1A* mRNA is inversely correlated with the methylation levels of *PPARGC1A* promoter, and also with the status of peripheral insulin resistance, suggesting that methylation of certain points in the gene promoter efficiently repressed its transcriptional activity.[38] Finally, mitochondrial biogenesis is reduced in the liver of NAFLD patients and is associated with peripheral insulin resistance and *PPARGC1A* promoter methylation status. These changes can be observed in the umbilical cord of small- and large-for-gestational-age newborns,[46,47] which may explain the fetal origin of adult disease by metabolic programming, as originally proposed by Barker and recently reviewed by Dyer and Rosenfeld.[48]

To conclude, after the description by Romeo et al[6] of the association of the I148M variant with fatty liver, we replicated the findings for the first time and extended the association to disease severity in biopsy-proven NAFLD patients,[49] which was replicated in a series of different studies.[7] These findings, as shown here, may open new opportunities for the understanding of the disease pathophysiology and the design of new therapies.

REFERENCES

1. Hernaez R. Genetic factors associated with the presence and progression of nonalcoholic fatty liver disease: a narrative review. Gastroenterol Hepatol 2012; 35(1):32–41.
2. Sookoian S, Castano G, Gianotti TF, et al. Genetic variants in STAT3 are associated with nonalcoholic fatty liver disease. Cytokine 2008;44(1):201–6.
3. Sookoian S, Castano GO, Burgueno AL, et al. The nuclear receptor PXR gene variants are associated with liver injury in nonalcoholic fatty liver disease. Pharmacogenet Genomics 2010;20(1):1–8.
4. Carulli L, Canedi I, Rondinella S, et al. Genetic polymorphisms in non-alcoholic fatty liver disease: interleukin-6-174G/C polymorphism is associated with non-alcoholic steatohepatitis. Dig Liver Dis 2009;41(11):823–8.
5. Namikawa C, Shu-Ping Z, Vyselaar JR, et al. Polymorphisms of microsomal triglyceride transfer protein gene and manganese superoxide dismutase gene in non-alcoholic steatohepatitis. J Hepatol 2004;40(5):781–6.
6. Romeo S, Kozlitina J, Xing C, et al. Genetic variation in PNPLA3 confers susceptibility to nonalcoholic fatty liver disease. Nat Genet 2008;40(12):1461–5.
7. Sookoian S, Pirola CJ. Meta-analysis of the influence of I148M variant of patatin-like phospholipase domain containing 3 gene (PNPLA3) on the susceptibility and histological severity of nonalcoholic fatty liver disease. Hepatology 2011;53(6):1883–94.
8. Bambha K, Belt P, Abraham M, et al. Ethnicity and nonalcoholic fatty liver disease. Hepatology 2012;55(3):769–80.
9. Huang Y, Cohen JC, Hobbs HH. Expression and characterization of a PNPLA3 protein isoform (I148M) associated with nonalcoholic fatty liver disease. J Biol Chem 2011;286(43):37085–93.
10. Prentki M, Madiraju SR. Glycerolipid metabolism and signaling in health and disease. Endocr Rev 2008;29(6):647–76.
11. Zechner R, Strauss JG, Haemmerle G, et al. Lipolysis: pathway under construction. Curr Opin Lipidol 2005;16(3):333–40.
12. Kienesberger PC, Oberer M, Lass A, et al. Mammalian patatin domain containing proteins: a family with diverse lipolytic activities involved in multiple biological functions. J Lipid Res 2009;50(Suppl):S63–8.
13. Warde-Farley D, Donaldson SL, Comes O, et al. The GeneMANIA prediction server: biological network integration for gene prioritization and predicting gene function. Nucleic Acids Res 2010;38(Web Server issue):W214–20.
14. Puri P, Wiest MM, Cheung O, et al. The plasma lipidomic signature of nonalcoholic steatohepatitis. Hepatology 2009;50(6):1827–38.

15. Basantani MK, Sitnick MT, Cai L, et al. Pnpla3/Adiponutrin deficiency in mice does not contribute to fatty liver disease or metabolic syndrome. J Lipid Res 2011;52(2):318–29.

16. Chen W, Chang B, Li L, et al. Patatin-like phospholipase domain-containing 3/adiponutrin deficiency in mice is not associated with fatty liver disease. Hepatology 2010;52(3):1134–42.

17. Yang LY, Kuksis A, Myher JJ, et al. Origin of triacylglycerol moiety of plasma very low density lipoproteins in the rat: structural studies. J Lipid Res 1995;36(1):125–36.

18. Jenkins CM, Mancuso DJ, Yan W, et al. Identification, cloning, expression, and purification of three novel human calcium-independent phospholipase A2 family members possessing triacylglycerol lipase and acylglycerol transacylase activities. J Biol Chem 2004;279(47):48968–75.

19. Turban S, Hajduch E. Protein kinase C isoforms: mediators of reactive lipid metabolites in the development of insulin resistance. FEBS Lett 2011;585(2):269–74.

20. Li ZZ, Berk M, McIntyre TM, et al. Hepatic lipid partitioning and liver damage in nonalcoholic fatty liver disease: role of stearoyl-CoA desaturase. J Biol Chem 2009;284(9):5637–44.

21. Carabelli J, Burgueno AL, Rosselli MS, et al. High fat diet-induced liver steatosis promotes an increase in liver mitochondrial biogenesis in response to hypoxia. J Cell Mol Med 2011;15(6):1329–38.

22. Sookoian S, Gianotti TF, Rosselli MS, et al. Liver transcriptional profile of atherosclerosis-related genes in human nonalcoholic fatty liver disease. Atherosclerosis 2011;218(2):378–85.

23. Baulande S, Lasnier F, Lucas M, et al. Adiponutrin, a transmembrane protein corresponding to a novel dietary- and obesity-linked mRNA specifically expressed in the adipose lineage. J Biol Chem 2001;276(36):33336–44.

24. D'Eon TM, Souza SC, Aronovitz M, et al. Estrogen regulation of adiposity and fuel partitioning. Evidence of genomic and non-genomic regulation of lipogenic and oxidative pathways. J Biol Chem 2005;280(43):35983–91.

25. Rosselli MS, Burgueno AL, Pirola CJ, et al. Cyclooxygenase inhibition up-regulates liver carnitine palmitoyltransferase 1A expression and improves fatty liver. Hepatology 2011;53(6):2143–4.

26. Aerts S, Lambrechts D, Maity S, et al. Gene prioritization through genomic data fusion. Nat Biotechnol 2006;24(5):537–44.

27. Sookoian S, Gianotti TF, Schuman M, et al. Gene prioritization based on biological plausibility over genome wide association studies renders new loci associated with type 2 diabetes. Genet Med 2009;11(5):338–43.

28. Lefebvre P, Cariou B, Lien F, et al. Role of bile acids and bile acid receptors in metabolic regulation. Physiol Rev 2009;89(1):147–91.

29. Knop FK. Bile-induced secretion of glucagon-like peptide-1: pathophysiological implications in type 2 diabetes? Am J Physiol Endocrinol Metab 2010;299(1):E10–3.

30. Ding X, Saxena NK, Lin S, et al. Exendin-4, a glucagon-like protein-1 (GLP-1) receptor agonist, reverses hepatic steatosis in ob/ob mice. Hepatology 2006; 43(1):173–81.

31. Byrne CD. Hypoxia and non-alcoholic fatty liver disease. Clin Sci (Lond) 2010; 118(6):397–400.

32. Nath B, Szabo G. Hypoxia and hypoxia inducible factors: diverse roles in liver diseases. Hepatology 2012;55(2):622–33.

33. Sookoian S, Gemma C, Pirola CJ. Influence of hepatocyte nuclear factor 4alpha (HNF4alpha) gene variants on the risk of type 2 diabetes: a meta-analysis in 49,577 individuals. Mol Genet Metab 2010;99(1):80–9.

34. Rosselli MS, Burgueno AL, Carabelli J, et al. Losartan reduces liver expression of plasminogen activator inhibitor-1 (PAI-1) in a high fat-induced rat nonalcoholic fatty liver disease model. Atherosclerosis 2009;206(1):119–26.

35. Sanyal AJ, Chalasani N, Kowdley KV, et al. Pioglitazone, vitamin E, or placebo for nonalcoholic steatohepatitis. N Engl J Med 2010;362(18):1675–85.

36. Rapavi E, Kocsis I, Feher E, et al. The effect of citrus flavonoids on the redox state of alimentary-induced fatty liver in rats. Nat Prod Res 2007;21(3):274–81.

37. Gnoni GV, Paglialonga G, Siculella L. Quercetin inhibits fatty acid and triacylglycerol synthesis in rat-liver cells. Eur J Clin Invest 2009;39(9):761–8.

38. Sookoian S, Rosselli MS, Gemma C, et al. Epigenetic regulation of insulin resistance in nonalcoholic fatty liver disease: impact of liver methylation of the peroxisome proliferator-activated receptor gamma coactivator 1alpha promoter. Hepatology 2010;52(6):1992–2000.

39. Smoliga JM, Baur JA, Hausenblas HA. Resveratrol and health—a comprehensive review of human clinical trials. Mol Nutr Food Res 2011;55(8):1129–41.

40. Kotronen A, Peltonen M, Hakkarainen A, et al. Prediction of non-alcoholic fatty liver disease and liver fat using metabolic and genetic factors. Gastroenterology 2009;137(3):865–72.

41. Adams LA, Feldstein AE. Non-invasive diagnosis of nonalcoholic fatty liver and nonalcoholic steatohepatitis. J Dig Dis 2011;12(1):10–6.

42. Sookoian S, Castano G, Burgueno AL, et al. A diagnostic model to differentiate simple steatosis from nonalcoholic steatohepatitis based on the likelihood ratio form of Bayes theorem. Clin Biochem 2009;42(7–8):624–9.

43. He S, McPhaul C, Li JZ, et al. A sequence variation (I148M) in PNPLA3 associated with nonalcoholic fatty liver disease disrupts triglyceride hydrolysis. J Biol Chem 2010;285(9):6706–15.

44. Bamshad MJ, Ng SB, Bigham AW, et al. Exome sequencing as a tool for Mendelian disease gene discovery. Nat Rev Genet 2011;12(11):745–55.

45. Yuan X, Waterworth D, Perry JR, et al. Population-based genome-wide association studies reveal six loci influencing plasma levels of liver enzymes. Am J Hum Genet 2008;83(4):520–8.

46. Gemma C, Sookoian S, Alvarinas J, et al. Mitochondrial DNA depletion in small- and large-for-gestational-age newborns. Obesity (Silver Spring) 2006;14(12):2193–9.

47. Gemma C, Sookoian S, Alvarinas J, et al. Maternal pregestational BMI is associated with methylation of the PPARGC1A promoter in newborns. Obesity (Silver Spring) 2009;17(5):1032–9.

48. Dyer JS, Rosenfeld CR. Metabolic imprinting by prenatal, perinatal, and postnatal overnutrition: a review. Semin Reprod Med 2011;29(3):266–76.

49. Sookoian S, Castaño GO, Burgueño AL, et al. A nonsynonymous gene variant in the adiponutrin gene is associated with nonalcoholic fatty liver disease severity. J Lipid Res 2009;50(10):2111–6.

The Relevance of Liver Histology to Predicting Clinically Meaningful Outcomes in Nonalcoholic Steatohepatitis

Mangesh R. Pagadala, MD[a],*, Arthur J. McCullough, MD[b]

KEYWORDS

- Nonalcoholic steatohepatitis • Fibrosis • Steatosis • Liver-related mortality
- Cardiovascular morbidity

KEY POINTS

- The natural course of nonalcoholic fatty liver disease (NAFLD) has yet to be precisely defined, due in large part to the difficulty in establishing the exact disease burden of NAFLD in the general population and identifying those NAFLD patients at risk for increased morbidity and mortality.
- Based on the data available and review of the current literature, particularly in general population studies, it appears that NAFLD, including nonalcoholic steatohepatitis (NASH) but not simple steatosis, is associated with worse outcomes compared with the general population. However, despite these observations, the differences in all-cause mortality between no NASH and NASH are not significant.
- Given the recent evidence supporting the importance of fibrosis in disease progression, prospective studies are required to compare the outcomes among NASH patients with and without fibrosis to identify the 25% patients with NASH who will progress to advanced liver disease.
- The presence of NASH on liver biopsy, especially among those having any degree of fibrosis, should necessitate enhanced surveillance for cardiovascular disease and malignancies, aggressive management of comorbidities, and referral (if possible) to a medical center with expertise in NAFLD.

Funding: Dr Pagadala is supported by NIH grant T32 DK061917. Dr McCullough is supported in part by NIH grant 5 U01 DK 061732.
[a] Department of Gastroenterology and Hepatology, Cleveland Clinic, 9500 Euclid Avenue, A30, Cleveland, OH 44195, USA; [b] Department of Gastroenterology and Hepatology, Cleveland Clinic Lerner College of Medicine at Case Western Reserve University, Cleveland Clinic, 9500 Euclid Avenue, Cleveland, OH 44195, USA
* Corresponding author.
E-mail address: pagadam@ccf.org

INTRODUCTION

Nonalcoholic fatty liver disease (NAFLD) has emerged as the most prevalent chronic liver disease. Population-based studies in the United States estimate that the prevalence of NAFLD is between 17% and 30% in the general population and as high as 80% in obese individuals undergoing weight-loss surgery.[1,2] NAFLD represents a histopathologic spectrum ranging from steatosis alone, to necroinflammation, an entity described as nonalcoholic steatohepatitis (NASH); the latter having an increased risk for the progression to advanced fibrosis and cirrhosis. The prevalence of NASH is between 12% and 17%, with the highest rates observed in Hispanics (19%) and diabetics (22%).[3,4] Approximately 15% to 25% of individuals with NASH can progress to cirrhosis.[5] NASH cirrhosis is now the third most common cause of liver transplantation in the United States.[6] It is associated with an increased risk for hepatocellular carcinoma and mortality in patients awaiting orthotopic liver transplant,[7] and can recur posttransplant.[8] Recently NAFLD has also been linked to an increased risk of cardiovascular morbidity, which further predisposes these individuals to increased mortality from non–liver-related deaths.[9] Several biomarkers and algorithms continue to be evaluated as noninvasive markers for the diagnosis and progression of NASH.[10] Although there is ongoing extensive research in the development of biomarkers, liver biopsy remains the gold standard in diagnosing and predicting the severity of NAFLD.[10,11] Despite the limitations of liver biopsy,[12,13] a few studies have identified specific histologic findings that are able to predict NAFLD-related mortality. These data suggest a more benign course for individuals with steatosis alone, but increased morbidity and mortality among those with advanced histologic findings of NASH and fibrosis.[14–17] Most of these studies have been limited to tertiary centers, and information from population-based studies on long-term outcomes in NAFLD are clearly lacking. Despite many studies and much discussion, the natural history of this disease remains ill defined. This article reviews the data that have evaluated the natural history of NAFLD and discusses the relevance of histology to predicting meaningful outcomes in NASH. Although NAFLD in children is also associated with increased morbidity and mortality,[18] only adult NAFLD is reviewed here.

HISTOLOGIC PROGRESSION OF NAFLD

The spectrum of NAFLD (**Fig. 1**) begins initially with simple fatty liver (steatosis) but can progress to necroinflammation (NASH) in a subgroup of patients. Progressive fibrosis as a result of the necroinflammation can lead to cirrhosis, the last and most severe form of the NAFLD spectrum. Of patients with NASH, 25% to 50% develop progressive fibrosis over a period of 4 to 6 years.[14,15,19–22] Fewer than 1% to 4% of patients with simple steatosis progress to a more advanced fibrosis.[15,20] By contrast, 15% to 25% of individuals with NASH can progress to cirrhosis.[5] In a cohort of biopsy-proven NAFLD patients, 37% of patients had progression of fibrosis, whereas 34% remained stable and 29% had some regression of fibrosis over 3 to 6 years.[23] In another study with a mean follow-up of 13 years, 13.3% of NASH patients with mild to moderate fibrosis (F1–F2) and 50% of patients with stage 3 fibrosis developed cirrhosis.[14]

HISTOLOGIC SCORING SYSTEMS

Accumulation of greater than 5% of fat, particularly in the form of triglycerides, is generally considered to be the minimal requirement in the histologic diagnosis of NAFLD.[24] Since the original description of Ludwig and colleagues,[25] the histologic criteria for diagnosing NAFLD have evolved, and several grading systems have

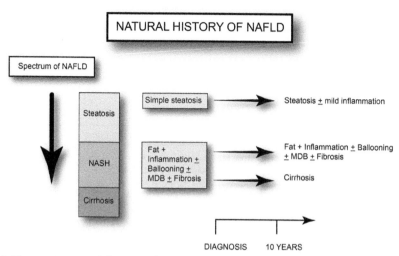

Fig. 1. The spectrum and the natural progression of nonalcoholic fatty liver disease. MDB, Mallory-Denk bodies. (*Courtesy of* Cleveland Clinic Foundation, Cleveland, OH; with permission.)

been proposed to assess histologic severity.[15,24,26,27] Based on previously validated scoring systems,[28] in 1999 Matteoni and colleagues[15] characterized histologic subtypes that correlated with clinical outcomes (**Table 1**). In 2005, the NAFLD activity score was developed by the NASH Clinical Research Network (CRN), supported by the National Institute of Diabetes and Digestive and Kidney Diseases.[24] It consists of weighted sums of each of the following: steatosis, lobular inflammation, and the presence of hepatocytes ballooning (**Table 2**), which comprise the NASH activity score (NAS). There is a separate classification for fibrosis used by NASH CRN (**Table 3**). Recently Younossi and colleagues[17] proposed a new classification to define NASH, which included steatosis with the presence of centrolobular ballooning and/or Mallory-Denk bodies (MDBs) or fibrosis. According to these criteria (**Table 4**), a diagnosis of NASH was made if there was (1) any degree of steatosis along with centrilobular ballooning and/or MDBs, or if there was (2) any degree of steatosis along with centrilobular, pericellular/perisinusoidal fibrosis, or bridging fibrosis in the absence of other identifiable causes.[17]

Table 1
Classification of nonalcoholic fatty liver disease (NAFLD) by subtype

NAFLD Subtype	Pathology	Clinicopathologic Correlation
Type 1	Simple steatosis alone	No NASH
Type 2	Steatosis + lobular inflammation only	No NASH
Type 3	Steatosis + hepatocellular ballooning	NASH without fibrosis
Type 4	Steatosis, ballooning, Mallory bodies, or fibrosis	NASH with fibrosis

Data from Matteoni CA, Younossi ZM, Gramlich T, et al. Nonalcoholic fatty liver disease: a spectrum of clinical and pathological severity. Gastroenterology 1999;116(6):1413–9.

Table 2 Classification of nonalcoholic fatty liver disease by NAFLD activity score (NASH Clinical Research Network)	
Histologic Finding	**Grade**
Steatosis	0–3
Lobular inflammation	0–3
Hepatocellular ballooning	0–2
Maximum score	8
NASH requires a score of $\geq$4 with at least 1 point from ballooning injury[a]	

[a] Used in some clinical studies to diagnose NASH. However, it was developed as a scoring system to be used in clinical trials not to diagnose NASH based on a number.[32]

Data from Kleiner DE, Brunt EM, Van Natta M, et al. Design and validation of a histological scoring system for nonalcoholic fatty liver disease. Hepatology 2005;41(6):1313–21.

The major differences between the NAFLD Scoring System[24] and the 2 scoring systems that used NAFLD subtype categories[15,17] are that the latter 2 incorporate fibrosis and nonfibrotic lesions into each subtype. More importantly, they provide a better prediction of long-term liver-related mortality in these patients.[17] Therefore, it is important to carefully consider the similarities and differences among the published scoring systems, as well as the importance of individual histologic lesions, when assessing disease severity, the accuracy of biomarkers, and the different imaging modalities for the histologic diagnosis, and most importantly the prognosis, of NAFLD patients.[29]

ROLE OF SPECIFIC HISTOLOGIC FEATURES IN PROGNOSTICATION

There are several individual histologic features that are essential both in the diagnosis of NASH and the prediction of clinical outcomes.

Ballooning

Hepatocellular ballooning is a key feature of NASH and typically denotes hepatocyte injury from steatohepatitis, and is considered a marker for apoptosis.[30] The characteristic ballooned hepatocytes are typically large round cells with a reticulated

Table 3 Classification of fibrosis in NAFLD by NASH Clinical Research Network	
Fibrosis Type[a]	**Score**
None	0
Perisinusoidal Zone 3	
Mild	1A
Moderate	1B
Portal/periportal	1C
Perisinusoidal and portal/periportal	2
Bridging	3
Cirrhosis	4

[a] Not a prerequisite for diagnosis of NASH in this scoring system.

Data from Kleiner DE, Brunt EM, Van Natta M, et al. Design and validation of a histological scoring system for nonalcoholic fatty liver disease. Hepatology 2005;41(6):1313–21.

Table 4	
Classification of NAFLD by subtype	
Pathology	**Clinicopathologic Correlation**
Simple steatosis alone	No NASH
Steatosis + lobular inflammation only	No NASH
Steatosis with centrilobular ballooning and/or Mallory-Denk bodies	NASH
Any steatosis with centrilobular pericellular/perisinusoidal or bridging fibrosis	NASH

Data from Younossi ZM, Stepanova M, Rafiq N, et al. Pathologic criteria for nonalcoholic steatohepatitis: interprotocol agreement and ability to predict liver-related mortality. Hepatology 2011; 53(6):1874–82.

cytoplasm.[31] More than 99% of patients with definitive NASH have some degree of ballooning, which is considered the most important histologic feature for predicting steatohepatitis.[32] Therefore it is not surprising that ballooning degeneration ($\geq$2) was associated with an increased liver-related mortality (hazard ratio [HR] 5.32; $P =$ .0015).[17] However, the findings of ballooning may be subtle and difficult to diagnose consistently even by a trained pathologist, as noted in a study that reported a poor to fair reliability among pathologists to diagnose inflammation, balloon degeneration, and MDBs.[33] In addition, the irregularity in distribution of ballooning degeneration and MDBs could lead to underreporting of NASH. A study of 51 NAFLD patients with paired liver biopsies taken simultaneously from the right lobe reported a low to moderate interbiopsy agreement for various liver lesions: lobular inflammation −0.13 (poor), ballooning degeneration −0.45 (moderate), Mallory bodies −0.27 (poor), and acidophilic bodies −0.07 (poor).[34]

Mallory-Denk Bodies

MDBs, also known as Mallory bodies, are cytoplasmic inclusion bodies in the hepatocyte of patients with chronic liver disease containing an abnormal keratin protein that has been ubiquinated.[35] Both ballooning degeneration and the presence of MDBs can trigger the development of apoptosis. MDBs are not specific to NASH and can be found in several other diseases, including chronic hepatitis C.[35–38] The presence of MDBs is a pathologic lesion that has been incorporated into various definitions to describe the severity of steatohepatitis,[15,17,24] and has been associated with endoplasmic reticulum stress and oxidative stress.[39,40] However, the clinical significance and prognostic value of MDBs in disease progression and outcomes in NAFLD is not completely understood. Several studies in the past have alluded to the presence of MDBs as being associated with disease severity and unfavorable outcomes in both alcoholic liver disease and NASH.[15,41,42] While the presence of MDBs is associated with the presence of ballooned hepatocytes, it can also form in their absence, making them less interchangeable. Matteoni and colleagues[15] were the first to report the importance of Mallory bodies in disease progression, and suggest a possible prognostic role in steatohepatitis. In a subsequent study comparing long-term survival between patients with NASH and those with alcoholic steatohepatitis, patients with nonalcoholic steatohepatitis had a better survival. However, a subgroup of NASH patients with moderate to severe Mallory bodies and fibrosis had a significantly worse survival.[42] In a recent study, Younossi and colleagues[17] observed that in patients with NASH who had an associated liver-related mortality (LRM) (28%), the presence of

MDBs was noted in 89% of the biopsy samples, with 56% of these having at least moderate to severe Mallory bodies (grade ≥ 2). The presence of MDBs (grade ≥ 2; HR = 4.21, P = .002) was significantly associated with liver-related mortality.

Even though there appears to be a role for MDBs in disease progression and outcomes, their presence is not considered a prerequisite to diagnose NASH.[32] The presence of MDBs is descriptively mentioned in the NAS scoring system but does not carry any weight in terms of the overall score,[24] and additional data will be required to determine their prognostic importance. Apoptosis has been validated as an accurate marker for diagnosis of NASH based on immunochemistry in liver tissue.[43] This aspect is of particular interest because serum level of CK-18, a biomarker of apoptosis, has been validated to differentiate NASH from no NASH.[44]

Fibrosis

Although fibrosis predicts clinical outcomes in NASH, it is not included in all the currently published scoring systems. While evaluating 103 sequential liver biopsies in NAFLD subjects, Adams and colleagues[23] noted an interesting observation linking fibrosis progression and pathologic lesions in NASH. A significant overall reduction in steatosis, inflammation, ballooning, Mallory hyaline, and progression of fibrosis was noted between interval liver biopsies over a period of 3 years. It should be emphasized that reduction in steatosis but not the other NASH lesions correlated with fibrosis progression. It has been reported in previous studies that up to 47% of NAFLD patients without fibrosis at baseline developed fibrosis on subsequent follow-up liver biopsy.[14] Approximately 37% to 41% of the NAFLD subjects have fibrosis progression over 3 to 10 years.[14,23] A higher body mass index (BMI), the presence of diabetes, and a low initial fibrosis stage are associated with higher rates of fibrosis progression.[23] Based on this information, it appears that with disease progression over time there is a decrease in the NAS simultaneously with the worsening fibrosis, thereby decreasing the accuracy for diagnosing NASH (based on NAS CRN score). This issue was illustrated in a recent study by Soderberg and colleagues,[45] who reported no differences in survival between NASH and no NASH, based on the NAS. An increased presence of fibrosis (72%) was noted even in the group classified as no NASH/borderline, and additionally the presence of fibrosis (stage 1–4) was more common in NAFLD patients who died than in those who survived (90% vs 75%, respectively). In the same study, if one reclassified those patients who had any type of fibrosis as NASH and those with steatosis and inflammation without fibrosis as no-NASH, both overall and liver-related mortality in the NASH group would be significantly higher than in the no-NASH group. Absence of periportal fibrosis has a high negative predictive value (100%) in predicting liver-related outcomes.[14] The lack of difference in survival among the NASH and no-NASH groups in previous studies lacked the prognostic utility for key pathologic lesions in NASH, as they were not adjusted for fibrosis.[16,45] However, in a subsequent study it was clearly shown that the presence of advanced fibrosis is the only histologic lesion to be associated with liver-related mortality. Neither steatosis, inflammation, ballooning, nor Mallory hyaline was associated with liver-related mortality after adjusting for the presence of fibrosis.[17] The inclusion of fibrosis could explain, in part, why the classifications for NASH used by Younossi and Matteoni, and not the NAS, independently correlated with liver-related mortality.[17] Furthermore, fibrosis is the histologic feature in NASH with the best inter- and intra-agreements among pathologists.[33] Using this observation one can make an argument that NAFLD in the presence of fibrosis, especially in those who have NASH, portends a higher risk of death.

NAFLD-RELATED MORTALITY
All-Cause Mortality

There are several hospital-based and community-based studies comparing overall and liver-related outcomes in NAFLD patients with that of the general population (**Table 5**), with some studies lacking a histologic diagnosis of NAFLD.[19,46–49] A community-based study that used ultrasonography to compare outcomes between NAFLD patients and the general population had higher all-cause mortality in the former group (standardized mortality ratio [SMR] = 1.34; P = .03).[46] Similar findings were reported in females with NAFLD, and no differences were observed between males and females (HR = 1.2 vs 0.92).[47] More recently, in a study with a 15-year follow-up that used the Fatty Liver Index (FLI) as a surrogate marker for fatty liver, the FLI was independently associated with increased all-cause mortality compared with the general population.[48] Similar observations were also noted in studies that used histologic criteria for diagnosing NAFLD.[14,16,45] In a small Swedish cohort, there was a significantly decreased overall survival among biopsy-proven NAFLD patients (78% vs 84%) compared with the reference population.[14] Another recent study by Soderberg and colleagues[45] validated these observations with higher all-cause mortality in NAFLD patients followed for at least 21 years compared with the general population (SMR = 1.7; 95% confidence interval [CI] 1.24–2.25). In these studies, there is an incremental increase in overall mortality rates among subjects with biopsy-proven NAFLD from 50% in the first decade of follow-up to as high as 70% by the second decade.[14,45,46] NAFLD patients with metabolic syndrome, particularly those with diabetes mellitus and insulin resistance, have more advanced fibrosis and are prone to a more rapid progression of their fibrosis.[23,50] NAFLD patients with type 2 diabetes can double the risk of overall mortality in comparison with the general population who have diabetes without NAFLD (HR = 2.2).[51] Compared with patients with alcoholic liver disease or viral hepatitis, NAFLD patients have lower risk of death but are at higher risk than patients with autoimmune and genetic disorders.[45]

Within the NAFLD spectrum, patients with histologic evidence of steatosis alone in the absence of NASH appear to generally follow a more benign course. In a Danish cohort of 109 subjects with bland steatosis, there was no difference in survival compared with the general population.[20] These findings have been corroborated by many other histology-based studies on NAFLD.[14,16,45,52] By contrast, the presence of histologic NASH is associated with worse outcomes in comparison with the general population.[14,45] In a national registry–based cohort of 129 patients with elevated liver enzymes and biopsy-proven NAFLD followed for 13 years, Ekstedt and colleagues[14] found a significant increase in all-cause mortality in patients with NASH compared with the reference population. The overall survival of patients with NASH was significantly lower (70% vs 80%, respectively, P = .01). The poor outcomes in this cohort were attributed to the presence of increased cardiovascular morbidity and, to a lesser degree, liver-related mortality. Similarly, in another study with a 28-year follow-up, the overall mortality was higher in NASH patients compared with the general population (SMR = 1.9; 95% CI 1.19–2.76; P = .007).[45] In the same study all-cause mortality in NASH patients remained significantly higher even after exclusion of those patients with stage-3 and stage-4 fibrosis.

There are only a few studies that have directly compared outcomes among patients with NASH and no-NASH patients (**Table 6**). Matteoni and colleagues[15] were the first group to analyze the long-term outcomes of NAFLD patients in relation to their histologic subtypes. A series of NAFLD patients were divided based on their

Table 5
Studies on long-term mortality in NAFLD patients in comparison with the general population

Authors[Ref.]	Year	Population (N)	Follow-Up (Years)	Comparison Group	Diagnosis	All-Cause Mortality	Liver-Related Mortality	Cardiovascular Mortality
Jespen et al[19]	2003	1804	6.4	Age- and sex-matched general population	Medical records	SMR = 2.26 (2.4–2.9)[a]	SMR = 19.7 (15.3–25.5)[a]	SMR = 2.1 (1.8–2.5)[a]
Dam-Larsen et al[20]	2009	109	16.7	General population	Biopsy	No differences between both groups	NR	NR
Adam et al[46]	2005	420	7.6	Age- and sex-matched general population	Imaging/biopsy	SMR = 1.3 (1.00–1.76)[a]	NR	NR
Ekstedt et al[14]	2006	129	13.7	Age- and sex-matched general population	Biopsy	22% vs 16%[a] 30% vs 20%[a,b]	2.8% vs 0.2% (NASH)[a,b]	15.5% vs 7.5% (NASH)[a,b]
Ong et al[59]	2008		8.7	General population	Ultrasound	HR = 1.038 (1.036–1.041)[a]	HR = 9.32 (9.21–9.43)[a]	25% vs 35%
Haring et al[47]	2009	4160	7.3	General population	Ultrasound	Men: HR = 0.92 (0.7–1.2) Women: HR = 1.2 (0.8–1.8)	NR	Men: HR 6.22 (1.22–31.62)[e]
Soderberg et al[45]	2010	118	21	Age- and sex-matched general population	Biopsy	SMR = 1.7 (1.2–2.2)[a] SMR = 1.86 (1.19–2.76)[a,b] SMR = 1.55 (0.98–2.32)[c]	NR	NR
Adams et al[51]	2010	337	10.9	Type 2 DM without NAFLD	Imaging/biopsy	HR = 2.2 (1.1–4.2)[a]	NR	HR = 0.9 (0.3–2.4)
Calori et al[48]	2011	2011	15	General population	Fatty Liver Index	HR = 1.004 (1.004–1.007)[a]	HR = 1.04 (1.02–1.05)[a]	HR = 1.006 (1.00–1.01)[d]
Lazo et al[49]	2011	11371	NR	General population	Ultrasound/LFT	Normal LFT-HR = 0.92 (0.78–1.09) Abnormal LFT-HR = 0.80 (0.52–1.22)	Normal LFT-HR = 0.64 (0.12–3.59) Abnormal LFT-HR = 1.17 (0.15–8.93)	Normal LFT-HR = 0.86 (0.67–1.12) Abnormal LFT-HR = 0.59 (0.29–1.2)

SMR and HR are given as ratio (95% confidence interval).

Abbreviations: DM, diabetes mellitus; HR, hazard ratio; LFT, liver function test; NR, not reported; SMR, standardized mortality ratio.

[a] P<.05.
[b] Comparisons made between NASH patients and the general population.
[c] Comparisons made between no-NASH patients and the general population.
[d] Not significant in the presence of insulin resistance.
[e] In the presence of elevated γ-glutamyl transpeptidase.

Table 6
Studies comparing the overall and cause-specific mortality in no-NASH compared with NASH

Authors[Ref.]	Year	Population (N)	Follow-Up (Years)	Comparison Groups	Histology Classification	All-Cause Mortality (%)	Liver-Related Mortality (%)	Cardiovascular Mortality (%)	Cancer-Related Mortality (%)
Matteoni et al[15]	1999	132	18	NASH vs steatosis ± inflammation	Matteoni	39.7 vs 32.2[b]	10.9 vs 1.69[c]	NR	NR
Ekstedt et al[14]	2006	129	13.7	NASH vs steatosis ± nonspecific inflammation	Brunt	26.7 vs 12[b]	2.8 vs none[b]	15.5 vs 8.6[b]	5.6 vs 1.7[b]
Rafiq et al[16]	2009	173	18.5	NASH vs steatosis ± nonspecific inflammation	Matteoni	No differences between both groups (P = .30)	17.5 vs 2.5[a]	NR	NR
Soderberg et al[45]	2010	118	45	NASH vs simple steatosis	Kleiner	47 vs 34.3[b]	5.8 vs 8.9[b]	13.7 vs 10.4[b]	15.6 vs 7.4[b]
Younossi et al[17]	2011	209	12	NASH vs no NASH	Younossi	30.5 vs 30.8[c]	13 vs 1.3[a]	NR	NR

Abbreviation: NR, not reported.
[a] P<.05.
[b] Significance not reported.
[c] Not significant.

histology into 4 distinct subtypes: types 1 & 2 (steatosis ± lobular inflammation) and types 3 & 4 (steatosis + ballooning degeneration ± Mallory-Denk ± fibrosis). In a mean follow-up of 18 years, those with type 3 & 4 histology (NASH) had higher rates of cirrhosis and liver-related mortalities (30.8% vs 5.6%) compared with type 1 & 2 histology (no NASH), but the overall survival was not different between the two groups.[15] Findings from this study pioneered the need to study liver histology for prognostic information on long-term survival among patients with steatohepatitis. The same group reported that the presence of diabetes mellitus decreased survival in these patients.[15,16] In the study by Ekstedt and colleagues,[14] although NASH and no-NASH were not directly compared, those patients with no NASH had a better survival than patients with NASH in comparison with the general population. However, there were no differences in overall mortality between the two groups in other studies.[16,17,45] In one study, the presence of any fibrosis in NAFLD was associated with an increased all-cause mortality compared with those patients without any fibrosis.[45] NAFLD-related advanced fibrosis is associated with an overall death rate of 13% to 28% (**Table 7**) but is lower than that for other chronic liver diseases.[53–56]

Cardiovascular-Related Mortality

NAFLD patients have a higher risk for cardiovascular morbidity and mortality compared with a general population controlled for age and gender.[57] Both hospital-based and community-based studies have established cardiovascular complications as one of the leading causes of death in the NAFLD cohort.[14–16,19,46,58] The death from cardiovascular disease in NAFLD ranges from 13% to 30% and is the most common cause of mortality, followed by malignancy (6%–28%) and liver-related deaths (2.8%–19%).[14,16,45,46,59] The prevalence of cardiovascular disease is higher in NASH than in other chronic liver diseases other than alcoholic liver disease.[45] Furthermore, cardiovascular deaths remain significantly higher in patients with NASH cirrhosis (the second highest cause of mortality) compared with patients with hepatitis C virus–related

Table 7
Comparison of outcomes for NAFLD cirrhosis with those for hepatitis C virus (HCV)-related cirrhosis

Authors[Ref.]	Year	Cirrhosis Population with NASH (N)	Follow-Up (Years)	Comparison Groups	All-Cause Mortality (%)	Liver-Related Mortality (%)	Cardiovascular Mortality (%)
Hui et al[55]	2003	23	7	NASH vs HCV (total)	26 vs 39.1[d]	21.7 vs 30.4[d]	0 vs 2.2[d]
Sanyal et al[53]	2006	152	10	NASH vs HCV	19.1 vs 29.3[a]	14.5 vs 28[b]	5.2 vs 0.6[a]
Yatsuji et al[54]	2009	68	5	NASH vs HCV	27.9 vs 40.6[d]	22 vs 37.6[d]	None in both groups
Bhala et al[56]	2011	247	7	NASH vs HCV	13.4 vs 9.4[c]	5.7 vs 7.9[c]	No differences

[a] P<.05.
[b] P<.05 for Child A but not Child B & Child C.
[c] Not significant.
[d] Significance not reported.

cirrhosis (sixth leading cause).[53] These findings are not surprising, given that 41% to 58% of subjects who undergo coronary angiography have NAFLD on imaging; furthermore, the presence of NAFLD was also an independent predictor of coronary artery calcification.[60,61] The risk of death from cardiovascular events among the histologic subtypes has shown variable results.[14,15,45] Ekstedt and colleagues[14] reported higher death rates from cardiovascular disease in patients with NASH compared with the general population (15.5% vs 7.5%, $P = .04$) as well as those with no NASH (15.5% vs 8.6%); a similar but nonsignificant trend was noted in a Swedish cohort.[45] However, more recent data suggest that patients with NASH do not have an increased risk of cardiovascular disease in comparison with no-NASH patients.[62] Several large population-based studies that have used nonhistologic modalities of diagnosis have reported no difference in cardiovascular mortality among patients with NAFLD compared with the general population.[48,49,51] In a large population-based cohort of patients with diabetes mellitus, NAFLD with diabetes was associated with increased overall mortality including deaths from malignancy, but not with cardiovascular disease, compared with those without NAFLD.[51] Moreover, the presence of NAFLD is also an independent predictor for cardiovascular mortality. Therefore, whether cardiovascular mortality is related to NASH independently of the comorbidities in the metabolic syndrome remains to be determined.[58,63] While the rate of cardiovascular disease is higher in both NAFLD and NASH patients than in the general population, the differences in mortality between NASH and no-NASH patients has yet to be clearly ascertained.

Liver-Related Mortality

NASH is associated with progression to advanced fibrosis and cirrhosis, leading to the development of liver-related complications and deaths.[64,65] In addition, cirrhosis can also predispose to the development of hepatocellular cancer and need for transplantation. Whereas liver disease is the third leading cause of death in NAFLD patients, it is the 11th and 13th cause of death in obese patients without fatty liver and in the general population, respectively.[16,59] Liver-related deaths are significantly higher in patients with NASH (13%–17.5%) than in those with simple steatosis and no NASH (1.3%–2.5%).[16,17] Among the causes of liver-related death, hepatocellular carcinoma is the most common occurrence.[14,16,45] Besides NASH, the presence of NASH-related fibrosis including both mild fibrosis (F1–F2) and advanced fibrosis (F3–F4) have significantly higher liver-related mortality rates than simple steatosis.[21] The ability of the NASH subtype classification to predict LRM outcomes in NASH was tested in a cohort of 209 biopsy-proven NAFLD patients followed for a median of 146 months.[17] The liver-related mortality was significantly higher in NASH (13%) than in no NASH (1.3%). After adjusting for confounding variables, the proposed scoring of NASH had a Cox-adjusted HR of 4.43 (95% CI 0.97–20.20; $P = .05$) as a predictor of LRM. Assessment of individual components of pathologic features found that advanced fibrosis of grade 3 or more (stage 3 fibrosis and cirrhosis), but not grades of steatosis, lobular inflammation, or ballooning degeneration, predicted an increased risk of LRM in NASH. The overall liver-related mortality rate in patients with NASH and advanced fibrosis is as high as 22% (see **Table 7**) but is lower than that for other chronic liver diseases.[53–55] More recently, a large study with mean follow-up of 85.6 months comparing outcomes between NAFLD and hepatitis C–related cirrhosis showed fewer liver-related complications, deaths, and transplant rates in the NAFLD group.[56] However, most studies comparing NAFLD cirrhosis with other chronic liver diseases are hampered by small size and variability in duration of follow-up.

NASH-Related Posttransplant Outcomes

Liver transplantation is an effective therapy for chronic end-stage liver disease, with greater than 90% and 70% survival at 1 year and 5 years, respectively.[66] The percentage of patients undergoing a liver transplant for NASH in the last decade has increased from 1.2% to 9.7%. NASH is now the third most common indication for liver transplantation in the United States behind hepatitis C and alcoholic liver disease, and is the only liver-related indication that continues to increase.[6] Patients after transplantation can develop several well-recognized complications, including infection, graft rejection, cardiovascular disorders, renal insufficiency, diabetes, hypertension, chronic rejection, dyslipidemia, and certain types of malignancies.[8] A common link in the development of cardiovascular, renal disorders and malignancies is the presence of posttransplant metabolic syndrome (PTMS). The prevalence of PTMS after transplant is approximately 50% and is most often associated with development of insulin resistance in the setting of immunosuppression.[67] It is not surprising that the development of metabolic disorders after orthotopic liver transplant can result in de novo steatosis and NASH in up to 70% and 30% of patients, respectively, with a minority developing cirrhosis.[68,69] Patients with recurrent NASH did not develop allograft failure or require retransplantation at 3 years.[68] The overall posttransplant survival rates of patients with NASH at 1 and 3 years are as high as 84% and 78%, respectively, compared with 87% and 78% for other indications ($P = .67$).[6] More recently the 5-year survival was reported as 76.4%, with cardiovascular mortality (26%) being the second highest cause of death after sepsis.[69,70] Among those transplanted for NASH cirrhosis, a combination of older age, a higher BMI, diabetes, and hypertension have an associated mortality rate of at least 50%.[71]

HISTOLOGIC FEATURES AND CLINICAL OUTCOMES

Data from several large population-based and hospital-based studies have confirmed that the presence of NAFLD by using either histology or abnormal liver imaging is associated with an increased all-cause and liver-related mortality compared with the age-matched and sex-matched general population.[14,19,45,46,51,59] In these studies, the all-cause mortality from NAFLD increased by 50% in the first 10 years and peaked to 70% in the second decade.[14,45,46,51] The presence of diabetes in NAFLD patients doubles the risk of disease progression and is prognostic for higher all-cause mortality in NAFLD patients.[16,51] However, NAFLD includes the presence of simple steatosis and steatohepatitis, and one must exercise caution while extrapolating these results to the entire spectrum of disease. The long-term outcomes vary across the disease stage and are based on histologic severity among NAFLD subtypes. Although NAFLD by itself has significantly poorer outcomes than age-matched and sex-matched general populations, studies reported to date have uniformly concluded that the presence of simple steatosis, either alone or with minimal inflammation, in the absence of ballooning degeneration or fibrosis are associated with similar outcomes to those of the age-matched and gender-matched general population without NAFLD.[14,20,45] However, one aspect that has clearly stood out is the lack of difference within the spectrum of NASH, with no differences in all-cause mortality between NASH and no NASH.[16,17,45] Given that NASH is a more histologically severe form of NAFLD, with an increased predisposition to cirrhosis, one should have expected findings to the contrary. Several different possibilities may explain this discrepancy, including (1) difficulty in establishing a true definition for NASH,[72] (2) determining the exact role of pathologic features including fibrosis in NASH outcomes, and (3) limitations in the role of liver biopsy in NAFLD-related outcome studies.[28]

Lack of Consensus for a True Definition of NASH

The definition of NASH is still evolving. Several different histologic definitions have been reported, which makes it difficult to establish a universally accepted diagnosis of histologic NASH that can predict meaningful clinical outcomes.[15,17,24,32,73] For example, a recent study that included a cohort of 257 patients with NAFLD proposed a new histologic definition of NASH and compared this definition interprotocol agreement with 3 other existing classifications, including the Brunt classification, NAS $\geq$5, and the Matteoni subtypes, which have been discussed earlier in this article. The reported measure of interprotocol agreement of the definition (κ statistic = 0.896) was in almost perfect agreement with the Matteoni classification in regard of distinguishing NASH. The agreement between the proposed definition and the now widely used NAS $\geq$5 and Brunt classification was moderate (κ = 0.511) and at best fair (κ = 0.365), respectively. Lowering NAS to 4 or less resulted in better agreement between the NAS and the new NAFLD subtype classification.[17] The results are not surprising, as both the NASH definitions that had the best interprotocol agreement have some key similarities in their definitions.[15,17] This study also compared the association of LRM with the existing NASH definitions in 209 NAFLD patients followed over a median period of 12 years. After adjusting for various confounders, the diagnosis of NASH using the Younossi and Matteoni definitions showed significant associations with LRM. However, NASH defined by the NAS $\geq$5 and the original Brunt criteria did not reach statistical significance.[17] As recently emphasized, however, the NAS CRN scoring system was developed as a tool for descriptive purposes to measure changes in NAFLD during therapeutic trials, and not to diagnose NASH.[32] The diagnosis should not be made based on a NAS-calculated number, but rather on the pathologist's overall evaluation of histologic patterns and individual lesions on the liver biopsy. Using 934 biopsies taken from the NASH CRN network database, the use of NAS cutoffs ($\geq$5 vs $\leq$4) for histologic diagnosis of steatohepatitis versus borderline/no NASH did not provide sufficient sensitivity and specificity to support their use for NASH diagnosis.[32] These results do not in any way suggest a superiority of one definition over another but rather emphasize the need for uniformity across studies, especially concerning outcomes-related studies on NAFLD.

Variability in Diagnosing Individual Pathologic Lesions in NASH

Another possible reason for the lack of differences in mortality within the NAFLD spectrum could be explained in part by the heterogeneity in distribution of individual pathologic lesions in the liver, and intraobserver variability using these lesions to define NASH on a biopsy. By far the highest variability in intraobserver and interobserver agreement has been for lobular inflammation, ballooning degeneration, and presence of certain intracytoplasmic inclusions[28,33,34] that are central to the diagnosis of histologic steatohepatitis[24] already discussed.

Limitations of Liver Biopsy in Outcome Studies

NAFLD is essentially an asymptomatic disease, discovered incidentally by the presence of elevated liver enzymes during routine blood work and abnormal imaging done for a variety of reasons.[74] Liver biopsy continues to remain the gold standard to assess severity in NAFLD, making it logistically difficult to use this method in the general population because of the invasive nature of the procedure and related complications.[75] Furthermore, the chronicity of NAFLD would require many years of follow-up to reach the hard end points of cardiovascular and liver-related

Table 8				
Liver biopsy in NAFLD with minimum criteria for size of biopsy				
Authors[Ref.]	Year	Size (mm)	Portal Tract (n)	Aim
Goldstein et al[77]	2005	$\geq$16	—	Stage
Arun et al[78]	2007	$\geq$25	8	Diagnosis
Merriman et al[13]	2006	$\geq$28	18	Grade/Stage
Ratziu et al[34]	2005	$\geq$40	33	Grade/Stage

morbidity/mortality, resulting in the paucity of population-based data that elucidate the natural history of NAFLD.[76] In addition, regardless of the scoring system used, the presence of sampling error, adequacy of sample size for grading and staging (**Table 8**), and interobserver variability among pathologists who diagnose NAFLD remains an important limitation for clinical care, investigative trials, and outcome studies.[13,34,77,78]

SUMMARY

Unfortunately, the natural course of NAFLD has yet to be precisely defined, in large part due to the difficulty in establishing the exact disease burden of NAFLD in the general population and identifying those NAFLD patients at risk for increased morbidity and mortality. Based on the data available and review of the current literature, particularly in general population studies, it appears that NAFLD, including NASH but not simple steatosis, is associated with worse outcomes in comparison with the general population. However, despite these observations, the differences in all-cause mortality between no-NASH and NASH are not significantly different. Recently, there also has been increasing interest in the association between NAFLD and cardiovascular disease.[9] Whereas histologic severity in NAFLD was associated with an increased LRM, cardiovascular mortality did not significantly differ between the NAFLD despite it being a leading cause of death in NAFLD. Potential explanations for this include (1) early death from liver disease and cancer, (2) overlapping comorbid risk factor for heart disease, and (3) had small sample sizes in most studies that investigated this issue. In addition, the relevance of histologic severity to predicting outcomes is also confounded by the presence of certain metabolic derangements, especially diabetes mellitus and dyslipidemia. Therefore, additional large, prospective, randomized, multicenter trials are needed to determine the precise role of NAFLD histology in the morbidity and mortality of both liver-related and cardiovascular outcomes. Given the recent evidence supporting the importance of fibrosis in disease progression, prospective studies are required to compare the outcomes among NASH patients with and without fibrosis to identify the 25% patients with NASH who will progress to advanced liver disease. Additional work is also required to (1) form a consensus of the histologic diagnosis of NASH, (2) increase the accuracy among pathologists to identify the key pathologic lesions in NASH, (3) clarify the role of fibrosis across the spectrum of NAFLD, and (4) identify biomarkers that can accurately stage NAFLD and obviate repeat liver biopsy in these patients. Until such data are available, it seems reasonable to consider that the stage of disease is a critical determinant in the overall prognosis of NAFLD. The presence of NASH on liver biopsy, especially among those having any degree of fibrosis, should necessitate enhanced surveillance for cardiovascular disease and malignancies, aggressive management of comorbidities, and referral (if possible) to a medical center with expertise in NAFLD.

REFERENCES

1. Browning JD, Szczepaniak LS, Dobbins R, et al. Prevalence of hepatic steatosis in an urban population in the United States: impact of ethnicity. Hepatology 2004; 40(6):1387–95.
2. Luyckx FH, Desaive C, Thiry A, et al. Liver abnormalities in severely obese subjects: effect of drastic weight loss after gastroplasty. Int J Obes Relat Metab Disord 1998;22(3):222–6.
3. Bambha K, Belt P, Abraham M, et al. Ethnicity and nonalcoholic fatty liver disease. Hepatology 2012;55(3):769–80.
4. Williams CD, Stengel J, Asike MI, et al. Prevalence of nonalcoholic fatty liver disease and nonalcoholic steatohepatitis among a largely middle-aged population utilizing ultrasound and liver biopsy: a prospective study. Gastroenterology 2011;140(1):124–31.
5. McCullough AJ. Pathophysiology of nonalcoholic steatohepatitis. J Clin Gastroenterol 2006;40(Suppl 1):S17–29.
6. Charlton MR, Burns JM, Pedersen RA, et al. Frequency and outcomes of liver transplantation for nonalcoholic steatohepatitis in the United States. Gastroenterology 2011;141(4):1249–53.
7. Hashimoto E, Tokushige K. Hepatocellular carcinoma in non-alcoholic steatohepatitis: Growing evidence of an epidemic? Hepatol Res 2012;42(1):1–14.
8. Pagadala M, Dasarathy S, Eghtesad B, et al. Posttransplant metabolic syndrome: an epidemic waiting to happen. Liver Transpl 2009;15(12):1662–70.
9. Targher G, Day CP, Bonora E. Risk of cardiovascular disease in patients with nonalcoholic fatty liver disease. N Engl J Med 2010;363(14):1341–50.
10. Wieckowska A, Feldstein AE. Diagnosis of nonalcoholic fatty liver disease: invasive versus noninvasive. Semin Liver Dis 2008;28(4):386–95.
11. Adams LA, Angulo P. Role of liver biopsy and serum markers of liver fibrosis in non-alcoholic fatty liver disease. Clin Liver Dis 2007;11(1):25–35, viii.
12. Janiec DJ, Jacobson ER, Freeth A, et al. Histologic variation of grade and stage of non-alcoholic fatty liver disease in liver biopsies. Obes Surg 2005;15(4):497–501.
13. Merriman RB, Ferrell LD, Patti MG, et al. Correlation of paired liver biopsies in morbidly obese patients with suspected nonalcoholic fatty liver disease. Hepatology 2006;44(4):874–80.
14. Ekstedt M, Franzen LE, Mathiesen UL, et al. Long-term follow-up of patients with NAFLD and elevated liver enzymes. Hepatology 2006;44(4):865–73.
15. Matteoni CA, Younossi ZM, Gramlich T, et al. Nonalcoholic fatty liver disease: a spectrum of clinical and pathological severity. Gastroenterology 1999;116(6):1413–9.
16. Rafiq N, Bai C, Fang Y, et al. Long-term follow-up of patients with nonalcoholic fatty liver. Clin Gastroenterol Hepatol 2009;7(2):234–8.
17. Younossi ZM, Stepanova M, Rafiq N, et al. Pathologic criteria for nonalcoholic steatohepatitis: interprotocol agreement and ability to predict liver-related mortality. Hepatology 2011;53(6):1874–82.
18. Feldstein AE, Charatcharoenwitthaya P, Treeprasertsuk S, et al. The natural history of non-alcoholic fatty liver disease in children: a follow-up study for up to 20 years. Gut 2009;58(11):1538–44.
19. Jepsen P, Vilstrup H, Mellemkjaer L, et al. Prognosis of patients with a diagnosis of fatty liver—a registry-based cohort study. Hepatogastroenterology 2003; 50(54):2101–4.

20. Dam-Larsen S, Becker U, Franzmann MB, et al. Final results of a long-term, clinical follow-up in fatty liver patients. Scand J Gastroenterol 2009;44(10):1236–43.
21. Musso G, Gambino R, Cassader M, et al. Meta-analysis: natural history of non-alcoholic fatty liver disease (NAFLD) and diagnostic accuracy of non-invasive tests for liver disease severity. Ann Med 2011;43(8):617–49.
22. Angulo P, Keach JC, Batts KP, et al. Independent predictors of liver fibrosis in patients with nonalcoholic steatohepatitis. Hepatology 1999;30(6):1356–62.
23. Adams LA, Sanderson S, Lindor KD, et al. The histological course of nonalcoholic fatty liver disease: a longitudinal study of 103 patients with sequential liver biopsies. J Hepatol 2005;42(1):132–8.
24. Kleiner DE, Brunt EM, Van Natta M, et al. Design and validation of a histological scoring system for nonalcoholic fatty liver disease. Hepatology 2005;41(6): 1313–21.
25. Ludwig J, Viggiano TR, McGill DB, et al. Nonalcoholic steatohepatitis: Mayo Clinic experiences with a hitherto unnamed disease. Mayo Clin Proc 1980; 55(7):434–8.
26. Mendler MH, Kanel G, Govindarajan S. Proposal for a histological scoring and grading system for non-alcoholic fatty liver disease. Liver Int 2005;25(2):294–304.
27. Brunt EM, Janney CG, Di Bisceglie AM, et al. Nonalcoholic steatohepatitis: a proposal for grading and staging the histological lesions. Am J Gastroenterol 1999;94(9):2467–74.
28. Younossi ZM, Gramlich T, Liu YC, et al. Nonalcoholic fatty liver disease: assessment of variability in pathologic interpretations. Mod Pathol 1998;11(6):560–5.
29. Adams LA, Feldstein AE. Non-invasive diagnosis of nonalcoholic fatty liver and nonalcoholic steatohepatitis. J Dig Dis 2011;12(1):10–6.
30. Malhi H, Gores GJ, Lemasters JJ. Apoptosis and necrosis in the liver: a tale of two deaths? Hepatology 2006;43(2 Suppl 1):S31–44.
31. Lackner C, Gogg-Kamerer M, Zatloukal K, et al. Ballooned hepatocytes in steatohepatitis: the value of keratin immunohistochemistry for diagnosis. J Hepatol 2008;48(5):821–8.
32. Brunt EM, Kleiner DE, Wilson LA, et al. Nonalcoholic fatty liver disease (NAFLD) activity score and the histopathologic diagnosis in NAFLD: distinct clinicopathologic meanings. Hepatology 2011;53(3):810–20.
33. Fukusato T, Fukushima J, Shiga J, et al. Interobserver variation in the histopathological assessment of nonalcoholic steatohepatitis. Hepatol Res 2005;33(2): 122–7.
34. Ratziu V, Charlotte F, Heurtier A, et al. Sampling variability of liver biopsy in nonalcoholic fatty liver disease. Gastroenterology 2005;128(7):1898–906.
35. Zatloukal K, French SW, Stumptner C, et al. From Mallory to Mallory-Denk bodies: what, how and why? Exp Cell Res 2007;313(10):2033–49.
36. Zhong B, Strnad P, Selmi C, et al. Keratin variants are overrepresented in primary biliary cirrhosis and associate with disease severity. Hepatology 2009;50(2): 546–54.
37. Rakoski MO, Brown MB, Fontana RJ, et al. Mallory-Denk bodies are associated with outcomes and histologic features in patients with chronic hepatitis C. Clin Gastroenterol Hepatol 2011;9(10):902–909.e1.
38. Omary MB, Ku NO, Strnad P, et al. Toward unraveling the complexity of simple epithelial keratins in human disease. J Clin Invest 2009;119(7):1794–805.
39. Hanada S, Strnad P, Brunt EM, et al. The genetic background modulates susceptibility to mouse liver Mallory-Denk body formation and liver injury. Hepatology 2008;48(3):943–52.

40. Hanada S, Snider NT, Brunt EM, et al. Gender dimorphic formation of mouse Mallory-Denk bodies and the role of xenobiotic metabolism and oxidative stress. Gastroenterology 2010;138(4):1607–17.
41. Gramlich T, Kleiner DE, McCullough AJ, et al. Pathologic features associated with fibrosis in nonalcoholic fatty liver disease. Hum Pathol 2004;35(2):196–9.
42. Cortez-Pinto H, Baptista A, Camilo ME, et al. Nonalcoholic steatohepatitis— a long-term follow-up study: comparison with alcoholic hepatitis in ambulatory and hospitalized patients. Dig Dis Sci 2003;48(10):1909–13.
43. Feldstein AE, Wieckowska A, Lopez AR, et al. Cytokeratin-18 fragment levels as noninvasive biomarkers for nonalcoholic steatohepatitis: a multicenter validation study. Hepatology 2009;50(4):1072–8.
44. Machado MV, Cortez-Pinto H. Cell death and nonalcoholic steatohepatitis: where is ballooning relevant? Expert Rev Gastroenterol Hepatol 2011;5(2):213–22.
45. Soderberg C, Stal P, Askling J, et al. Decreased survival of subjects with elevated liver function tests during a 28-year follow-up. Hepatology 2010;51(2):595–602.
46. Adams LA, Lymp JF, St Sauver J, et al. The natural history of nonalcoholic fatty liver disease: a population-based cohort study. Gastroenterology 2005;129(1): 113–21.
47. Haring R, Wallaschofski H, Nauck M, et al. Ultrasonographic hepatic steatosis increases prediction of mortality risk from elevated serum gamma-glutamyl transpeptidase levels. Hepatology 2009;50(5):1403–11.
48. Calori G, Lattuada G, Ragogna F, et al. Fatty liver index and mortality: the Cremona study in the 15th year of follow-up. Hepatology 2011;54(1):145–52.
49. Lazo M, Hernaez R, Bonekamp S, et al. Non-alcoholic fatty liver disease and mortality among US adults: prospective cohort study. BMJ 2011;343:d6891.
50. Angulo P, Alba LM, Petrovic LM, et al. Leptin, insulin resistance, and liver fibrosis in human nonalcoholic fatty liver disease. J Hepatol 2004;41(6):943–9.
51. Adams LA, Harmsen S, St Sauver JL, et al. Nonalcoholic fatty liver disease increases risk of death among patients with diabetes: a community-based cohort study. Am J Gastroenterol 2010;105(7):1567–73.
52. Teli MR, James OF, Burt AD, et al. The natural history of nonalcoholic fatty liver: a follow-up study. Hepatology 1995;22(6):1714–9.
53. Sanyal AJ, Banas C, Sargeant C, et al. Similarities and differences in outcomes of cirrhosis due to nonalcoholic steatohepatitis and hepatitis C. Hepatology 2006; 43(4):682–9.
54. Yatsuji S, Hashimoto E, Tobari M, et al. Clinical features and outcomes of cirrhosis due to non-alcoholic steatohepatitis compared with cirrhosis caused by chronic hepatitis C. J Gastroenterol Hepatol 2009;24(2):248–54.
55. Hui JM, Kench JG, Chitturi S, et al. Long-term outcomes of cirrhosis in nonalcoholic steatohepatitis compared with hepatitis C. Hepatology 2003;38(2): 420–7.
56. Bhala N, Angulo P, van der Poorten D, et al. The natural history of nonalcoholic fatty liver disease with advanced fibrosis or cirrhosis: an international collaborative study. Hepatology 2011;54(4):1208–16.
57. Treeprasertsuk S, Leverage S, Adams LA, et al. The Framingham risk score and heart disease in nonalcoholic fatty liver disease. Liver Int 2012;32(6):945–50.
58. Stepanova M, Younossi ZM. Independent association between nonalcoholic fatty liver disease and cardiovascular disease in the US population. Clin Gastroenterol Hepatol 2012;10(6):646–50.
59. Ong JP, Pitts A, Younossi ZM. Increased overall mortality and liver-related mortality in non-alcoholic fatty liver disease. J Hepatol 2008;49(4):608–12.

60. Chen CH, Nien CK, Yang CC, et al. Association between nonalcoholic fatty liver disease and coronary artery calcification. Dig Dis Sci 2010;55(6):1752–60.

61. Wong VW, Wong GL, Yip GW, et al. Coronary artery disease and cardiovascular outcomes in patients with non-alcoholic fatty liver disease. Gut 2011;60(12): 1721–7.

62. Domanski JP, Park SJ, Harrison SA. Cardiovascular disease and nonalcoholic Fatty liver disease: does histologic severity matter? J Clin Gastroenterol 2012; 46(5):427–30.

63. Targher G, Bertolini L, Padovani R, et al. Increased prevalence of cardiovascular disease in Type 2 diabetic patients with non-alcoholic fatty liver disease. Diabet Med 2006;23(4):403–9.

64. Farrell GC, Larter CZ. Nonalcoholic fatty liver disease: from steatosis to cirrhosis. Hepatology 2006;43(2 Suppl 1):S99–112.

65. Rinella ME. Will the increased prevalence of nonalcoholic steatohepatitis (NASH) in the age of better hepatitis C virus therapy make NASH the deadlier disease? Hepatology 2011;54(4):1118–20.

66. Roberts MS, Angus DC, Bryce CL, et al. Survival after liver transplantation in the United States: a disease-specific analysis of the UNOS database. Liver Transpl 2004;10(7):886–97.

67. Laish I, Braun M, Mor E, et al. Metabolic syndrome in liver transplant recipients: prevalence, risk factors, and association with cardiovascular events. Liver Transpl 2011;17(1):15–22.

68. Malik SM, Devera ME, Fontes P, et al. Recurrent disease following liver transplantation for nonalcoholic steatohepatitis cirrhosis. Liver Transpl 2009;15(12): 1843–51.

69. Bhagat V, Mindikoglu AL, Nudo CG, et al. Outcomes of liver transplantation in patients with cirrhosis due to nonalcoholic steatohepatitis versus patients with cirrhosis due to alcoholic liver disease. Liver Transpl 2009;15(12):1814–20.

70. Afzali A, Berry K, Ioannou GN. Excellent posttransplant survival for patients with nonalcoholic steatohepatitis in the United States. Liver Transpl 2012;18(1):29–37.

71. Malik SM, deVera ME, Fontes P, et al. Outcome after liver transplantation for NASH cirrhosis. Am J Transplant 2009;9(4):782–93.

72. Brunt EM, Kleiner DE, Behling C, et al. Misuse of scoring systems. Hepatology 2011;54(1):369–70 [author reply: 370–1].

73. Promrat K, Lutchman G, Uwaifo GI, et al. A pilot study of pioglitazone treatment for nonalcoholic steatohepatitis. Hepatology 2004;39(1):188–96.

74. Vuppalanchi R, Chalasani N. Nonalcoholic fatty liver disease and nonalcoholic steatohepatitis: selected practical issues in their evaluation and management. Hepatology 2009;49(1):306–17.

75. Piccinino F, Sagnelli E, Pasquale G, et al. Complications following percutaneous liver biopsy. A multicentre retrospective study on 68,276 biopsies. J Hepatol 1986;2(2):165–73.

76. Sanyal AJ, Brunt EM, Kleiner DE, et al. Endpoints and clinical trial design for nonalcoholic steatohepatitis. Hepatology 2011;54(1):344–53.

77. Goldstein NS, Hastah F, Galan MV, et al. Fibrosis heterogeneity in nonalcoholic steatohepatitis and hepatitis C virus needle core biopsy specimens. Am J Clin Pathol 2005;123(3):382–7.

78. Arun J, Jhala N, Lazenby AJ, et al. Influence of liver biopsy heterogeneity and diagnosis of nonalcoholic steatohepatitis in subjects undergoing gastric bypass. Obes Surg 2007;17(2):155–61.

Mechanisms of Simple Hepatic Steatosis: Not So Simple After All

Scott C. Matherly, MD, Puneet Puri, MBBS, MD*

KEYWORDS

- Nonalcoholic fatty liver disease • Triglycerides • Hepatic steatosis
- Nonalcoholic steatohepatitis

KEY POINTS

- Hepatic steatosis is the result of a complex interplay between the diet, the metabolic system, and host responses at the level of adipose tissue, muscle, pancreas, and the liver.
- The disruption of normal insulin signaling in the hepatocyte and increased abundance of fatty acids leads to disordered lipid metabolism.
- Dietary factors such as high carbohydrate intake, high fat intake, and fructose all worsen insulin sensitivity and increase hepatic steatosis.
- The extreme complexity of this system explains the inherent difficulty in treating it.
- Effective therapies and prevention based on understanding of the pathogenesis are the key in curbing this epidemic.

Nonalcoholic fatty liver disease (NAFLD) is fast becoming an epidemic in the world. It was estimated in 2000 that there were as many as 30.1 million Americans with hepatic steatosis,[1] and the prevalence is rising. The histologic spectrum of NAFLD ranges from hepatic steatosis to nonalcoholic steatohepatitis (NASH), which is characterized by the additional presence of inflammation and cell injury. NASH can lead to cirrhosis in up to 15% to 20% of individuals. Hepatic steatosis is the hallmark of NAFLD and represents excessive accumulation of fat, mainly in the form of triglycerides (TGs) within the cytoplasm of hepatocytes. Recent studies indicate that NAFLD is just not accumulating TG but a variety of other biologically active lipids that contribute to disease phenotype in NAFLD. Unlike other species, humans do not use the liver as a fat storage organ. Fat is typically stored in adipose tissue in the form of TGs. Their high caloric density (9 kcal/g) and inert nature make TGs the ideal energy storage molecule. The deposition of TGs in the liver is the result of an imbalance between the amount of energy taken in and the amount used. This balance is maintained by a complex interplay between the dietary intake of nutrients, the hormonal response to the nutrients, and their effect on

Division of Gastroenterology, Hepatology and Nutrition, Department of Internal Medicine, Virginia Commonwealth University Medical Center, Box 980341, Richmond, VA 23298, USA
* Corresponding author.
E-mail address: ppuri@mcvh-vcu.edu

both the liver and adipose tissue. Disruption of this system is what leads to the development of steatosis and is the focus of this article.

METABOLIC CHANGES LEADING TO THE DEVELOPMENT OF HEPATIC STEATOSIS

In the hepatocyte during periods of energy excess, nutrient sources such as glucose, free fatty acids (FFAs), and dietary fats are stored as glycogen or shunted into de novo lipogenesis (DNL) pathways. DNL is the process by which hepatocytes create new fatty acids that are ultimately stored as TGs, packaged into very low density lipoproteins (VLDL) for export or used for the production of other cellular components such as phospholipids. Hepatic steatosis occurs when there is sustained excess delivery of fatty acids to the liver in combination with insulin resistance. Fatty acids are available to the liver from 3 sources: the nonesterified fatty acid (NEFA) pool, DNL, and dietary fats. The lipid handling by the liver is shown in **Fig. 1**. The metabolism and transport of fatty acids are affected strongly by diet and the hormonal response to diet. When fatty acids are absorbed by the enterocyte, they are esterified into TGs, packaged into chylomicrons, and released into the circulation via lymphatics.[2] Approximately 80% of the TGs in the chylomicrons are hydrolyzed by lipoprotein lipase (LPL), allowing FFAs to be taken up by adipose tissue.[3] The remaining TGs are transported in chylomicron remnants and taken up by the liver after binding the apolipoprotein E receptor. In the fasting state, TGs stored in adipocytes undergo lipolysis by adipose TG lipase and hormone-sensitive lipase.[4] The released fatty acids join the NEFA and are transported to the liver bound to albumin. This process occurs during the postabsorptive state under the influence of glycogen, epinephrine, and norepinephrine.[4] In the hepatocyte, the fatty acids can be oxidized by mitochondria to create energy and ketone bodies, used to build other lipids such as phospholipids, added to apolipoproteins for secretion as VLDL, or transformed back into TGs and stored. In order for fatty acids to move into the β-oxidation pathway for use as energy, they must be transported from the cytoplasm into the mitochondria. This crucial step is catalyzed by the enzyme carnitine palmitoyl transferase 1 (CPT-1) on the outer mitochondrial membrane. CPT-1 activity is inhibited by increasing levels of malonyl-coenzyme A (CoA), a key intermediary in DNL.[5] In patients with NAFLD, isotope studies have shown that 59% of hepatic fat is from the NEFA, 26% from DNL, and 15% from the diet.[6] This finding is summarized in **Fig. 2**, which

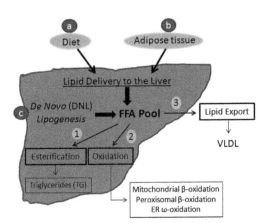

Fig. 1. Lipid handling in the liver. The fat is delivered to the liver from 3 sources: diet, adipose tissue lipolysis, and DNL. Hepatic lipid homeostasis is maintained by a fine balance between delivery of fat to the liver, its utilization either by esterification or oxidation, and turnover.

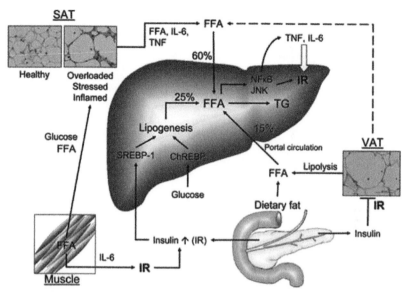

Fig. 2. Interorgan cross talk in the development of insulin resistance: interactions between visceral and subcutaneous adipose tissues, muscle, and liver contributing to the pathogenesis of insulin resistance. Most FFA pool in insulin-resistant state is a result of lipolysis from subcutaneous adipose tissue (60%), whereas DNL, dietary, and visceral adipose tissue contribute the rest. IR, insulin resistance; SAT, subcutaneous adipose tissue; VAT, visceral adipose tissue. (*From* Larter CZ, Chitturi S, Heydet D, et al. A fresh look at NASH pathogenesis. Part 1: the metabolic movers. J Gastroenterol Hepatol 2010;25:683; with permission.)

shows the role of liver, adipose tissue, muscle, and pancreas in glucose and lipid metabolism.

Carbohydrate intake can also affect fatty acid metabolism in the liver. Glucose is used by the liver in several ways. Under the influence of insulin, excess glucose is stored in the form of glycogen. When the glycogen stores of the liver are replete, any further glucose is used to produce fatty acids, which are further esterified into TGs or VLDLs.[7] Glucose is converted to pyruvate, which enters the Krebs cycle. Citrate produced in this way is moved into the cytoplasm, where it is used to create acetyl-CoA (**Fig. 3**). Acetyl-CoA carboxylase 1 (ACC-1) then produces malonyl-CoA, which is further converted by fatty acid synthase (FAS) into the saturated fatty acid, palmitate (C16:0). From this base, the enzymes stearyl-CoA desaturase (SCD) and long chain fatty acid elongase are used to create other fatty acids such as palmitoleic acid (C16:1), stearic acid (C18:0), or oleic acid (C18:1).[8] In the normal postabsorptive state, DNL is believed to contribute to less than 5% of fatty acid, TG, and VLDL synthesis.[9] As mentioned by Donnelly and colleagues,[6] DNL in patients with NAFLD can represent up to 26% of hepatic fat. This finding suggests that there is significant stimulation of DNL or inhibition of fatty acid β-oxidation in patients with hepatic steatosis. Accumulation of excessive amounts of the end product of DNL, oleic acid, in humans with steatosis is further evidence of increased hepatic lipogensis.[10,11] The process of DNL is under complex transcriptional control, mainly under the influence of insulin and glucose.

METABOLIC, TRANSCRIPTIONAL, AND INFLAMMATORY FACTORS IN THE GENERATION OF HEPATIC STEATOSIS

Insulin controls lipogenesis primarily through the actions of a transcription factor called the sterol regulatory element-binding protein 1c (SREBP-1c). There are 3 isoforms of

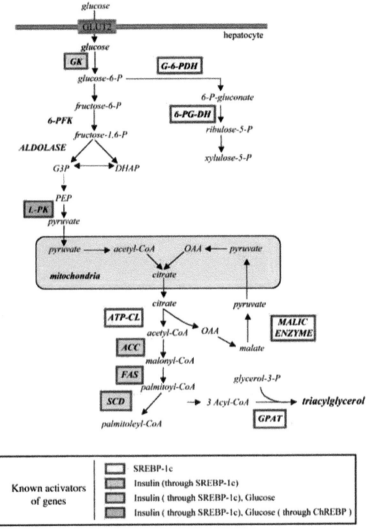

Fig. 3. The glycolytic and lipogenic pathways in the liver, and the role of SREBP-1c in the regulation of hepatic lipid metabolism. The enzymes indicated are induced at a transcriptional level by a high carbohydrate diet. The known activators of their transcription are indicated at the bottom. ATP-CL, adenosine triphosphate citrate-lyase; DHAP, dihydroxyacetone 3-phosphate; G-6-PDH, glucose-6-phosphate dehydrogenase; G3P, glyceraldehyde 3-phosphate; L-PK, liver pyruvate kinase; OAA, oxaloacetate; 6-PG-DH, 6-phosphogluconate dehydrogenase; PEP, phosphoenolpyruvate; P, phosphate; 6-PFK, 6-phosphofructo-1-kinase. (*From* Foufelle F, Ferre P. New perspectives in the regulation of hepatic glycolytic and lipogenic genes by insulin and glucose: a role for the transcription factor sterol regulatory element binding protein-1c. Biochem J 2002;366:379; with permission.)

the SREBP family of basic helix-loop-helix-leucine zipper transcription factors but only SREBP-1c plays a role in DNL.[12] SREBP-1c promotes the production of several enzymes important to DNL. These enzymes include ACC-1, FAS, SCD, and long chain elongase (see **Fig. 3**).[13,14] TG synthesis is also affected by increasing levels of glycerol

3-phosphate acyltransferase (GPAT) and VLDL secretion is inhibited by decreasing expression of microsomal transfer protein.[15,16] Gluconeogenesis is also diminished secondary to SREBP-1c inhibition of phosphoenoylpyruvate carboxykinase.[17] The net result is increased DNL, decreased packaging, and secretion of VLDL and decreased gluconeogenesis. When SREBP-1c is overexpressed in mice they develop hepatic steatosis.[18] Saturated fats and sterols increase SREBP-1c production, whereas polyunsaturated fats decrease levels of SREBP-1c in the nucleus.[19]

Glucose directly stimulates lipogenesis through the activation of another basic helix-loop-helix-leucine zipper transcription factor known as the carbohydrate response element binding protein (ChREBP).[20] High levels of glucose in the cytoplasm cause ChREBP to be translocated from the cytoplasm to the nucleus.[21] The ChREBP binds to the carbohydrate-responsive element in the promoter region of certain lipogenic genes.[22] The primary enzyme upregulated by this process is liver pyruvate kinase, which catalyzes the conversion of phosphoenolpyruvate to pyruvate. This pyruvate can then be converted to citrate through the Krebs cycle, which can then act as a substrate for DNL (see **Fig. 3**).[8] Studies in ChREBP knockout mice revealed that the presence of other enzymes associated with DNL was significantly decreased, suggesting that ChREBP had a role in transcriptional control of different enzymes.[23] Subsequent investigations have revealed that ChREBP can affect the expression of ACC-1, FAS, SCD1, and GPAT as well as other proteins associated with packaging and secretion of VLDLs.[24]

SREBP-1c and ChREBP have significant transcriptional control over the production of enzymes in the DNL pathway, but current evidence suggests that another receptor can affect the activity and prevalence of both. Liver X receptors (LXRs) are nuclear hormone receptors that act as transcription factors when bound to their ligands. LXRα is found mostly in hepatocytes, adipose tissue, and macrophages, whereas LXRβ is more widespread.[25] As mentioned earlier, SREBP-1c is strongly induced by insulin. The metabolic pathway leading to this situation is not fully understood but involves increased levels of AKT, which seem to act through the mammalian target of rapamycin 1 complex to increase SREBP-1c.[26] LXRα null mice show substantially decreased SREBP-1c activity and hence lipogenesis.[27] The ChREBP has also been shown to be a target gene of LXRs.[28] In addition, LXR has been shown to directly induce the important DNL enzymes ACC1, FAS, and SCD1.[29] Oxysterols are known ligands of LXRs, which is consistent with their role in cholesterol and bile salt metabolism. They can be activated indirectly by the action of insulin and glucose as well.[30]

Other nuclear receptors have effects on lipid metabolism that can cause or alter hepatic steatosis. Chief among these are the peroxisome proliferator-activated receptors (PPAR). Three PPAR isotypes have been described: PPARα, PPARβ/δ, and PPARγ (**Table 1**).[31] Much like LXR, PPARs are ligand-inducible transcription factors. PPARα is heavily expressed in the liver, where is acts to promote use of fatty acids. When stimulated by long chain fatty acids and oxidized phospholipids, it promotes the transcription of genes for movement of fatty acids into the cell and mitochondria including fatty acid transport protein and CPT1. Key enzymes in the β-oxidation pathway are upregulated as well as enzymes related to apolipoprotein B (apoB) metabolism.[32] The result of PPARα activation in the liver is increased fatty acid uptake and oxidation, lipolysis, and clearance of ApoB-containing lipoproteins. When PPARα knockout mice were developed, they manifested with hepatic steatosis, dyslipidemia, and obesity.[33] PPARα agonists include the fenofibrates, which improve TG profiles but have weak affinity for the enzyme; research is ongoing to produce more potent PPARα agonists.[34] PPARβ/δ is found predominantly in tissues that have an active role in metabolizing lipids such as muscle, heart, small intestine, and adipose tissue.[35] The role of PPARβ/δ in hepatic steatosis has not been defined but it seems to play

Table 1
A summary of PPAR-related metabolic changes in major organs

	PPARα	PPARβ/δ	PPARγ
Liver	Increased fatty acid uptake Increased fatty acid oxidation Increased high density apolipoproteins Decreased very low density lipoprotein production	Deceases glucose production	Increased lipogenesis Increased insulin sensitivity
Muscle	Increased fatty acid uptake Increased fatty acid oxidation Increased TG lipolysis Increased glucose intolerance Decreased glucose utilization	Increased during starvation Increased fatty acid oxidation Increased fatty acid transport Increased thermogenesis	Increased insulin sensitivity
Adipose tissue	Increased lipolysis during starvation	Increased fatty acid oxidation Increased fatty acid transport Increased thermogenesis	Increases adipocyte differentiation Increased adipocyte survival Increased lipogenesis Increased insulin sensitivity Increased adiponectin secretion
Pancreas	Decreased β-cell lipotoxicity Increased glucose-stimulated	Not known	Not known

a role in fatty acid transportation, oxidation, and thermogenesis. PPARγ is most strongly expressed in adipose tissue and macrophages with low levels in the normal liver. Murine models have shown significantly increased levels of PPARγ in the livers of mice with fatty liver and insulin resistance, suggesting that the receptor may be upregulated in this condition.[36] Monounsaturated fatty acids, polyunsaturated fatty acids, and eicosanoid fatty acid derivatives act as the ligands for PPARγ, suggesting it works as a fatty acid sensor.[37] SREBP-1 plays a role in the activation of PPARγ through the production of an endogenous ligand.[38] The major pharmaceutical ligand of PPARγ is the thiazolidinediones (rosiglitazone and pioglitazone). PPARγ mainly works in the adipocytes to increase fatty acid uptake, storage, and increased insulin sensitivity. Activation causes fat to be redistributed from the viscera including the liver into the subcutaneous fat. In the liver, PPARγ decreases gluconeogenesis and increases insulin sensitivity.[39] PPARγ increases production of the adipokine, adiponectin, which has significant effects on insulin sensitivity and fatty acid oxidation.[40]

Another important mediator of fatty acid metabolism is adenosine monophosphate (AMP)-activated protein kinase (AMPK). As energy is expended in cells, there is an accumulation of AMP. The increased levels of AMP in the cells activate AMPK. In this way, AMPK serves as a sensor of intracellular energy levels.[41] AMPK stimulates pathways designed to create more adenosine triphosphate. Metformin has been shown to be an activator of AMPK. When activated, AMPK causes decreased activity of ACC, increased β-oxidation of fatty acids, and decreased expression of SREBP-1.[42] AMPK has also been shown to directly phosphorylate and thereby deactivate ChREBP.[43]

Peripheral insulin resistance is considered the primary driving force behind the development of hepatic steatosis. Using a hyperinsulinemic/euglycemic clamp, it has been shown that patients with hepatic steatosis and NASH have peripheral insulin resistance.[44] In addition to insulin resistance, patients with hepatic steatosis have a compensatory increase in insulin secretion from the pancreas, leading to hyperinsulinemia.[45] The strong relationship between hepatic steatosis and insulin resistance holds up even for lean individuals with NASH.[46] The pathophysiology of insulin resistance is complex and multifactorial. The insulin resistance also happens at the level of the adipose tissue, muscle, and the liver.

Adipose tissue is a complex metabolically active endocrine organ that has profound effects on insulin resistance and hepatic steatosis. The normal effects of insulin on the adipose tissue are shown in **Fig. 4**. It has been shown that as obesity increases, there is an increase in macrophage infiltration of adipose tissue. These activated macrophages secrete inflammatory cytokines such as interleukin 6 (IL-6) and tumor necrosis factor α (TNF-α).[47] This situation leads to a chronic inflammatory state within the adipose tissue and release of both cytokines and adipokines, which have effects on other peripheral tissues, including the liver.[48] Obese rats fed a high-fat diet have significant reductions in IL-6 and TNF-α levels after undergoing roux-en-Y gastric bypass and weight loss, suggesting that this effect is reversible.[49] The substances secreted by both adipose tissue and the macrophages can work toward either increased insulin resistance or improved insulin responsiveness. TNF-α, IL-6, monocyte chemoattractant

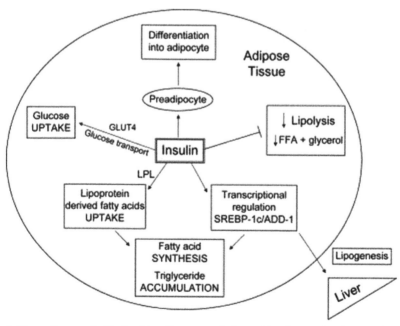

Fig. 4. The actions and effects of insulin on regulation of fat depots: insulin stimulates differentiation of preadipocytes to adipocytes. In mature adipocytes, insulin promotes lipogenesis by stimulating the uptake of glucose and lipoprotein-derived fatty acid. It is also involved in the transcriptional regulation by inducing SREBP-1c/adipocyte determination and differentiation-dependent factor 1 (ADD-1), which regulates genes promoting fatty acid synthesis and lipogenesis. Insulin diminishes TG breakdown by inhibiting lipolysis. GLUT4, glucose transporter 4. (*Adapted from* Puri P, Sanyal AJ. Role of obesity, insulin resistance, and steatosis in hepatitis C virus infection. Clin Liver Dis 2006;10(4):796; with permission.)

protein 1 (MCP-1), Plasminogen activator inhibitor 1 (PAI-1), retinol binding protein 4 (RBP-4), and resistin are some of the key cytokines and adipokines secreted by the adipose tissue/macrophage interaction that lead to increased insulin resistance. Adiponectin and leptin are adipokines with potent insulin-sensitizing effects. Significant dysregulation of these adipokines has been reported in obesity, diabetes, and the metabolic syndrome.[50]

TNF-α is expressed more in visceral fat than in subcutaneous fat and is mostly produced by activated macrophages.[51] TNF-α works via activation of 2 proinflammatory signaling pathways: the nuclear factor (NF)-κB pathway and the c-Jun NH2-terminal kinase (JNK) pathway.[52] JNK-mediated phosphorylation of insulin receptor substrate 1 (IRS-1) disrupts insulin signaling and is the main cause of TNF-α–induced insulin resistance.[53] TNF-α also causes increased production of other proinflammatory cytokines (including itself) via the NF-κB pathway, worsening the inflammation. Increased levels of TNF-α have been reported in patients with steatosis.[54] Proposed mechanisms of TNF-α–mediated effects leading to insulin resistance are shown in **Fig. 5**. In mice fed a high-fat diet, the anti-TNF-α molecule infliximab led to decreased inflammation and decreased hepatic fat deposition/fibrosis as well as improved insulin signaling.[55] IL-6 is produced by multiple cell types in the body, including adipocytes, and levels are increased in obesity.[56] An increased IL-6 level in mice induces hepatic insulin resistance.[53] The mechanism for increased insulin resistance is believed to involve induction of a protein called suppressor of cytokine signaling 3, which directly inactivates the insulin receptor and targets IRS proteins for removal.[53] IL-6 seems to increase insulin sensitivity in skeletal muscle, suggesting a different effect depending on the levels of the cytokine and duration of exposure.[57] MCP-1 is a chemokine important for the migration of macrophages into adipose tissue. It is expressed more in visceral fat than subcutaneous fat and has been shown to be increased in obesity.[58] MCP-1 knockout mice show a decreased inflammatory profile with decreased insulin resistance and hepatic steatosis.[59] PAI-1 is

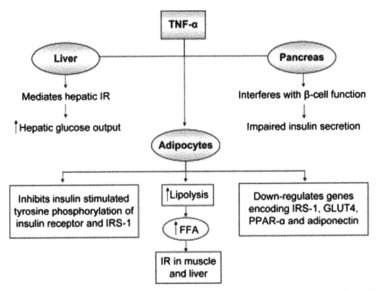

Fig. 5. Diverse mechanisms by which TNF-α contributes to the development of insulin resistance. GLUT4, glucose transporter 4; IR, insulin resistance. (*Adapted from* Puri P, Sanyal AJ. Role of obesity, insulin resistance, and steatosis in hepatitis C virus infection. Clin Liver Dis 2006;10(4):799; with permission.)

produced in multiple tissues, including the liver and adipocytes. Its role in the development of insulin resistance and hepatic steatosis is not yet clear but seems potent. PAI-1 levels increase with obesity and it has been implicated in the development of insulin resistance, diabetes, and atherothrombosis.[60] Mice with a PAI-1 knockout do not become obese on a high-fat diet and have improved insulin sensitivity.[61] RBP-4 is a transport protein for vitamin A produced by adipose tissue. Data in humans have been conflicting, but when RBP-4 is injected or overexpressed in mice it leads to insulin resistance by disrupting insulin and increasing hepatic gluconeogenesis through induction of phosphoenolpyruvate carboxykinase.[62] Increased levels of RBP-4 have been detected in patients with hepatic steatosis.[63] The cytokine resistin has also been shown to have increased levels in NAFLD and NASH, which parallel the severity of the disease but do not closely correlate with insulin resistance.[64]

Adipokines that act against insulin resistance and hepatic steatosis include adiponectin and leptin. Adiponectin is a protein created by mature fat cells that has strong effects on the development of fatty liver. It acts through 2 receptors (adipoR1 and adipoR2) to modulate lipid metabolism and decrease inflammation primarily through the AMPK and PPARα pathways,[65] which is summarized in **Fig. 6**. Stimulation of AMPK and PPARα leads to enhanced β-oxidation of fatty acids and inhibition of ACC, and therefore lipogenesis. Adiponectin has potent insulin-sensitizing effects that are the result of an AMPK-mediated decrease in hepatic gluconeogenesis and improved fatty acid oxidation.[66] Adiponectin levels decrease as obesity increases. This finding is related to the increased inflammation seen in adipose tissue because both TNF-α and IL-6 have been shown to decrease its levels.[67] Conversely, adiponectin has been shown to have antiinflammatory effects. Through a cyclic AMP-dependent pathway, it has been shown to inhibit TNF-α activation of NF-κB.[68] It has also been

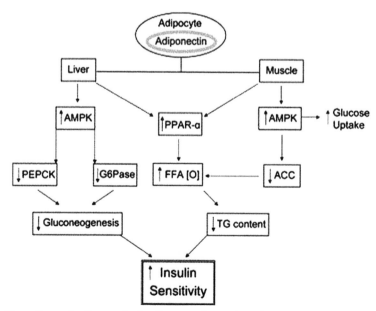

Fig. 6. The actions of adiponectin, leading to enhanced insulin sensitivity in the muscle and the liver. FFA [O], free fatty acid oxidation; G6Pase, glucose-6-phosphatase; PEPCK, phosphoenol pyruvate carboxylase. (*Adapted from* Puri P, Sanyal AJ. Role of obesity, insulin resistance, and steatosis in hepatitis C virus infection. Clin Liver Dis 2006;10(4):798; with permission.)

shown to decrease superoxide radical generation in cells treated with oxidized LDL.[69] Patients with NAFLD have been reported to have low adiponectin levels, and mice with steatosis treated with recombinant adiponectin have improved insulin sensitivity, decreased steatosis, and lowered levels of TNF-α.[70,71] Leptin is another hormone secreted from adipose tissue that may have a significant role in the development of hepatic steatosis. Leptin-deficient (ob/ob) mice are noted to become massively obese, diabetic, and to develop fatty livers. Similar to adiponectin, leptin works through AMPK signaling to increase fatty acid oxidation, increase glucose uptake, limit ectopic lipid storage, and improve insulin sensitivity.[72] Unlike murine models, most patients with obesity, diabetes, and NAFLD have increased leptin levels, and resistance to leptin may be the problem. Supporting this theory is the discovery of single nucleotide polymorphisms in the leptin receptor, which occur in greater frequency in patients with hepatic steatosis compared with controls.[73]

Insulin resistance leads to increased fatty acid delivery to the hepatocyte, decreased inhibition of gluconeogenesis, and amplification of DNL. It is a combination of these effects that leads to hepatic steatosis. In patients with NAFLD, insulin does not suppress lipolysis normally, leading to increased delivery of FFA to the liver via the NEFA pool.[44,74] Increased FFA levels in the liver typically lead to increased β-oxidation through the effects of PPARα and by a complex between PPARγ coactivator 1 (PPARγC1) and forkhead box protein a2 (FOXa2).[75] FOXa2 is part of the insulin-signaling pathway that is disrupted in insulin resistance. The result is the inability of FOXa2 to associate with PPARγC1, allowing fatty acids to be shunted from the β-oxidation pathway into DNL pathways.[76] FFAs alone may impair insulin signaling and increase hepatic gluconeogenesis, although this needs further study because the exact mechanisms are not clear.[77] What is clear is that lipid metabolites can cause insulin resistance. Diacylglycerol (DAG) is an intermediate in the conversion of the fatty acid oleate into TG. Excess DAG has been shown to directly cause insulin resistance through activation of an isoform of protein kinase C, which binds the insulin receptor and inhibits its activity.[78] The disruption in insulin signaling in the hepatocyte is not balanced. Pathways inactivating gluconeogenesis are disrupted, whereas pathways leading to DNL such as SREBP1c continue to be stimulated.[79] This situation leads to the development of hyperglycemia, worsening steatosis, and insulin resistance. A summary of interorgan cross talk in the development of hepatic steatosis caused by insulin resistance is highlighted in **Fig. 7**.

GENETICS

Genetic factors also play a role in the development of hepatic steatosis. This finding is shown by genetic studies that estimate the heritability of hepatic steatosis to approach 39%.[80] People with similar amounts and distributions of fat can have differing degrees of hepatic steatosis. Sex and ethnicity have also been shown to affect the prevalence of NAFLD. Men develop hepatic steatosis at a higher rate than women until the age of 60 years, when the trend reverses.[81] The same population-based study reported a higher rate of hepatic steatosis in people of Hispanic descent (45%) when compared with whites (33%) and African Americans (24%).[81] Asian Indians have also been discovered to have a higher risk of hepatic steatosis. In a study of young lean individuals of different ethnic groups, Asian Indian males had a 3-fold to 4-fold higher prevalence of insulin resistance, a 2-fold increase in hepatic TG content, and increased levels of IL-6 when compared with white men.[82] Efforts are being undertaken to discover the genetic susceptibility for hepatic steatosis. One missense mutation {I148M} in the patatinlike phospholipase domain-containing 3 gene (PNPLA3) has been associated with the

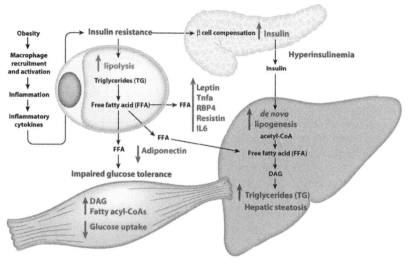

Fig. 7. Three links between adipocyte biology and metabolic syndrome. Obesity leads to the recruitment by adipocytes of macrophages. These macrophages are activated to produce inflammatory cytokines, which blunt insulin signaling. In adipocytes, insulin resistance leads to an impaired ability of insulin to suppress lipolysis, leading to an increased flux of FFAs from adipocytes to other tissues. In muscle, increased fatty acid flux leads to impaired glucose uptake, leading to whole-body impaired glucose tolerance. In the liver, the increased flux of FFA contributes to increased TG synthesis and hepatic steatosis. Insulin resistance causes pancreatic β cells to compensate with increased insulin production, leading to hyperinsulinemia. This situation in turn stimulates DNL in the liver, contributing to the pool of FFAs available for TG production. Obesity also alters the balance of adipokines produced by adipocytes, with an increase in leptin, TNF-α, RBP-4, resistin, and IL-6, and a decrease in adiponectin. This altered balance contributes to impaired glucose tolerance and insulin resistance. (*Adapted from* Attie AD, Scherer PE. Adipocyte metabolism and obesity. J Lipid Res 2009;50:S398; with permission.)

development of NAFLD.[83] The prevalence of this mutation may explain the differences in susceptibility to NAFLD seen between different ethnicities.[84] The protein product PNPLA3 is induced by insulin through pathways controlled by LXR and SREBP1c.[85] How this mutation leads to hepatic steatosis is not fully understood. Experiments in mice and hepatocyte cell culture suggest that the I148M missense mutation leads to decreased TG hydrolase activity and development of steatosis.[86] Other genome-wide studies have turned up other genetic regions that confer risk of development of hepatic steatosis, including NCAN, PPP1R3B, and in Asian Indians, apolipoprotein C3, but further study needs to be performed to understand their clinical relevance.[3]

DIETARY FACTORS IN THE GENESIS OF HEPATIC STEATOSIS

Dietary habits can affect the incidence of hepatic steatosis. A high-fat diet leads to increased endocannabinoid activity. Endocannabinoids are lipid mediators that act via cannabinoid receptors to affect lipid metabolism. Although found throughout the body, cannabinoid receptor 1 (CB1) has effects on both adipose and hepatic tissue. CB1 and the endocannabinoid, arachidonoyl ethanolamide, show increased expression with a high-fat diet.[87] Stimulation of CB1 leads to increased fatty acid release from adipose tissue, decreased adiponectin levels, increased insulin resistance, and decreased fatty acid β-oxidation.[88] Intake of fructose is another possible cause behind the increasing incidence of hepatic steatosis. Fructose consumption is increasing dramatically in the United States. In the early twentieth century, Americans consumed on average 15 g of fructose per day, which represented 4% of total daily calories. Current estimates put fructose consumption at 73 g per day in teenagers, which represents 12% of daily calories.[89] In a study in which human individuals were given drinks sweetened with either glucose or fructose for 10 weeks, the fructose group had higher levels of DNL, more visceral adiposity, more altered lipid metabolism, and decreased insulin sensitivity when compared with the glucose group.[90] Fructose is taken up by the liver and metabolized in a process separate from glycolysis. Most of the fructose is shunted in a reverse fashion through the glycolysis pathway to create glucose and glycogen. A small but significant portion of fructose is used as substrate for DNL. Fructose has been shown in cell culture and in mice to alter expression of

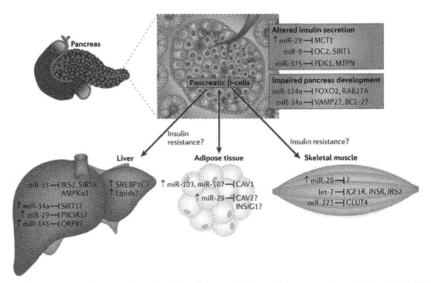

Fig. 8. miRNA regulation of insulin signaling and glucose homeostasis: miRNAs that affect diverse parts of insulin signaling in the pancreas, liver, muscle, and adipose tissue. In the pancreas: miR-124a and miR-34a are involved in pancreatic development (through effects on FOXO2 (forkhead box protein O2), RAB27A, VAMP2 (vesicle-associated membrane protein 2), and BCL-2 (B cell lymphoma 2)). miR-29, miR-9, and miR-375 are involved in insulin secretion (miR-29 activates insulin secretion, whereas miR-9 and miR-375 inhibit insulin secretion), acting through MCT1 (monocarboxylate transporter 1), OC2 (1 cut homeobox 2), SIRT1 (sirtuin 1), PDK1 (phosphoinositide-dependent kinase 1), and MTPN (myotrophin). In the liver: miR-33, miR-34a, miR-29, and miR-143 act in the liver on targets involved in insulin signaling and its regulation (such as IRS-2, SIRT6, AMPKα1 (AMP-activated protein kinase-α subunit 1), SIRT1, PIK3R1 (phosphatidylinositol 3-kinase subunit-α), and ORP8 (oxysterol-binding protein-related protein 8)). In the adipose tissue: insulin signaling in adipose tissue is modulated by miR-103 and miR-107 (through CAV1 [caveolin 1]) and miR-29 (through INSIG1 [insulin-induced gene 1] and CAV2). In the muscle: the miR-29, let-7 and miR-223 miRNAs may act in muscle to modulate insulin signaling (IGF1R [insulinlike growth factor receptor 1], INSR [insulin receptor] and IRS2) and glucose uptake (GLUT4 [glucose transporter type 4]). Known and predicted targets that lack in vivo evidence are marked with a question mark. In disease conditions, such as impaired insulin secretion or insulin resistance, several miRNAs are upregulated (*arrow*). (*Adapted from* Rottiers V, Näär AM. MicroRNAs in metabolism and metabolic disorders. Nat Rev Mol Cell Biol 2012;13(5):243; with permission.)

glucose-stimulated enzymes associated with lipid metabolism (activated acetyl-CoA carboxylase, hormone-sensitive lipase, and adipose TG lipase), leading to increased DNL in cell culture and development of steatosis in mice.[91]

MICRO-RNA REGULATION OF INSULIN SIGNALING AND GLUCOSE HOMEOSTASIS

Micro-RNAs (miRNAs) are 21-nucleotide-long to 23-nucleotide-long non–protein-coding, single-stranded RNAs that regulate gene expression via messenger RNA (mRNA) degradation by binding with imperfect complementarity to the 3′ untranslated region of their targets and preventing translation, mechanisms of which remain unclear. The expression of miRNAs is both organ-specific and dependent on the stage of development. MiRNAs regulate important cellular processes such as metabolism. We showed that NASH is associated with altered hepatic miRNA expression and that altered lipid metabolism implicated in the pathogenesis of NASH is potentially caused by the underexpression of miR-122.[92] In a recent review, the role of miRNAs affecting insulin handling and its potential implications in glucose and lipid metabolism contributing to hepatic steatosis are discussed in detail, which is beyond the scope of this review.[93] Pancreatic β cells secrete insulin in response to feeding. Insulin increases glucose uptake, decreases glucose production, and facilitates lipid synthesis and storage. These actions of insulin happen at the level of liver, adipose tissue, and muscle.

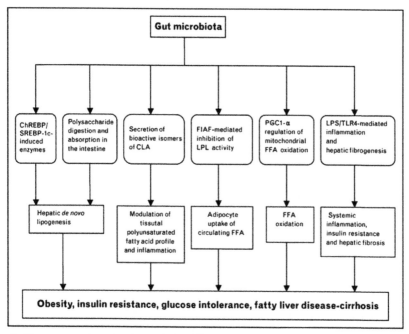

Fig. 9. The proposed mechanisms of the effects of gut microbiota on host metabolic and inflammatory processes contributing to obesity, insulin resistance, and fatty liver disease. ChREBP, carbohydrate-responsive element-binding protein; CLA, conjugated linoleic acid; FIAF, fasting-induced adipose factor; LPL, lipoprotein lipase; LPS, lipopolysaccharide; PGC1-α, peroxisomal proliferator-activated receptor coactivator 1α; SREBP-1C, sterol-responsive element binding protein-1c; TLR-4, toll-like receptor 4. (*Adapted from* Musso G, Gambino R, Cassader M. Gut microbiota as a regulator of energy homeostasis and ectopic fat deposition: mechanisms and implications for metabolic disorders. Curr Opin Lipidol 2010;21(1):77; with permission.)

The emerging role of miRNAs in the regulation of insulin-mediated effects and its dys-regulation contributing to insulin resistance and metabolic derangements leading to increased hepatic steatosis as a result of increased lipogenesis is depicted in **Fig. 8**.[93]

GUT MICROBIOTA AND FATTY LIVER DISEASE

The human gut harbors a diverse and dynamic bacterial ecosystem, which is important to human health. The human gut has an estimated 500 to 1000 distinct bacterial species, with the total number of bacteria approaching 10^{14} cells and containing 100 times as many genes as the human genome. Obesity and fatty liver disease are global health prob-lems and have recently been linked to alterations of gut microbiota and its metabolic effects. The gut microbiota regulates host energy homeostasis, as shown by the

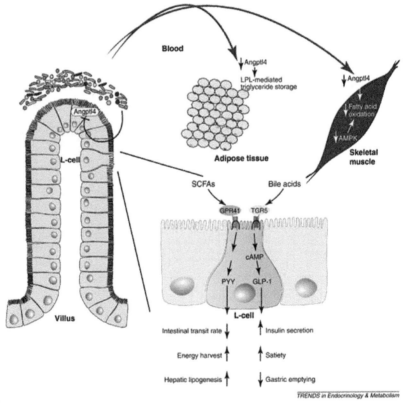

Fig. 10. Gut microbiota regulation of host metabolism. The gut microbiota suppresses enter-ocyte expression of Angptl4; this alleviates LPL inhibition and promotes LPL-mediated TG storage in adipose tissue. In addition, reduced Angptl4 levels together with diminished activa-tion of AMPK reduce fatty acid oxidation in skeletal muscle. The gut microbiota also has direct effects on enteroendocrine L cells: microbially generated short-chain fatty acids (SCFAs) bind to the G-protein-coupled receptor (GPCR) Gpr41, which stimulates secretion of the gut hormone PYY. Secretion of PYY leads to reduced intestinal transit, increased energy harvest, and stimulates hepatic lipogenesis. The gut microbiota generates secondary bile acids that are the major ligands for the GPCR TGR5. Stimulation of TGR5 enhances GLP-1 secretion, and this promotes increased insulin secretion, satiety, and reduced gastric emptying. (*Adapted from* Greiner T, Bäckhed F. Effects of the gut microbiota on obesity and glucose homeostasis. Trends Endocrinol Metab 2011;22(4):119; with permission.)

pioneering works of Gordon and colleagues.[94] They noticed that germ-free (ie, raised in the absence of microorganisms) mice had 40% less total body fat than mice with a normal gut microbiota, even although the latter ate 30% less calories than did the germ-free animals.[94] When germ-free mice were exposed to gut microbiota harvested from the cecum of a normal mouse, within 2 weeks they developed insulin resistance and had a 60% increase in body fat despite a significant lower food intake. The weight gain was a result of increased intestinal glucose absorption and energy extraction from the undigestible food component with concomitant development of hyperglycemia and hyperinsulinemia. The germ-free mice had increased expression of ACC and FAS, the 2 key lipogenic enzymes promoting hepatic de novo lipogenesis after a 2-week exposure to the normal mice flora. Also, the hepatic TG content was increased by 2-fold, accompanied by an increased hepatic mRNA expression of SREBP-1 and ChREBP, 2 nuclear regulators of lipogenic enzymes.[94,95] The exposure of germ-free mice to normal mice flora also induced a systemic increase in LPL activity, the enzyme catalyzing the release of FFAs and triacylglycerol from circulating TG-rich lipoproteins to adipose tissue and muscle. This finding was believed to be related to the suppression of fasting-induced adipose factor (FIAF) in the gut. FIAF inhibits the LPL activity. This finding showed for the first time that an environmental factor such as gut microbiota can regulate energy storage. The proposed gut microbiota-related pathophysiologic changes in obesity and fatty liver disease are shown in **Fig. 9**. Subsequent studies have linked gut microbiota in the pathogenesis of obesity.[96] A recent review[97] highlighted the integrative role of gut microbiota and host metabolism (**Fig. 10**).

SUMMARY

Hepatic steatosis is the result of a complex interplay between the diet, the metabolic system, and host responses at the level of adipose tissue, muscle, pancreas, and the liver. Increasing adiposity leads to an inflammatory milieu, which causes the release of proinflammatory cytokines such as TNF-α and IL-6, whereas beneficial adipokines such as adiponectin become suppressed. This situation leads to the development of peripheral insulin resistance and hyperinsulinemia and increased fatty acid delivery to the hepatocyte. The disruption of normal insulin signaling in the hepatocyte and increased abundance of fatty acids leads to disordered lipid metabolism. Transcriptional factors such as SREBP-1c, ChREBP, and LXR are overactivated, causing more fatty acid and glucose products to be shunted into DNL pathways. β-Oxidation in the mitochondria is inhibited because malonyl-CoA inhibits the crucial fatty acid transporter CPT-1. VLDL packaging and export are inhibited, leading to buildup of TGs in the hepatocytes. End products of fatty acid metabolism also accumulate, such as DAG, which leads to even more insulin resistance in a positive feedback loop. Gluconeogenesis is not suppressed despite hyperinsulinemia in the insulin-resistant hepatocyte, and increased glucose levels provide more substrate for DNL. Dietary factors such as high carbohydrate intake, high fat intake and fructose all worsen insulin sensitivity and increase hepatic steatosis. The contribution of genetic susceptibility is only now becoming clear but may play a role in future treatments or prognosis. The extreme complexity of this system explains the inherent difficulty in treating it. Correction of 1 problem or pathway is overcome by other redundant pathways. This situation explains why promising therapies such as thiazolidenediones, fenofibrates, and metformin often fall short in clinical practice. Continued research into the pathogenesis of hepatic steatosis is important because NAFLD and NASH are rapidly increasing in prevalence and have become a burgeoning health care crisis. Effective therapies and prevention based on understanding of the pathogenesis are the key in curbing this epidemic.

REFERENCES

1. Angulo P. Nonalcoholic fatty liver disease. N Engl J Med 2002;346:1221–31.
2. Mansbach CM 2nd, Gorelick F. Development and physiological regulation of intestinal lipid absorption. II. Dietary lipid absorption, complex lipid synthesis, and the intracellular packaging and secretion of chylomicrons. Am J Physiol Gastrointest Liver Physiol 2007;293:G645–50.
3. Cohen JC, Horton JD, Hobbs HH. Human fatty liver disease: old questions and new insights. Science 2011;332:1519–23.
4. Macfarlane DP, Forbes S, Walker BR. Glucocorticoids and fatty acid metabolism in humans: fuelling fat redistribution in the metabolic syndrome. J Endocrinol 2008;197:189–204.
5. McGarry JD, Mannaerts GP, Foster DW. A possible role for malonyl-CoA in the regulation of hepatic fatty acid oxidation and ketogenesis. J Clin Invest 1977; 60:265–70.
6. Donnelly KL, Smith CI, Schwarzenberg SJ, et al. Sources of fatty acids stored in liver and secreted via lipoproteins in patients with nonalcoholic fatty liver disease. J Clin Invest 2005;115:1343–51.
7. Postic C, Girard J. Contribution of de novo fatty acid synthesis to hepatic steatosis and insulin resistance: lessons from genetically engineered mice. J Clin Invest 2008;118:829–38.
8. Browning JD, Horton JD. Molecular mediators of hepatic steatosis and liver injury. J Clin Invest 2004;114:147–52.
9. Diraison F, Beylot M. Role of human liver lipogenesis and reesterification in triglycerides secretion and in FFA reesterification. Am J Physiol 1998;274:E321–7.
10. Araya J, Rodrigo R, Videla LA, et al. Increase in long-chain polyunsaturated fatty acid n - 6/n - 3 ratio in relation to hepatic steatosis in patients with non-alcoholic fatty liver disease. Clin Sci (Lond) 2004;106:635–43.
11. Puri P, Baillie RA, Wiest MM, et al. A lipidomic analysis of nonalcoholic fatty liver disease. Hepatology 2007;46:1081–90.
12. Brown MS, Goldstein JL. The SREBP pathway: regulation of cholesterol metabolism by proteolysis of a membrane-bound transcription factor. Cell 1997;89:331–40.
13. Horton JD, Shah NA, Warrington JA, et al. Combined analysis of oligonucleotide microarray data from transgenic and knockout mice identifies direct SREBP target genes. Proc Natl Acad Sci U S A 2003;100:12027–32.
14. Moon YA, Shah NA, Mohapatra S, et al. Identification of a mammalian long chain fatty acyl elongase regulated by sterol regulatory element-binding proteins. J Biol Chem 2001;276:45358–66.
15. Gonzalez-Baro MR, Lewin TM, Coleman RA. Regulation of triglyceride metabolism. II. Function of mitochondrial GPAT1 in the regulation of triacylglycerol biosynthesis and insulin action. Am J Physiol Gastrointest Liver Physiol 2007; 292:G1195–9.
16. Sato R, Miyamoto W, Inoue J, et al. Sterol regulatory element-binding protein negatively regulates microsomal triglyceride transfer protein gene transcription. J Biol Chem 1999;274:24714–20.
17. Chakravarty K, Leahy P, Becard D, et al. Sterol regulatory element-binding protein-1c mimics the negative effect of insulin on phosphoenolpyruvate carboxykinase (GTP) gene transcription. J Biol Chem 2001;276:34816–23.
18. Shimomura I, Bashmakov Y, Horton JD. Increased levels of nuclear SREBP-1c associated with fatty livers in two mouse models of diabetes mellitus. J Biol Chem 1999;274:30028–32.

19. Jump DB. Dietary polyunsaturated fatty acids and regulation of gene transcription. Curr Opin Lipidol 2002;13:155–64.
20. Yamashita H, Takenoshita M, Sakurai M, et al. A glucose-responsive transcription factor that regulates carbohydrate metabolism in the liver. Proc Natl Acad Sci U S A 2001;98:9116–21.
21. Kawaguchi T, Takenoshita M, Kabashima T, et al. Glucose and cAMP regulate the L-type pyruvate kinase gene by phosphorylation/dephosphorylation of the carbohydrate response element binding protein. Proc Natl Acad Sci U S A 2001;98:13710–5.
22. Towle HC. Glucose as a regulator of eukaryotic gene transcription. Trends Endocrinol Metab 2005;16:489–94.
23. Iizuka K, Bruick RK, Liang G, et al. Deficiency of carbohydrate response element-binding protein (ChREBP) reduces lipogenesis as well as glycolysis. Proc Natl Acad Sci U S A 2004;101:7281–6.
24. Ma L, Robinson LN, Towle HC. ChREBP*Mlx is the principal mediator of glucose-induced gene expression in the liver. J Biol Chem 2006;281:28721–30.
25. Liu Y, Qiu de K, Ma X. Liver X receptors bridge hepatic lipid metabolism and inflammation. J Dig Dis 2012;13:69–74.
26. Laplante M, Sabatini DM. An emerging role of mTOR in lipid biosynthesis. Curr Biol 2009;19:R1046–52.
27. Repa JJ, Liang G, Ou J, et al. Regulation of mouse sterol regulatory element-binding protein-1c gene (SREBP-1c) by oxysterol receptors, LXRalpha and LXRbeta. Genes Dev 2000;14:2819–30.
28. Cha JY, Repa JJ. The liver X receptor (LXR) and hepatic lipogenesis. The carbohydrate-response element-binding protein is a target gene of LXR. J Biol Chem 2007;282:743–51.
29. Vacca M, Degirolamo C, Mariani-Costantini R, et al. Lipid-sensing nuclear receptors in the pathophysiology and treatment of the metabolic syndrome. Wiley Interdiscip Rev Syst Biol Med 2011;3:562–87.
30. Mitro N, Mak PA, Vargas L, et al. The nuclear receptor LXR is a glucose sensor. Nature 2007;445:219–23.
31. Wang YX. PPARs: diverse regulators in energy metabolism and metabolic diseases. Cell Res 2010;20:124–37.
32. Rogue A, Renaud MP, Claude N, et al. Comparative gene expression profiles induced by PPARgamma and PPARalpha/gamma agonists in rat hepatocytes. Toxicol Appl Pharmacol 2011;254:18–31.
33. Costet P, Legendre C, More J, et al. Peroxisome proliferator-activated receptor alpha-isoform deficiency leads to progressive dyslipidemia with sexually dimorphic obesity and steatosis. J Biol Chem 1998;273:29577–85.
34. Nissen SE, Nicholls SJ, Wolski K, et al. Effects of a potent and selective PPAR-alpha agonist in patients with atherogenic dyslipidemia or hypercholesterolemia: two randomized controlled trials. JAMA 2007;297:1362–73.
35. Barish GD, Narkar VA, Evans RM. PPAR delta: a dagger in the heart of the metabolic syndrome. J Clin Invest 2006;116:590–7.
36. Chao L, Marcus-Samuels B, Mason MM, et al. Adipose tissue is required for the antidiabetic, but not for the hypolipidemic, effect of thiazolidinediones. J Clin Invest 2000;106:1221–8.
37. Krey G, Braissant O, L'Horset F, et al. Fatty acids, eicosanoids, and hypolipidemic agents identified as ligands of peroxisome proliferator-activated receptors by coactivator-dependent receptor ligand assay. Mol Endocrinol 1997;11:779–91.
38. Kim JB, Wright HM, Wright M, et al. ADD1/SREBP1 activates PPARgamma through the production of endogenous ligand. Proc Natl Acad Sci U S A 1998;95:4333–7.

39. Shulman AI, Mangelsdorf DJ. Retinoid x receptor heterodimers in the metabolic syndrome. N Engl J Med 2005;353:604–15.
40. Maeda N, Takahashi M, Funahashi T, et al. PPARgamma ligands increase expression and plasma concentrations of adiponectin, an adipose-derived protein. Diabetes 2001;50:2094–9.
41. Hardie DG. Minireview: the AMP-activated protein kinase cascade: the key sensor of cellular energy status. Endocrinology 2003;144:5179–83.
42. Zhou G, Myers R, Li Y, et al. Role of AMP-activated protein kinase in mechanism of metformin action. J Clin Invest 2001;108:1167–74.
43. Kawaguchi T, Osatomi K, Yamashita H, et al. Mechanism for fatty acid "sparing" effect on glucose-induced transcription: regulation of carbohydrate-responsive element-binding protein by AMP-activated protein kinase. J Biol Chem 2002; 277:3829–35.
44. Sanyal AJ, Campbell-Sargent C, Mirshahi F, et al. Nonalcoholic steatohepatitis: association of insulin resistance and mitochondrial abnormalities. Gastroenterology 2001;120:1183–92.
45. Pagano G, Pacini G, Musso G, et al. Nonalcoholic steatohepatitis, insulin resistance, and metabolic syndrome: further evidence for an etiologic association. Hepatology 2002;35:367–72.
46. Chitturi S, Abeygunasekera S, Farrell GC, et al. NASH and insulin resistance: insulin hypersecretion and specific association with the insulin resistance syndrome. Hepatology 2002;35:373–9.
47. Weisberg SP, McCann D, Desai M, et al. Obesity is associated with macrophage accumulation in adipose tissue. J Clin Invest 2003;112:1796–808.
48. Xu H, Barnes GT, Yang Q, et al. Chronic inflammation in fat plays a crucial role in the development of obesity-related insulin resistance. J Clin Invest 2003;112: 1821–30.
49. Ramos EJ, Xu Y, Romanova I, et al. Is obesity an inflammatory disease? Surgery 2003;134:329–35.
50. Maury E, Brichard SM. Adipokine dysregulation, adipose tissue inflammation and metabolic syndrome. Mol Cell Endocrinol 2010;314:1–16.
51. Fain JN, Bahouth SW, Madan AK. TNFalpha release by the nonfat cells of human adipose tissue. Int J Obes Relat Metab Disord 2004;28:616–22.
52. Cawthorn WP, Sethi JK. TNF-alpha and adipocyte biology. FEBS Lett 2008;582: 117–31.
53. Sabio G, Das M, Mora A, et al. A stress signaling pathway in adipose tissue regulates hepatic insulin resistance. Science 2008;322:1539–43.
54. Hui JM, Hodge A, Farrell GC, et al. Beyond insulin resistance in NASH: TNF-alpha or adiponectin? Hepatology 2004;40:46–54.
55. Barbuio R, Milanski M, Bertolo MB, et al. Infliximab reverses steatosis and improves insulin signal transduction in liver of rats fed a high-fat diet. J Endocrinol 2007;194:539–50.
56. Bastard JP, Lagathu C, Caron M, et al. Point-counterpoint: interleukin-6 does/ does not have a beneficial role in insulin sensitivity and glucose homeostasis. J Appl Physiol 2007;102:821–2 [author reply: 825].
57. Pedersen BK, Fischer CP. Physiological roles of muscle-derived interleukin-6 in response to exercise. Curr Opin Clin Nutr Metab Care 2007;10:265–71.
58. Bruun JM, Lihn AS, Pedersen SB, et al. Monocyte chemoattractant protein-1 release is higher in visceral than subcutaneous human adipose tissue (AT): implication of macrophages resident in the AT. J Clin Endocrinol Metab 2005;90: 2282–9.

59. Kanda H, Tateya S, Tamori Y, et al. MCP-1 contributes to macrophage infiltration into adipose tissue, insulin resistance, and hepatic steatosis in obesity. J Clin Invest 2006;116:1494–505.

60. Alessi MC, Poggi M, Juhan-Vague I. Plasminogen activator inhibitor-1, adipose tissue and insulin resistance. Curr Opin Lipidol 2007;18:240–5.

61. Ma LJ, Mao SL, Taylor KL, et al. Prevention of obesity and insulin resistance in mice lacking plasminogen activator inhibitor 1. Diabetes 2004;53:336–46.

62. Yang Q, Graham TE, Mody N, et al. Serum retinol binding protein 4 contributes to insulin resistance in obesity and type 2 diabetes. Nature 2005;436:356–62.

63. Wu H, Jia W, Bao Y, et al. Serum retinol binding protein 4 and nonalcoholic fatty liver disease in patients with type 2 diabetes mellitus. Diabetes Res Clin Pract 2008;79:185–90.

64. Pagano C, Soardo G, Pilon C, et al. Increased serum resistin in nonalcoholic fatty liver disease is related to liver disease severity and not to insulin resistance. J Clin Endocrinol Metab 2006;91:1081–6.

65. Yamauchi T, Hara K, Kubota N, et al. Dual roles of adiponectin/Acrp30 in vivo as an anti-diabetic and anti-atherogenic adipokine. Curr Drug Targets Immune Endocr Metabol Disord 2003;3:243–54.

66. Kadowaki T, Yamauchi T, Kubota N, et al. Adiponectin and adiponectin receptors in insulin resistance, diabetes, and the metabolic syndrome. J Clin Invest 2006;116:1784–92.

67. Ouchi N, Walsh K. Adiponectin as an anti-inflammatory factor. Clin Chim Acta 2007;380:24–30.

68. Ouchi N, Kihara S, Arita Y, et al. Adiponectin, an adipocyte-derived plasma protein, inhibits endothelial NF-kappaB signaling through a cAMP-dependent pathway. Circulation 2000;102:1296–301.

69. Motoshima H, Wu X, Mahadev K, et al. Adiponectin suppresses proliferation and superoxide generation and enhances eNOS activity in endothelial cells treated with oxidized LDL. Biochem Biophys Res Commun 2004;315:264–71.

70. Matsubara M. Plasma adiponectin decrease in women with nonalcoholic fatty liver. Endocr J 2004;51:587–93.

71. Xu A, Wang Y, Keshaw H, et al. The fat-derived hormone adiponectin alleviates alcoholic and nonalcoholic fatty liver diseases in mice. J Clin Invest 2003;112:91–100.

72. Oral EA, Simha V, Ruiz E, et al. Leptin-replacement therapy for lipodystrophy. N Engl J Med 2002;346:570–8.

73. Swellam M, Hamdy N. Association of nonalcoholic fatty liver disease with a single nucleotide polymorphism on the gene encoding leptin receptor. IUBMB Life 2012;64:180–6.

74. Lewis GF, Carpentier A, Adeli K, et al. Disordered fat storage and mobilization in the pathogenesis of insulin resistance and type 2 diabetes. Endocr Rev 2002;23:201–29.

75. Wolfrum C, Stoffel M. Coactivation of Foxa2 through Pgc-1beta promotes liver fatty acid oxidation and triglyceride/VLDL secretion. Cell Metab 2006;3:99–110.

76. Wolfrum C, Asilmaz E, Luca E, et al. Foxa2 regulates lipid metabolism and ketogenesis in the liver during fasting and in diabetes. Nature 2004;432:1027–32.

77. Kabir M, Catalano KJ, Ananthnarayan S, et al. Molecular evidence supporting the portal theory: a causative link between visceral adiposity and hepatic insulin resistance. Am J Physiol Endocrinol Metab 2005;288:E454–61.

78. Samuel VT, Liu ZX, Qu X, et al. Mechanism of hepatic insulin resistance in nonalcoholic fatty liver disease. J Biol Chem 2004;279:32345–53.

79. Brown MS, Goldstein JL. Selective versus total insulin resistance: a pathogenic paradox. Cell Metab 2008;7:95–6.
80. Schwimmer JB, Celedon MA, Lavine JE, et al. Heritability of nonalcoholic fatty liver disease. Gastroenterology 2009;136:1585–92.
81. Browning JD, Szczepaniak LS, Dobbins R, et al. Prevalence of hepatic steatosis in an urban population in the United States: impact of ethnicity. Hepatology 2004; 40:1387–95.
82. Petersen KF, Dufour S, Feng J, et al. Increased prevalence of insulin resistance and nonalcoholic fatty liver disease in Asian-Indian men. Proc Natl Acad Sci U S A 2006;103:18273–7.
83. Speliotes EK, Butler JL, Palmer CD, et al. PNPLA3 variants specifically confer increased risk for histologic nonalcoholic fatty liver disease but not metabolic disease. Hepatology 2010;52:904–12.
84. Romeo S, Kozlitina J, Xing C, et al. Genetic variation in PNPLA3 confers susceptibility to nonalcoholic fatty liver disease. Nat Genet 2008;40:1461–5.
85. Huang Y, He S, Li JZ, et al. A feed-forward loop amplifies nutritional regulation of PNPLA3. Proc Natl Acad Sci U S A 2010;107:7892–7.
86. He S, McPhaul C, Li JZ, et al. A sequence variation (I148M) in PNPLA3 associated with nonalcoholic fatty liver disease disrupts triglyceride hydrolysis. J Biol Chem 2010;285:6706–15.
87. Osei-Hyiaman D, DePetrillo M, Pacher P, et al. Endocannabinoid activation at hepatic CB1 receptors stimulates fatty acid synthesis and contributes to diet-induced obesity. J Clin Invest 2005;115:1298–305.
88. Tam J, Liu J, Mukhopadhyay B, et al. Endocannabinoids in liver disease. Hepatology 2011;53:346–55.
89. Lustig RH. Fructose: metabolic, hedonic, and societal parallels with ethanol. J Am Diet Assoc 2010;110:1307–21.
90. Stanhope KL, Schwarz JM, Keim NL, et al. Consuming fructose-sweetened, not glucose-sweetened, beverages increases visceral adiposity and lipids and decreases insulin sensitivity in overweight/obese humans. J Clin Invest 2009; 119:1322–34.
91. Huang D, Dhawan T, Young S, et al. Fructose impairs glucose-induced hepatic triglyceride synthesis. Lipids Health Dis 2011;10:20.
92. Cheung O, Puri P, Eicken C, et al. Nonalcoholic steatohepatitis is associated with altered hepatic microRNA expression. Hepatology 2008;48:1810–20.
93. Rottiers V, Naar AM. MicroRNAs in metabolism and metabolic disorders. Nat Rev Mol Cell Biol 2012;13:1.
94. Backhed F, Ding H, Wang T, et al. The gut microbiota as an environmental factor that regulates fat storage. Proc Natl Acad Sci U S A 2004;101:15718–23.
95. Musso G, Gambino R, Cassader M. Recent insights into hepatic lipid metabolism in non-alcoholic fatty liver disease (NAFLD). Prog Lipid Res 2009;48:1–26.
96. Turnbaugh PJ, Ley RE, Mahowald MA, et al. An obesity-associated gut microbiome with increased capacity for energy harvest. Nature 2006;444:1027–31.
97. Greiner T, Backhed F. Effects of the gut microbiota on obesity and glucose homeostasis. Trends Endocrinol Metab 2011;22:117–23.

A Myriad of Pathways to NASH

Soledad Larrain, MD, Mary E. Rinella, MD*

KEYWORDS

- Nonalcoholic fatty liver disease • Nonalcoholic steatohepatitis • NASH • Drug
- Nutrition • Endocrine • Metabolism

KEY POINTS

- There is substantial heterogeneity in the nonalcoholic steatohepatitis (NASH) population.
- Several drugs can lead to NASH or exacerbate preexisting disease, primarily through their effects on hepatic lipid metabolism.
- Endocrine disorders, such as growth hormone deficiency and hypothyroidism, should be considered when evaluating patients with NASH.
- Several genetic, metabolic and nutritional disease states should be considered in patients with an atypical presentation, particularly because diseases such as Wilson disease can be catastrophic if not treated.

INTRODUCTION

Nonalcoholic steatohepatitis (NASH), the progressive phenotype of nonalcoholic fatty liver disease (NAFLD), represents the end product of a myriad of pathogenic mechanisms with insulin resistance at its core. Other important factors that contribute to the liver injury include lipid peroxidation, endoplasmic reticulum stress, and alterations in innate immune function. These factors promote a proinflammatory state leading to the development of cell death and fibrosis. Histologically, NASH is characterized by specific features, including steatosis, cellular ballooning, and inflammation with varying degrees of fibrosis.[1,2] In the absence of alcohol abuse, this hepatic ailment most often occurs in overweight patients with concomitant features of the metabolic syndrome (MetS). Overall, patients with NASH are a heterogeneous group. Even among patients with NASH with MetS, rate of progression and response to therapy are often unpredictable and variable. Environmental influences and their interplay

The authors have no conflicts of interest pertinent to this study.

This research was supported by investigator-initiated funds.

Division of Gastroenterology & Hepatology, Department of Medicine, Northwestern University Feinberg School of Medicine, 676 North St Clair, 14-005, Chicago, IL 60611, USA

* Corresponding author.

E-mail address: m-rinella@northwestern.edu

Clin Liver Dis 16 (2012) 525–548

doi:10.1016/j.cld.2012.05.009

1089-3261/12/$ – see front matter © 2012 Elsevier Inc. All rights reserved.

with genetic factors, most of which remain unknown, likely play a role in these discrepancies.

Although many mechanisms contribute to the development of NASH, the contribution of each is variable in a given patient. Furthermore, external factors can promote or exacerbate underlying steatosis or steatohepatitis. For this reason, defining NASH as a diagnosis of exclusion is fitting. Perhaps instead of attempting to treat the condition with an intervention targeting one or more mechanisms generalizable to the NASH population, we should consider what the appropriate therapy is for each specific patient with NASH. The most effective pharmacologic treatments for NASH to date have been successful in less than 50% of patients enrolled in clinical trials.[3-5] Until we have a better understanding of the various subgroups within NASH, attempting to avoid a non-name will prove challenging. In this review, the authors discuss acquired or intrinsic disease states, nutritional factors, and drugs that can either directly or indirectly lead to NASH (**Fig. 1**). By understanding these various pathophysiologic factors that may result in or exacerbate NASH, we will gain insight into how we can individualize the treatment of our patients.

DRUG-INDUCED STEATOHEPATITIS

Approximately 2% of NASH cases are estimated to be drug induced confirming that steatohepatitis is a rare manifestation of drug toxicity.[6] Awareness of specific drugs that cause or exacerbate this histologic lesion is important. Drugs can precipitate isolated hepatic steatosis (IHS) or NASH indirectly by promoting obesity and insulin

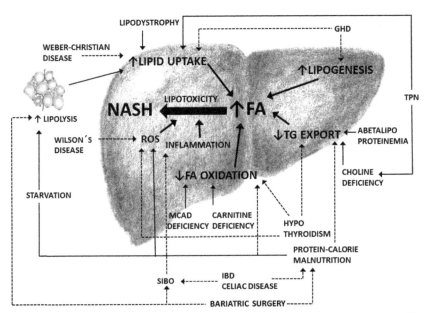

Fig. 1. Proposed mechanisms through which various conditions can promote or contribute to the development of steatohepatitis independent of insulin resistance. Solid arrows represent mechanisms for which there is significant evidence. Dashed arrows identify proposed mechanisms whereby there is less concrete evidence. FA, fatty acids; GHD, growth hormone deficiency; IBD, inflammatory bowel disease; MCAD, medium chain acyl coenzyme A dehydrogenase; ROS, reactive oxygen species; SIBO, small intestinal bacterial overgrowth; TG, triglyceride; TPN, total parenteral nutrition.

resistance (IR) or directly through alterations in lipid metabolism or through the promotion of oxidative injury. The last two are the most common culprits for most drugs. Several drugs have been reported to cause steatosis alone; however, this discussion is limited to those that have been associated with steatohepatitis. **Table 1** summarizes what is currently presumed to be the mechanistic link between each drug and the development of steatohepatitis.

Amiodarone

Amiodarone is a class III antiarrhythmic drug frequently prescribed since the 1960s. Amiodarone can induce hepatic steatosis, steatohepatitis, and even cirrhosis (**Fig. 2A**).[7–10] Furthermore, the drug can also cause asymptomatic elevation of aminotransferases (1.5–4 fold the upper limit of normal) in about 25% of patients,[11,12] symptomatic hepatitis (1–3%) and, rarely, severe cholestasis, a Reye's syndrome-like illness and fatal hepatocellular necrosis.[12–16] Although the mechanisms of steatohepatitis induced by amiodarone are not fully understood, mitochondrial dysfunction, decreased fatty acid β-oxidation, inhibition of respiratory chain enzymes, and oxidative stress all seem to play a role.[11–15] It is considered the most common cause of drug-induced steatohepatitis, with 1% to 3% of patients on chronic amiodarone developing steatohepatitis.[12,17] Amiodarone is one of the few drugs that cause true histologic NASH (as defined by Brunt and colleagues[1]): hepatic steatosis, cellular ballooning, Mallory Denk bodies (MDB), and pericellular fibrosis (see **Fig. 2**). Although the histologic changes have similarities to both alcohol and nonalcohol-induced steatohepatitis,[8,10] there are also characteristic features, such as phospholipid-laden lysosomal lamellae.[18,19] One study reported that in asymptomatic patients receiving amiodarone, steatohepatitis was present after 1 year of treatment.[8] Others have documented the development of phospholipidosis in patients treated for only 2 months.[18] Phospholipidosis may result from the inability of lysosomes to eliminate the drug or its metabolite, desethylamiodarone (caused by the inhibition of lysosomal phospholipases), thereby favoring its accumulation in the cytoplasm of the hepatocyte.[20,21] Furthermore, this cationic amphiphilic drug is concentrated in mitochondria where the benzofuran portion of the molecule may interrupt mitochondrial electron transport.[22–24] Amiodarone may also inhibit enzymes in the respiratory chain, depleting the cell of ATP,[22–25] and independently inhibit beta oxidation of fatty acids[22,24,26] via direct inhibition of carnitine palmitoyltransferase I (CPT-I) and long-chain acyl-CoA dehydrogenase.[22,27] Furthermore, a recent study demonstrated that it can increase hepatic de novo lipogenesis through increasing expression of sterol regulatory element binding protein 1c (SREBP-1c), fatty acid synthetase (FAS) and ATP citrate lyase lipogenic genes.[28] Thus, by several mechanisms, amiodarone can induce the generation of reactive oxygen species (ROS), lipid peroxidation, and fat accumulation in liver. The formation of MDBs in amiodarone-induced NASH seems to be the result of cell calcium increase by the drug with subsequent activation of tissue transglutaminase, which cross-links cytokeratin 8 (essential component of MDBs) to form a molecular scaffold (see **Fig. 2B**).[29] Malondialdehyde, the lipid peroxidation product, may also contribute to MDB formation through cross-linking cytokeratin 8 via an independent pathway.[29] The total daily amiodarone dose and duration of therapy seems to correlate with hepatotoxicity, and keeping the dosage less than 300 mg/d may protect from liver injury.[11,12] Importantly, because of its long half-life, hepatic injury can persist for weeks to months after drug discontinuation.[12,30]

Perhexiline Maleate and 4,4'-Diethylaminoethoxyhexestrol

Similar to amiodarone, perhexiline maleate and 4,4'-diethylaminoethoxyhexestrol (DEAEH) are cationic amphiphilic drugs that can also induce lysosomal

Table 1
Probable mechanisms of drug-induced steatohepatitis

Drug	Probable Mechanism	References
Amiodarone	Mitochondrial dysfunction, decreased FA beta oxidation, increased lipid peroxidation, ROS generation, and increased lipogenesis	Spaniol et al,[22] Berson et al,[24] Fromenty et al,[26] Antherieu et al[28]
Perhexiline and DEAEH	Mitochondrial dysfunction, decreased FA beta oxidation, lipid peroxidation, and ROS generation	Berson et al,[24] Deschamps et al,[34] Pessayre et al[35]
Tamoxifen	Increased TG synthesis, increased lipogenesis, and impaired FA beta oxidation	Gudbrandsen et al,[46] Cole et al,[47] Lelliott et al[48]
Methotrexate	Exacerbation of preexisting NASH, impaired FA beta oxidation, impaired TG export, ROS generation	Langman et al,[52] Huang et al,[54] Lee et al,[55] Deboyser et al[56]
Glucocorticoids	Association with MetS, impaired FA beta oxidation, impaired VLDL secretion, lipid peroxidation	Wang,[63] Letteron et al,[64] Letteron et al[65]
Irinotecan and oxaliplatin	Unknown	
NRTIs	Association with IR, mitochondrial injury	Brown et al,[72] Chen et al[78]
Stavudine	Inhibition of FA beta oxidation, increased de novo lipogenesis, impaired VLDL secretion	Igoudjil et al[77]
PI	Association with lipodystrophy	Carr et al,[73] Garg[74]
Ritonavir	Upregulation of de novo lipogenesis	Riddle et al[79]
Cannabis	Increased de novo lipogenesis, decreased FA beta oxidation, hyperphagia, association with insulin resistance	Osei-Hyiaman et al,[92] Osei-Hyiaman et al,[93] Cota et al,[94] Deveaux et al[95]
Stilboestrol	Impaired FA beta oxidation	Grimbert et al[203]
Calcium channel blockers	Unknown	
Petrochemicals	Unknown	
Vinyl chloride	Unknown	

Abbreviations: DEAEH, 4,4′-diethylaminoethoxyhexestrol; FA, fatty acids; IR, insulin resistance; MetS, metabolic syndrome; MTP, microsomal triglyceride transfer protein; NRTIs, nucleoside reverse transcriptase inhibitors; PI, protease inhibitor; ROS, reactive oxygen species; TG, triglycerides; VLDL, very-low-density lipoprotein.

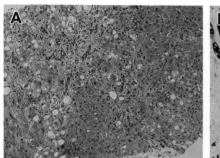
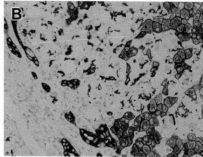

Fig. 2. Amiodarone. (*A*) In zone 3, there is marked hepatocyte ballooning and Mallory-Denk body formation. There is grade 1 macrovesicular steatosis and ductular reaction can be seen (hematoxylin-eosin, original magnification ×20). (*B*) The keratin (K) 8/18 immunohistochemical stain highlights the extent of zone 3 injury; the stained hepatocytes (*right*) and ductular cells (*left*) are surrounding hepatocytes that have lost K8/18 but in which clumped Mallory-Denk material is present and positive for the antibody (keratin 8/18 immunohistochemical stain, original magnification ×40).

phospholipidosis and steatohepatitis.[31,32] Both drugs, perhexiline maleate as an anti-anginal and DEAEH as coronary vasodilator, were widely used in Europe and Japan, respectively. Histologic liver lesions found in patients taking perhexiline or DEAEH include steatosis, MDBs, inflammatory infiltrate with polymorphonuclear leukocytes (PMNs), pericellular fibrosis, and phospholipidosis.[33] Because they share common chemical properties with amiodarone, these two drugs can cause steatosis and NASH through similar mechanisms.[24,34,35] Perhexiline and DEAEH also have a long half-life[33] and, in the case of perhexiline, this can be increased further in patients with a mutation in CYP2D6, an isoenzyme of cytochrome P450, impairing drug metabolism and thereby augmenting the risk for hepatotoxicity.[36] Severe steatohepatitis and even cirrhosis have been reported in patients taking perhexiline.[37]

Tamoxifen

Tamoxifen is associated with hepatic steatosis, steatohepatitis, and even cirrhosis.[38–40] This estrogen receptor ligand, with agonist and antagonist properties, is commonly prescribed for the treatment of breast cancer. In addition to NAFLD and NASH, there are limited reports of cholestasis, peliosis hepatis, acute hepatitis, and massive hepatic necrosis caused by tamoxifen treatment.[41] It was first associated with NASH in 1995.[41,42] Since then, several studies emerged showing the high frequency of tamoxifen-induced steatosis and attempting to elucidate its potential mechanisms of injury. About 33% to 43% of patients with breast cancer treated with the drug develop hepatic steatosis within the first 2 years of therapy.[43,44] Treatment with tamoxifen is suggested by some to be an independent predictor for the development NAFLD in obese and overweight women.[45] With drug discontinuation, steatosis reverses and NASH improves significantly.[39,43] The exact mechanism involved in tamoxifen-induced steatosis remains controversial. However, several pathways have been implicated, such as the upregulation of diacylglycerol acyltransferase, glycerol-3-phosphate acyltransferase,[46] and acetyl-CoA carboxylase (ACC) increasing de novo lipogenesis,[47] as well as the impairment of fatty acid beta oxidation.[48]

Methotrexate

Methotrexate (MTX) is a folate antagonist commonly used for autoimmune diseases, such as psoriasis and rheumatoid arthritis, connective tissue disorders, and as a chemotherapeutic agent in some malignancies. The most significant long-term side effect of chronic MTX is hepatic fibrosis leading to cirrhosis.[49] Known factors that predispose to liver injury are alcohol ingestion, obesity, type 2 diabetes, preexisting liver disease, and an age of more than 50 years.[6,50,51] Because these are also risk factors for fibrosis in NASH, some have suggested that preexisting NASH exacerbated by MTX may be an important mechanism of liver injury in patients on long-term therapy.[52] Reversible aminotransferase elevation has also been reported in 14% of these patients.[53] Patients on long-term MTX therapy can develop macrovesicular steatosis and other lesions characteristic of steatohepatitis.[49,52] One study showed that a NASH-like pattern was present in 17 of 24 patients with psoriasis treated with long-term MTX therapy. However, 13 patients had risk factors for NASH and the other 4 patients, without NASH risk factors, had a higher mean accumulated MTX dose. Although it is difficult to draw conclusions from such small numbers, this suggests that MTX could exacerbate or induce NASH, particularly at higher doses.[52] The mechanism by which MTX may cause or potentiate NASH is not clear yet, but several genes involved in hepatic fatty acid metabolism can be regulated by MTX leading to impaired fatty acid oxidation, triglyceride export,[54–56] and increased oxidative stress.[54]

Glucocorticoids

Although glucocorticoid-induced hepatic steatosis is well reported,[57] these agents have also been associated with steatohepatitis.[58–61] Rarely, NASH attributed to glucocorticoids has resulted in death from liver failure.[60,61] One study examined the prevalence of NASH in patients with systemic lupus erythematosus treated with either high- or low-dose glucocorticoids. Hepatic steatosis was present only in the high-dose group, 6% of whom had steatohepatitis. Importantly, the patients with NASH were not obese, diabetic, or hyperlipidemic.[62] Although steroids are known to cause hyperphagia, weight gain, and MetS,[63] thereby predisposing patients to IHS or NASH, there are also plausible independent mechanisms through which NASH could develop. For example, glucocorticoids can inhibit fatty acids beta oxidation and decrease very-low-density lipoprotein (VLDL) secretion, promoting hepatic lipid accumulation.[64] In experimental models, dexamethasone cannot only induce hepatic steatosis in mice but also increase lipid peroxidation.[65]

Chemotherapies

Chemotherapy-associated steatohepatitis was first reported after treatment with irinotecan or oxaliplatin as a neoadjuvant chemotherapy in patients with resectable hepatic colorectal metastases.[66] In that study, the investigators assessed NASH severity by histology scores. NASH scores were significantly higher in patients receiving irinotecan or oxaliplatin, especially in obese patients, compared with patients receiving only 5-fluorouacil or no chemotherapy.[66] In a larger study, irinotecan was associated with steatohepatitis regardless of body mass index (BMI). However, patients with a higher BMI and concurrent steatohepatitis had an increased perioperative risk of death.[67] Further studies are needed to support this association and to determine if chemotherapy-associated steatohepatitis results in liver injury that could be modified by drug or dose adjustment.

Antiretroviral Therapy

A total of 30% to 40% of patients with HIV are reported to have NAFLD[68]; however, studies documenting the prevalence of NASH are limited. In 3 recent studies, 20%, 53%, and 55% of patients with HIV with unexplained aminotransferase elevation had NASH on liver biopsy.[69–71] Although the mechanisms underlying the development of steatosis and steatohepatitis in the HIV population are likely multifactorial, antiretroviral therapy may have a role, especially the nucleoside reverse-transcriptase inhibitors (NRTIs), such as stavudine, and protease inhibitors (PIs), such as ritonavir. NRTIs are associated with insulin resistance[72] and may be an independent risk factor for the development of hepatic steatosis,[68] although this is debated.[69] Treatment with PIs has been associated with lipodystrophy,[73,74] which is clearly associated with insulin resistance and hyperlipidemia.[75,76] NRTIs can induce steatosis and steatohepatitis indirectly through mitochondrial injury or through direct inhibition of fatty acid oxidation.[77,78] Furthermore, stavudine can increase SREBP-1c gene expression and reduce microsomal triglyceride transfer protein expression in cultured rat hepatocytes. Ritonavir can increase the activation of SREBP-1 by promoting its nuclear translocation, suggesting these compounds may also cause steatosis by promoting de novo lipogenesis (DNL) and inhibiting triglyceride export.[77,79] Prospective studies are needed to assess the prevalence of NASH in the HIV population to determine the risk factors and mechanisms that predispose to liver injury.

Cannabis

Δ^9 tetrahydrocannabinol, the psychoactive component of cannabis sativa, acts through binding both cannabinoid 1 (CB1) and cannabinoid 2 receptors (CB2).[80,81] CB1 receptors are located in the human brain but also in lower concentrations in peripheral tissues, including hepatocytes and nonparenchymal cells, such as stellate cells and hepatic vascular endothelial cells.[82-84] CB2 receptors are expressed mostly in immune and hematopoietic cells,[85] although they are expressed in the liver in disease states, such as NAFLD,[86] liver fibrosis,[87] and hepatocellular carcinoma.[88] Mounting evidence demonstrates that the endocannabinoid system, cannabinoid receptors and their endogenous ligands, such as anandamide and 2-arachidonoyl glycerol, can lead to the development of hepatic steatosis and possibly steatohepatitis.[89-91]

There are several mechanisms through which activation of the cannabinoid system could contribute to the development of NAFLD and NASH. In particular, the cannabinoid system has direct effects on lipid metabolism, inflammation, and fibrogenesis. CB1 activation increases de novo lipogenesis, decreases fatty acid oxidation, and has orexigenic effects. Compared with CB1 $-/-$ mice, SREBP-1c, ACC, and FAS mRNA expression levels are increased in CB1 $+/+$ mice, and treatment with a CB1 agonist results in further upregulation of the same lipogenic genes.[92] Furthermore, CB1 agonists induce a decrease in CPT-I, the rate-limiting enzyme in mitochondrial beta oxidation, which can be prevented by rimonabant (a selective CB1 receptor antagonist).[93] CB1 receptor knockout mice are hypophagic and lose weight.[94] CB2 seems to be primarily involved in inflammation, fibrogenesis, and insulin resistance.[95] CB1 and CB2 are important mediators of hepatic fibrosis. CB1 expression is increased in both stellate cells and myofibroblasts in the cirrhotic human liver. Ablation of this receptor protects against fibrogenesis in mice by lowering transforming growth factor beta-1 and smooth muscle alpha-actin,[83] whereas the activation of CB2 receptors on hepatic stellate cells can exert an antifibrogenic effect.[87] Furthermore, in patients treated with rimonabant, adiponectin levels increased more than could be accounted for by weight loss alone.[96] Increased adiponectin levels could also improve insulin signaling and reduce hepatic steatosis, offering an additional mechanism through which the CB system could impact the development of steatohepatitis.

Despite animal and human data corroborating what has been observed in clinical practice, there is currently no published evidence showing the association between regular cannabis use and the development of NASH. Only one study has shown that daily cannabis smoking was an independent predictor of steatosis severity in patients with chronic hepatitis C.[97] However, based on the effects of the cannabinoid receptors in animal models and some human data, it is reasonable to consider cannabis use a possible contributing factor to the development of NAFLD/NASH, particularly in patients with atypical NASH. Patients should be questioned about cannabis use and informed that it could have untoward effects on the liver.

OCCUPATIONAL STEATOHEPATITIS

Even though several occupational chemicals have been associated with the development of hepatic steatosis,[98] only a few of them are likely to cause steatohepatitis. In a petrochemical plant in Northeastern Brazil, 20 workers chronically exposed to petrochemical products (benzene, xylene, ethylene, dimethylformamide, vinyl chloride, and others) were documented to have NASH on histology after excluding individuals with risk factors, such as obesity, diabetes, and heavy alcohol consumption. Ten of the patients were removed from their work environment with subsequent improvement in aminotransferases and liver histology after 1 year.[99] In another study, patients with NASH, for whom exposure to petrochemicals was the only risk factor, were compared with patients with NASH and metabolic risk factors (diabetes, dyslipidemia, and obesity) and to patients with NASH and both exposure to chemicals and metabolic risk factors. In this study, patients with NASH related to chemical exposure were younger than patients with NASH without petrochemical exposure. Moreover, metabolic factors did not seem to influence histologic or clinical presentation in exposed patients, suggesting that exposure to chemicals may be an independent risk factor in these patients. Curiously, cholestasis was a frequent finding on histology in these patients with NASH presumed secondary to petrochemicals.[100] The evaluation of insulin resistance among 40 petrochemical workers with NAFLD or NASH showed that IR was only present in 28% and 23% of patients with NAFLD and NASH, respectively, and 38% of these patients had no metabolic risks factors, which is in contrast to the extremely high prevalence of IR in patients with classic NASH.[101]

In addition to exposure to petrochemicals, exposure to vinyl chloride (VC) has been specifically associated with the development of NASH. In a study of 25 nonobese plastic workers with high exposure to VC (among other chemicals in less quantity) and normal liver enzymes, liver biopsy demonstrated NASH in 80%. Of these, 55% also had fibrosis and 16% hemangiosarcoma. Although patients were nonobese, they had insulin resistance and low adiponectin levels.[102] Here steatohepatitis was also associated with high levels of tumor necrosis factor (TNF) alpha, interleukin (IL)-1 beta, IL-6, IL-8, and cytokeratin 18. Due to its promise as a biomarker for the detection of NASH, cytokeratin-18 may have a role in the future for screening workers exposed to VC, although this has not been studied. If VC indeed leads to steatohepatitis, it is unclear if injury resolves with cessation of exposure. In a small study, 3 workers exposed to VC who had steatohepatitis developed progressive liver injury and fibrosis on subsequent liver biopsy even after they were removed from VC exposure.[102] VC has been associated with hepatic fibrosis,[103] hemangiosarcoma,[104] and hepatocellular carcinoma[105,106]; however, further studies are needed to better characterize steatohepatitis in patients exposed to VC. In studies linking exposure to petrochemical products with steatohepatitis mentioned previously, VC was also one of the chemical products that petrochemicals workers were exposed to.

GROWTH HORMONE DEFICIENCY

Growth hormone deficiency (GHD) presents with many features of the metabolic syndrome, such as insulin resistance, dyslipidemia, and truncal obesity. Not surprisingly, there is an association between GHD and the spectrum of NASH.[107–110] Both IHS and NASH can be found in patients with GHD, with the former being more common.[111] In one series, plasma levels of GH were lower among patients with NAFLD compared with those without it, suggesting that reduced levels of GH may have a role in NAFLD development.[112] Patients with hypothalamic or pituitary dysfunction may be at increased risk for excessive weight gain, impaired glucose tolerance, and dyslipidemia, with subsequent development of IHS, NASH, or even cirrhosis.[113] In a small study, fatty liver was detected more frequently in men with hypopituitarism compared with controls and the severity of GHD was associated with the severity of hepatic steatosis.[114]

Although the association between NAFLD/NASH and GHD may be a function of insulin resistance,[107,115,116] GH also has direct effects hepatic lipid metabolism, primarily through increased de novo lipogenesis and hepatic fatty acid uptake.[117–120] One study showed that human hepatocytes engrafted in chimeric mice that lack circulating human GH developed steatosis and this was prevented when the mice were treated with human GH.[118] Recent studies demonstrated the important role of the hepatic GH-signal transducer and activator of transcription 5 (STAT5) signaling. Liver-specific deletion of GH receptor and the deletion of STAT5 in mice increase SREBP-1c expression.[119,120] GH-induced STAT5 activation in vivo and in vitro administration of GH to human hepatocytes downregulate SREBP-1c and other lipogenic genes.[118,120] GH, via STAT5 signaling and upregulation of CD36, also seems to increase hepatic lipid uptake independent of increased lipolysis.[117] However, these results are still controversial.[121] Further studies are needed to substantiate these mechanisms and identify alternative pathways by which GHD could be involved with the development of steatohepatitis.

In conclusion, GHD can be a primary cause or a contributing factor for the development of NAFLD and NASH. Making the diagnosis can be challenging and varies according to the presence of concomitant pituitary hormone deficiencies. In patients with several ($\geq$3), documenting a low insulin-like growth factor-1 level can be sufficient, whereas in patients with 2 or less, a stimulation test is required.[122] Confirming the diagnosis when GHD is suspected is extremely important because GH-replacement therapy may significantly improve NASH and other features of the metabolic syndrome.[108,109] Therefore, it should be considered, particularly in patients with more severe disease than one would expect given their age or risk factors.

HYPOTHYROIDISM

The clinical observation that several patients with NASH also have hypothyroidism raised the question of an association. One study found that 15% of 174 patients with NASH had hypothyroidism, compared with 7% of controls, with no difference in weight between the groups.[123] A larger recent series supported this finding showing that hypothyroidism was more prevalent in patients with NAFLD (21%) compared with controls (9.5%) and patients with NASH had an even higher prevalence of hypothyroidism (25%).[124] Another study involving 4648 individuals showed an association between hypothyroidism and NAFLD independent of metabolic risk factors; NAFLD prevalence among patients with hypothyroidism was 30.2% compared with 19.5% in controls.[125] Also, thyroid-stimulating hormone (TSH) levels correlated with NAFLD prevalence, even when TSH was within the normal range.[125] The latter finding was supported by a series that showed that TSH levels were significantly higher, although within the normal range, in patients with NASH compared with patients with hepatic steatosis, raising the possibility that TSH levels at the upper limit of normal may predict NASH.[126] It is well known that hypothyroidism is related to obesity,[127] insulin resistance,[128] and hyperlipidemia,[129] which are important components of MetS; therefore, this may be an explanation for the NASH-hypothyroidism association. However, independent mechanisms through which hypothyroidism could directly induce or exacerbate IHS or NASH include impaired fatty acid oxidation and VLDL secretion.[129] Hypothyroidism may also directly lead to mitochondrial dysfunction,[130,131] oxidative stress, and lipid peroxidation,[132] which could contribute to the development of NASH. Further studies are needed to clarify whether or not hypothyroidism plays a meaningful role in the development of steatohepatitis.

NUTRITIONAL FACTORS

Unlike marasmus where all nutrients are deficient, patients with protein calorie malnutrition can develop hepatic steatosis and even NASH.[133–135] Patients with kwashiorkor characteristically have low protein intake, whereas carbohydrate intake may be adequate or increased, which can cultivate insulin resistance,[136] increased plasma free fatty acids (FFAs), and increased DNL.[134,137] Abnormal aminotransferases are reported in 26% to 56% of patients with anorexia nervosa (AN),[138,139] inversely related to BMI[138–140]; specifically, NASH on liver biopsy has been documented in patients with AN.[141] Although the precise mechanism of liver damage is incompletely understood, several mechanisms could be contributing. These mechanisms include increased lipolysis as an adaptive response to starvation with subsequent hepatic lipid loading, excessive production of ROS leading to oxidative injury, reduced synthesis of lipoproteins, and mitochondrial dysfunction resulting in impaired fatty acid beta oxidation.[141–143]

Specific nutrient deficiencies, such as carnitine and choline, may also lead to hepatic steatosis. Carnitine deficiency can be primary, caused by an autosomal recessive genetic disorder, or secondary, which occurs in relation to certain diseases, drug interactions, impaired nutrition, and aging.[144,145] Carnitine is essential for the translocation of long chain fatty acids across the inner mitochondrial membrane, thus carnitine deficiency can impair mitochondrial beta oxidation, favoring the accumulation of FFAs or other lipid subspecies that lead to lipotoxicity.[146,147]

Choline is a precursor of phospholipid biosynthesis, thus it is central to VLDL synthesis and, therefore, to hepatic triglyceride export. A choline-deficient diet in humans can cause elevated aminotransferase levels and hepatic steatosis,[148,149] which is likely related to impaired VLDL secretion.[150,151] Choline deficiency may induce DNA damage and apoptosis.[152,153] Choline deficiency is most commonly associated with long-term total parenteral nutrition (TPN)[154,155] but has also been described in malabsorption such as seen in short-bowel syndrome.[156] In some studies, patients on long-term TPN have low plasma-free choline concentrations that inversely correlate with AST and ALT levels.[154,155] Also, choline supplementation, either in the form of oral lecithin or intravenous choline, may reverse steatosis and normalize aminotransferase elevations in patients receiving TPN.[149,157,158]

INTESTINAL FACTORS
Bacterial Overgrowth and Liver Injury

Although jejunoileal (JI) bypass is no longer performed, current bariatric procedures can be associated with steatohepatitis that on occasion culminate in hepatic decompensation.[159,160] Furthermore, similar changes have been reported after extensive bowel resection.[161] There are several potential explanations for this, including increased FFA delivery, protein-calorie malnutrition, bacterial overgrowth, and the use of TPN. In the case of either surgically induced or disease-associated malabsorption, rapid weight loss can precipitate massive lipolysis that then floods the liver (**Fig. 3**). In the

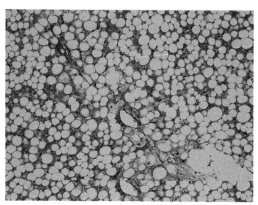

Fig. 3. Diffuse macrovesicular steatosis without ballooning, inflammation, or fibrosis in a patient with massive weight loss secondary to malabsorption (Masson trichrome stain, original magnification ×20).

setting of short bowel, the use of TPN can further exacerbate liver injury by way of excess lipid loading, calories, or nutrient deficiencies as detailed previously.

The notion that small intestinal bacterial overgrowth (SIBO) could play a role in liver injury emanated from studies showing improvement in liver injury in JI bypass patients treated with metronidazole.[162] However, NASH-like liver lesions can also be seen in the setting of intestinal bacterial overgrowth in the absence of an excluded bowel segment or diverticulosis.[163] In a small case control study, patients with NASH had a higher incidence of SIBO than controls (50% vs 22% respectively) as determined by ^{14}C-D-xylose and lactulose breath tests.[164] Unfortunately, the mechanisms responsible for this association were not clearly elucidated in that study because they were unable to show differences in intestinal permeability and systemic endotoxemia. Fatty livers are primed for endotoxin-related injury. Although systemic endotoxin levels are not reliable surrogates for portal levels, other bacterial products released into the portal circulation could be playing a role in the development of hepatic steatosis, inflammation, and fibrosis through the activation of the innate immune system.[165] TNF-alpha levels were also significantly higher in the NASH group.[165] TNF-alpha has a pathogenic role in NASH that may be related to impaired insulin signaling and the activation of several inflammatory pathways, including those triggered through innate immunity.[164] Another explanation for a higher prevalence of SIBO in patients with NASH is that obesity itself is associated with disordered small-bowel motility that can promote the development of SIBO.[166,167] Thus, dysregulation of intestinal barrier function permits the translocation of bacteria and proinflammatory cytokines into the portal system and subsequently to the liver. Intestine-derived LPS and bacterial products could then activate toll-like receptor 4 (TLR4) and TLR9, respectively, leading to hepatic inflammation, fibrogenesis, and potentially steatohepatitis. Another potential mechanism is the production of ethanol in the setting of bacterial overgrowth that can itself lead to steatosis or steatohepatitis. Although it is beyond the scope of this review, the emerging role of the intestinal microbiome is fascinating in that it may be an important contributor to metabolism, gut permeability, and endotoxemia.[168,169]

Inflammatory Bowel Disease

In the setting of inflammatory bowel disease (IBD), the most common cause of abnormal liver chemistry tests in a hepatocellular injury pattern is hepatic steatosis. The prevalence of hepatic steatosis in this setting ranges from 15% to 45%.[170–172] In a study of 511 patients with IBD, sonographic evidence of steatosis was noted in 35%.[173] Although both can be seen on liver biopsy, IHS is more frequent than NASH. Hepatic steatosis in some studies correlates with bowel disease severity in ulcerative colitis,[172] suggesting that increased intestinal permeability could be contributing. However other factors, such as use of steroids, TPN, weight loss, and poor nutrition, could also play a pathogenic role. Other pathogenic mechanisms to consider in the setting of IBD and Crohn disease are malabsorption, intestinal bacterial overgrowth, and changes in the microbiome that could alter intestinal barrier function leading to low-grade portal endotoxemia. Nevertheless, definitive evidence supporting a true association between IBD and NASH is lacking.

Celiac Disease

The prevalence of celiac disease (CD) in patients with NAFLD is estimated to be 2.6 to 3.4%, suggesting that CD may be a risk factor for the development of hepatic steatosis.[174–176] Few studies have examined the prevalence of CD in patients with NASH. In a small series, 4 (13%) of 30 patients with NASH were diagnosed with CD with positive antiendomysial antibodies and concordant duodenal histopathology. Among those with CD, aminotransferases normalized and ultrasonographic evidence of hepatic steatosis resolved after 1 year of a gluten-free diet. Unfortunately, weight loss was not reported in the study and could have accounted for these findings.[177] Some data suggest malabsorption and an increase in bowel permeability, with the development of SIBO, could be involved in liver injury in CD.[178] However, evidence supporting a true association between NASH and CD remains controversial.[179]

GENETIC AND OTHER METABOLIC DISEASES
Acquired or Inborn Errors of Metabolism

Medium-chain acyl-coenzyme A dehydrogenase (MCAD) deficiency is the most common inborn error of fatty acid oxidation, with a frequency estimated in the population of 1 in 15,000.[180] Because MCAD is one of the essential enzymes involved in mitochondrial fatty acid beta oxidation, a deficiency in this protein may cause an impairment of fatty acid metabolism leading to lipid accumulation in the liver. There are reported cases of this inherited autosomal recessive disorder with both microvesicular and macrovesicular hepatic steatosis[181–183]; however, there is no specific link with NASH.

Lysosomal acid lipase (LAL) deficiency has been also associated with hepatic steatosis. Deficient LAL activity can be caused by Wolman disease (WD), the severe clinical form, or cholesteryl ester storage disease (CESD), the milder late-onset form.[184] Because LAL catalyzes the hydrolysis of cholesteryl esters and triglycerides, its deficiency results in lipid accumulation in many organs, particularly in the liver. Both autosomal recessive disorders, WD and CESD, are characterized by the presence of hepatic steatosis[184–186]; however, NASH has not been reported.

Patients with hepatic copper overload, such in Wilson disease, Indian childhood cirrhosis, and idiopathic copper toxicosis, can develop histologic features of NASH, such as hepatocyte ballooning, inflammation, and MDB formation.[187,188] Unlike steatosis, which is a common feature, MDBs are less frequent in Wilson disease (25%) and they may be associated with liver failure and poorer prognosis.[189,190] It is important to distinguish these disorders of copper metabolism from NASH because misdiagnosis of Wilson disease as NASH can delay potentially lifesaving treatment.

Weber-Christian disease has been also associated with steatohepatitis on liver biopsy. This idiopathic acquired disorder is characterized by the presence of nodular subcutaneous panniculitis with involvement of other organs, including the liver, spleen, intestine, and heart.[191] Hepatic steatosis, MDBs, PMN infiltration, and pericellular fibrosis have been reported in patients with Weber-Christian disease.[192] The mechanism of liver injury is unknown but increased delivery of fatty acids from peripheral panniculitis lesions may be involved.[191]

Abetalipoproteinemia and familial hypobetalipoproteinemia are inherited disorders of lipid metabolism characterized by the deficiency of apolipoprotein B. Patients with these disorders typically present with low plasma cholesterol and triglyceride levels and gastrointestinal and neurologic manifestations. Fatty liver is frequently reported among these patients,[193,194] whereas steatohepatitis and cirrhosis are less common.[193,195] Here impaired hepatic triglyceride export seems to be the primary cause of hepatic lipid accumulation.[196]

Lipodystrophies

Lipodystrophies are a heterogeneous group of acquired or congenital disorders characterized by the partial or generalized loss of adipose tissue leading to ectopic triglyceride accumulation.[74] Patients frequently present with insulin resistance, dyslipidemia, and fatty liver disease. NASH has been associated with both partial and generalized lipodystrophy, whereas cirrhosis has been only described in the latter.[74,197] In one study, among 10 individuals with partial and generalized lipodystrophy, 8 had evidence of steatohepatitis on liver biopsy despite some of them having normal liver enzymes.[198] In another study, 14 patients with HIV, 9 with and 5 without lipodystrophy, underwent liver biopsy because of elevated aminotransferases. Among the patients with HIV who were lipodystrophic, 67% had NASH compared with 40% of the patients with HIV without lipodystrophy.[199] Congenital and acquired generalized lipodystrophies are characterized by low plasma leptin and adiponectin levels.[200] Even though insulin resistance and increased triglyceride flux to the liver are likely to play a central role in the development of hepatic steatosis and NASH, murine studies suggest that the impairment of fatty acid oxidation and increased de novo lipogenesis also contributes.[201,202] Whether these two proposed mechanisms are independent or a consequence of hyperinsulinemia is not yet clear.

SUMMARY

What we refer to as NASH is a complex, truly multifactorial process that is perhaps not one disease but a manifestation of several. Much remains to be learned about the nuances that distinguish various subpopulations within the context of NASH. From a practical perspective, it is important to appreciate which external or internal factors, including drugs, disease conditions, and individual genetic differences, can influence the development of steatohepatitis. Although a greater understanding of these contributing factors may not account for all individual differences in the NASH population, perhaps it will allow us to better define subpopulations and, thus, target more specific interventions.

ACKNOWLEDGMENTS

The authors would like to thank Elizabeth Brunt for contributing and interpreting the histology presented in this article.

REFERENCES

1. Brunt EM, Janney CG, Di Bisceglie AM, et al. Nonalcoholic steatohepatitis: a proposal for grading and staging the histological lesions. Am J Gastroenterol 1999;94(9):2467–74.
2. Kleiner DE, Brunt EM, Van Natta M, et al. Design and validation of a histological scoring system for nonalcoholic fatty liver disease. Hepatology 2005;41(6): 1313–21.
3. Sanyal AJ, Chalasani N, Kowdley KV, et al. Pioglitazone, vitamin E, or placebo for nonalcoholic steatohepatitis. N Engl J Med 2010;362(18):1675–85.
4. Zein CO, Yerian LM, Gogate P, et al. Pentoxifylline improves nonalcoholic steatohepatitis: a randomized placebo-controlled trial. Hepatology 2011;54(5): 1610–9.
5. Belfort R, Harrison SA, Brown K, et al. A placebo-controlled trial of pioglitazone in subjects with nonalcoholic steatohepatitis. N Engl J Med 2006;355(22): 2297–307.
6. Farrell GC. Drugs and steatohepatitis. Semin Liver Dis 2002;22(2):185–94.
7. Sung PS, Yoon SK. Amiodarone hepatotoxicity. Hepatology 2012;55(1):325–6.
8. Lewis JH, Mullick F, Ishak KG, et al. Histopathologic analysis of suspected amiodarone hepatotoxicity. Hum pathol 1990;21(1):59–67.
9. Raja K, Thung SN, Fiel MI, et al. Drug-induced steatohepatitis leading to cirrhosis: long-term toxicity of amiodarone use. Semin Liver Dis 2009;29(4):423–8.
10. Poucell S, Ireton J, Valencia-Mayoral P, et al. Amiodarone-associated phospholipidosis and fibrosis of the liver. Light, immunohistochemical, and electron microscopic studies. Gastroenterology 1984;86(5 Pt 1):926–36.
11. Hilleman D, Miller MA, Parker R, et al. Optimal management of amiodarone therapy: efficacy and side effects. Pharmacotherapy 1998;18(6 Pt 2):138S–45S.
12. Lewis JH, Ranard RC, Caruso A, et al. Amiodarone hepatotoxicity: prevalence and clinicopathologic correlations among 104 patients. Hepatology 1989;9(5): 679–85.
13. Morse RM, Valenzuela GA, Greenwald TP, et al. Amiodarone-induced liver toxicity. Ann Intern Med 1988;109(10):838–40.
14. Kalantzis N, Gabriel P, Mouzas J, et al. Acute amiodarone-induced hepatitis. Hepatogastroenterology 1991;38(1):71–4.
15. Gilinsky NH, Briscoe GW, Kuo CS. Fatal amiodarone hepatoxicity. Am J Gastroenterol 1988;83(2):161–3.
16. Jones DB, Mullick FG, Hoofnagle JH, et al. Reye's syndrome-like illness in a patient receiving amiodarone. Am J Gastroenterol 1988;83(9):967–9.
17. Rumessen JJ. Hepatotoxicity of amiodarone. Acta Med Scand 1986;219(2): 235–9.
18. Rigas B, Rosenfeld LE, Barwick KW, et al. Amiodarone hepatotoxicity. A clinicopathologic study of five patients. Ann Intern Med 1986;104(3):348–51.
19. Uchida T, Kao H, Quispe-Sjogren M, et al. Alcoholic foamy degeneration—a pattern of acute alcoholic injury of the liver. Gastroenterology 1983;84(4): 683–92.
20. Kannan R, Sarma JS, Guha M, et al. Amiodarone toxicity. II. Desethylamiodarone-induced phospholipidosis and ultrastructural changes during repeated administration in rats. Fundam Appl Toxicol 1991;16(1):103–9.
21. Hostetler KY, Reasor MJ, Walker ER, et al. Role of phospholipase A inhibition in amiodarone pulmonary toxicity in rats. Biochim Biophys Acta 1986;875(2): 400–5.

22. Spaniol M, Bracher R, Ha HR, et al. Toxicity of amiodarone and amiodarone analogues on isolated rat liver mitochondria. J Hepatol 2001;35(5):628–36.
23. Fromenty B, Fisch C, Berson A, et al. Dual effect of amiodarone on mitochondrial respiration. Initial protonophoric uncoupling effect followed by inhibition of the respiratory chain at the levels of complex I and complex II. J Pharmacol Exp Ther 1990;255(3):1377–84.
24. Berson A, De Beco V, Letteron P, et al. Steatohepatitis-inducing drugs cause mitochondrial dysfunction and lipid peroxidation in rat hepatocytes. Gastroenterology 1998;114(4):764–74.
25. Serviddio G, Bellanti F, Giudetti AM, et al. Mitochondrial oxidative stress and respiratory chain dysfunction account for liver toxicity during amiodarone but not dronedarone administration. Free Radic Biol Med 2011;51(12):2234–42.
26. Fromenty B, Fisch C, Labbe G, et al. Amiodarone inhibits the mitochondrial beta-oxidation of fatty acids and produces microvesicular steatosis of the liver in mice. J Pharmacol Exp Ther 1990;255(3):1371–6.
27. Kennedy JA, Unger SA, Horowitz JD. Inhibition of carnitine palmitoyltransferase-1 in rat heart and liver by perhexiline and amiodarone. Biochem Pharmacol 1996;52(2):273–80.
28. Antherieu S, Rogue A, Fromenty B, et al. Induction of vesicular steatosis by amiodarone and tetracycline is associated with up-regulation of lipogenic genes in HepaRG cells. Hepatology 2011;53(6):1895–905.
29. Robin MA, Descatoire V, Pessayre D, et al. Steatohepatitis-inducing drugs trigger cytokeratin cross-links in hepatocytes. Possible contribution to Mallory-Denk body formation. Toxicol In Vitro 2008;22(6):1511–9.
30. Brien JF, Jimmo S, Brennan FJ, et al. Distribution of amiodarone and its metabolite, desethylamiodarone, in human tissues. Can J Physiol Pharmacol 1987; 65(3):360–4.
31. Le Gall JY, Guillouzo A, Glaise D, et al. Perhexiline maleate toxicity on human liver cell lines. Gut 1980;21(11):977–84.
32. Kubo M, Hostetler KY. Metabolic basis of diethylaminoethoxyhexestrol-induced phospholipid fatty liver. Am J Phys 1987;252(3 Pt 1):E375–9.
33. Fromenty B, Pessayre D. Inhibition of mitochondrial beta-oxidation as a mechanism of hepatotoxicity. Pharmacol Ther 1995;67(1):101–54.
34. Deschamps D, DeBeco V, Fisch C, et al. Inhibition by perhexiline of oxidative phosphorylation and the beta-oxidation of fatty acids: possible role in pseudoalcoholic liver lesions. Hepatology 1994;19(4):948–61.
35. Pessayre D, Mansouri A, Haouzi D, et al. Hepatotoxicity due to mitochondrial dysfunction. Cell Biol Toxicol 1999;15(6):367–73.
36. Morgan MY, Reshef R, Shah RR, et al. Impaired oxidation of debrisoquine in patients with perhexiline liver injury. Gut 1984;25(10):1057–64.
37. Pessayre D, Bichara M, Degott C, et al. Perhexiline maleate-induced cirrhosis. Gastroenterology 1979;76(1):170–7.
38. Ogawa Y, Murata Y, Nishioka A, et al. Tamoxifen-induced fatty liver in patients with breast cancer. Lancet 1998;351(9104):725.
39. Saphner T, Triest-Robertson S, Li H, et al. The association of nonalcoholic steatohepatitis and tamoxifen in patients with breast cancer. Cancer 2009;115(14): 3189–95.
40. Oien KA, Moffat D, Curry GW, et al. Cirrhosis with steatohepatitis after adjuvant tamoxifen. Lancet 1999;353(9146):36–7.
41. Pinto HC, Baptista A, Camilo ME, et al. Tamoxifen-associated steatohepatitis–report of three cases. J Hepatol 1995;23(1):95–7.

42. Pratt DS, Knox TA, Erban J. Tamoxifen-induced steatohepatitis. Ann Intern Med 1995;123(3):236.

43. Nishino M, Hayakawa K, Nakamura Y, et al. Effects of tamoxifen on hepatic fat content and the development of hepatic steatosis in patients with breast cancer: high frequency of involvement and rapid reversal after completion of tamoxifen therapy. AJR Am J Roentgenol 2003;180(1):129–34.

44. Murata Y, Ogawa Y, Saibara T, et al. Unrecognized hepatic steatosis and non-alcoholic steatohepatitis in adjuvant tamoxifen for breast cancer patients. Oncol Rep 2000;7(6):1299–304.

45. Bruno S, Maisonneuve P, Castellana P, et al. Incidence and risk factors for non-alcoholic steatohepatitis: prospective study of 5408 women enrolled in Italian tamoxifen chemoprevention trial. BMJ 2005;330(7497):932.

46. Gudbrandsen OA, Rost TH, Berge RK. Causes and prevention of tamoxifen-induced accumulation of triacylglycerol in rat liver. J Lipid Res 2006;47(10): 2223–32.

47. Cole LK, Jacobs RL, Vance DE. Tamoxifen induces triacylglycerol accumulation in the mouse liver by activation of fatty acid synthesis. Hepatology 2010;52(4): 1258–65.

48. Lelliott CJ, Lopez M, Curtis RK, et al. Transcript and metabolite analysis of the effects of tamoxifen in rat liver reveals inhibition of fatty acid synthesis in the presence of hepatic steatosis. FASEB J 2005;19(9):1108–19.

49. Kanel GC. Histopathology of drug-induced liver disease. In: Kaplowitz N, DeLeve LD, editors. Drug-induced liver disease. New York: Marcel Dekker; 2003. p. 259–61.

50. Whiting-O'Keefe QE, Fye KH, Sack KD. Methotrexate and histologic hepatic abnormalities: a meta-analysis. Am J Med 1991;90(6):711–6.

51. Rosenberg P, Urwitz H, Johannesson A, et al. Psoriasis patients with diabetes type 2 are at high risk of developing liver fibrosis during methotrexate treatment. J Hepatol 2007;46(6):1111–8.

52. Langman G, Hall PM, Todd G. Role of non-alcoholic steatohepatitis in methotrexate-induced liver injury. J Gastroenterol Hepatol 2001;16(12):1395–401.

53. Berkowitz RS, Goldstein DP, Bernstein MR. Ten year's experience with metho-trexate and folinic acid as primary therapy for gestational trophoblastic disease. Gynecol Oncol 1986;23(1):111–8.

54. Huang Q, Jin X, Gaillard ET, et al. Gene expression profiling reveals multiple toxicity endpoints induced by hepatotoxicants. Mutat Res 2004;549(1–2): 147–67.

55. Lee MH, Hong I, Kim M, et al. Gene expression profiles of murine fatty liver induced by the administration of methotrexate. Toxicology 2008;249(1):75–84.

56. Deboyser D, Goethals F, Roberfroid M. Biochemical effects of methotrexate in isolated hepatocytes in relation to its steatogenic activity. Toxicol In Vitro 1992;6(2):129–32.

57. Matsumoto T, Yoshimine T, Shimouchi K, et al. The liver in systemic lupus eryth-ematosus: pathologic analysis of 52 cases and review of Japanese Autopsy Registry data. Hum Pathol 1992;23(10):1151–8.

58. Itoh S, Igarashi M, Tsukada Y, et al. Nonalcoholic fatty liver with alcoholic hyalin after long-term glucocorticoid therapy. Acta Hepatogastroenterol (Stuttg) 1977; 24(6):415–8.

59. Candelli M, Nista EC, Pignataro G, et al. Steatohepatitis during methylprednis-olone therapy for ulcerative colitis exacerbation. J Intern Med 2003;253(3): 391–2.

60. Nanki T, Koike R, Miyasaka N. Subacute severe steatohepatitis during prednisolone therapy for systemic lupus erythematosus. Am J Gastroenterol 1999; 94(11):3379.

61. Dourakis SP, Sevastianos VA, Kaliopi P. Acute severe steatohepatitis related to prednisolone therapy. Am J Gastroenterol 2002;97(4):1074–5.

62. Matsumoto T, Yamasaki S, Arakawa A, et al. Exposure to a high total dosage of glucocorticoids produces non-alcoholic steatohepatitis. Pathol Int 2007;57(6): 388–9.

63. Wang M. The role of glucocorticoid action in the pathophysiology of the metabolic syndrome. Nutr Metab (Lond) 2005;2(1):3.

64. Letteron P, Brahimi-Bourouina N, Robin MA, et al. Glucocorticoids inhibit mitochondrial matrix acyl-CoA dehydrogenases and fatty acid beta-oxidation. Am J Physiol 1997;272(5 Pt 1):G1141–50.

65. Letteron P, Fromenty B, Terris B, et al. Acute and chronic hepatic steatosis lead to in vivo lipid peroxidation in mice. J Hepatol 1996;24(2):200–8.

66. Fernandez FG, Ritter J, Goodwin JW, et al. Effect of steatohepatitis associated with irinotecan or oxaliplatin pretreatment on resectability of hepatic colorectal metastases. J Am Coll Surg 2005;200(6):845–53.

67. Vauthey JN, Pawlik TM, Ribero D, et al. Chemotherapy regimen predicts steatohepatitis and an increase in 90-day mortality after surgery for hepatic colorectal metastases. J Clin Oncol 2006;24(13):2065–72.

68. Guaraldi G, Squillace N, Stentarelli C, et al. Nonalcoholic fatty liver disease in HIV-infected patients referred to a metabolic clinic: prevalence, characteristics, and predictors. Clin Infect Dis 2008;47(2):250–7.

69. Crum-Cianflone N, Dilay A, Collins G, et al. Nonalcoholic fatty liver disease among HIV-infected persons. J Acquir Immune Defic Syndr 2009;50(5):464–73.

70. Akhtar MA, Mathieson K, Arey B, et al. Hepatic histopathology and clinical characteristics associated with antiretroviral therapy in HIV patients without viral hepatitis. Eur J Gastroenterol Hepatol 2008;20(12):1194–204.

71. Mohammed SS, Aghdassi E, Salit IE, et al. HIV-positive patients with nonalcoholic fatty liver disease have a lower body mass index and are more physically active than HIV-negative patients. J Acquir Immune Defic Syndr 2007;45(4):432–8.

72. Brown TT, Li X, Cole SR, et al. Cumulative exposure to nucleoside analogue reverse transcriptase inhibitors is associated with insulin resistance markers in the Multicenter AIDS Cohort Study. AIDS 2005;19(13):1375–83.

73. Carr A, Samaras K, Burton S, et al. A syndrome of peripheral lipodystrophy, hyperlipidaemia and insulin resistance in patients receiving HIV protease inhibitors. AIDS 1998;12(7):F51–8.

74. Garg A. Acquired and inherited lipodystrophies. N Engl J Med 2004;350(12): 1220–34.

75. Carr A. HIV protease inhibitor-related lipodystrophy syndrome. Clin Infect Dis 2000;30(Suppl 2):S135–42.

76. Walli R, Herfort O, Michl GM, et al. Treatment with protease inhibitors associated with peripheral insulin resistance and impaired oral glucose tolerance in HIV-1-infected patients. AIDS 1998;12(15):F167–73.

77. Igoudjil A, Massart J, Begriche K, et al. High concentrations of stavudine impair fatty acid oxidation without depleting mitochondrial DNA in cultured rat hepatocytes. Toxicol In Vitro 2008;22(4):887–98.

78. Chen CH, Vazquez-Padua M, Cheng YC. Effect of anti-human immunodeficiency virus nucleoside analogs on mitochondrial DNA and its implication for delayed toxicity. Mol Pharmacol 1991;39(5):625–8.

79. Riddle TM, Kuhel DG, Woollett LA, et al. HIV protease inhibitor induces fatty acid and sterol biosynthesis in liver and adipose tissues due to the accumulation of activated sterol regulatory element-binding proteins in the nucleus. J Biol Chem 2001;276(40):37514–9.

80. Bayewitch M, Avidor-Reiss T, Levy R, et al. The peripheral cannabinoid receptor: adenylate cyclase inhibition and G protein coupling. FEBS Lett 1995;375(1–2): 143–7.

81. Huffman JW. The search for selective ligands for the CB2 receptor. Curr Pharm Des 2000;6(13):1323–37.

82. Jeong WI, Osei-Hyiaman D, Park O, et al. Paracrine activation of hepatic CB1 receptors by stellate cell-derived endocannabinoids mediates alcoholic fatty liver. Cell Metab 2008;7(3):227–35.

83. Teixeira-Clerc F, Julien B, Grenard P, et al. CB1 cannabinoid receptor antagonism: a new strategy for the treatment of liver fibrosis. Nat Med 2006;12(6):671–6.

84. Batkai S, Jarai Z, Wagner JA, et al. Endocannabinoids acting at vascular CB1 receptors mediate the vasodilated state in advanced liver cirrhosis. Nat Med 2001;7(7):827–32.

85. Munro S, Thomas KL, Abu-Shaar M. Molecular characterization of a peripheral receptor for cannabinoids. Nature 1993;365(6441):61–5.

86. Mendez-Sanchez N, Zamora-Valdes D, Pichardo-Bahena R, et al. Endocannabinoid receptor CB2 in nonalcoholic fatty liver disease. Liver Int 2007;27(2):215–9.

87. Julien B, Grenard P, Teixeira-Clerc F, et al. Antifibrogenic role of the cannabinoid receptor CB2 in the liver. Gastroenterology 2005;128(3):742–55.

88. Xu X, Liu Y, Huang S, et al. Overexpression of cannabinoid receptors CB1 and CB2 correlates with improved prognosis of patients with hepatocellular carcinoma. Cancer Genet Cytogenet 2006;171(1):31–8.

89. Gary-Bobo M, Elachouri G, Gallas JF, et al. Rimonabant reduces obesity-associated hepatic steatosis and features of metabolic syndrome in obese Zucker fa/fa rats. Hepatology 2007;46(1):122–9.

90. Tam J, Liu J, Mukhopadhyay B, et al. Endocannabinoids in liver disease. Hepatology 2011;53(1):346–55.

91. Purohit V, Rapaka R, Shurtleff D. Role of cannabinoids in the development of fatty liver (steatosis). AAPS J 2010;12(2):233–7.

92. Osei-Hyiaman D, DePetrillo M, Pacher P, et al. Endocannabinoid activation at hepatic CB1 receptors stimulates fatty acid synthesis and contributes to diet-induced obesity. J Clin Invest 2005;115(5):1298–305.

93. Osei-Hyiaman D, Liu J, Zhou L, et al. Hepatic CB1 receptor is required for development of diet-induced steatosis, dyslipidemia, and insulin and leptin resistance in mice. J Clin Invest 2008;118(9):3160–9.

94. Cota D, Marsicano G, Tschop M, et al. The endogenous cannabinoid system affects energy balance via central orexigenic drive and peripheral lipogenesis. J Clin Invest 2003;112(3):423–31.

95. Deveaux V, Cadoudal T, Ichigotani Y, et al. Cannabinoid CB2 receptor potentiates obesity-associated inflammation, insulin resistance and hepatic steatosis. PLoS One 2009;4(6):e5844.

96. Despres JP, Golay A, Sjostrom L, et al. Effects of rimonabant on metabolic risk factors in overweight patients with dyslipidemia. N Engl J Med 2005;353(20): 2121–34.

97. Hezode C, Zafrani ES, Roudot-Thoraval F, et al. Daily cannabis use: a novel risk factor of steatosis severity in patients with chronic hepatitis C. Gastroenterology 2008;134(2):432–9.

98. Tolman KG. Occupational and environmental hepatotoxicity. In: Kaplowitz N, DeLeve LD, editors. Drug-induced liver disease. New York: Marcel Dekker; 2003. p. 727–32.
99. Cotrim HP, Andrade ZA, Parana R, et al. Nonalcoholic steatohepatitis: a toxic liver disease in industrial workers. Liver 1999;19(4):299–304.
100. Cotrim HP, De Freitas LA, Freitas C, et al. Clinical and histopathological features of NASH in workers exposed to chemicals with or without associated metabolic conditions. Liver Int 2004;24(2):131–5.
101. Cotrim HP, Carvalho F, Siqueira AC, et al. Nonalcoholic fatty liver and insulin resistance among petrochemical workers. JAMA 2005;294(13):1618–20.
102. Cave M, Falkner KC, Ray M, et al. Toxicant-associated steatohepatitis in vinyl chloride workers. Hepatology 2010;51(2):474–81.
103. Hsiao TJ, Wang JD, Yang PM, et al. Liver fibrosis in asymptomatic polyvinyl chloride workers. J Occup Environ Med 2004;46(9):962–6.
104. Falk H, Creech JL Jr, Heath CW Jr, et al. Hepatic disease among workers at a vinyl chloride polymerization plant. JAMA 1974;230(1):59–63.
105. Mastrangelo G, Fedeli U, Fadda E, et al. Increased risk of hepatocellular carcinoma and liver cirrhosis in vinyl chloride workers: synergistic effect of occupational exposure with alcohol intake. Environ Health Perspect 2004;112(11):1188–92.
106. Wong RH, Chen PC, Du CL, et al. An increased standardised mortality ratio for liver cancer among polyvinyl chloride workers in Taiwan. Occup Environ Med 2002;59(6):405–9.
107. Attanasio AF, Mo D, Erfurth EM, et al. Prevalence of metabolic syndrome in adult hypopituitary growth hormone (GH)-deficient patients before and after GH replacement. J Clin Endocrinol Metab 2010;95(1):74–81.
108. Takahashi Y, Iida K, Takahashi K, et al. Growth hormone reverses nonalcoholic steatohepatitis in a patient with adult growth hormone deficiency. Gastroenterology 2007;132(3):938–43.
109. Tai TS, Lin SY, Sheu WH. Metabolic effects of growth hormone therapy in an Alstrom syndrome patient. Horm Res 2003;60(6):297–301.
110. Johannsson G, Bengtsson BA. Growth hormone and the metabolic syndrome. J Endocrinol Invest 1999;22(Suppl 5):41–6.
111. Ichikawa T, Hamasaki K, Ishikawa H, et al. Non-alcoholic steatohepatitis and hepatic steatosis in patients with adult onset growth hormone deficiency. Gut 2003;52(6):914.
112. Lonardo A, Loria P, Leonardi F, et al. Growth hormone plasma levels in nonalcoholic fatty liver disease. Am J Gastroenterol 2002;97(4):1071–2.
113. Adams LA, Feldstein A, Lindor KD, et al. Nonalcoholic fatty liver disease among patients with hypothalamic and pituitary dysfunction. Hepatology 2004;39(4):909–14.
114. Hong JW, Kim JY, Kim YE, et al. Metabolic parameters and nonalcoholic fatty liver disease in hypopituitary men. Horm Metab Res 2011;43(1):48–54.
115. Johansson JO, Fowelin J, Landin K, et al. Growth hormone-deficient adults are insulin-resistant. Metabolism 1995;44(9):1126–9.
116. Verhelst J, Mattsson AF, Luger A, et al. Prevalence and characteristics of the metabolic syndrome in 2479 hypopituitary patients with adult-onset GH deficiency before GH replacement: a KIMS analysis. Eur J Endocrinol 2011;165(6):881–9.
117. Barclay JL, Nelson CN, Ishikawa M, et al. GH-dependent STAT5 signaling plays an important role in hepatic lipid metabolism. Endocrinology 2011;152(1):181–92.

118. Tateno C, Kataoka M, Utoh R, et al. Growth hormone-dependent pathogenesis of human hepatic steatosis in a novel mouse model bearing a human hepatocyte-repopulated liver. Endocrinology 2011;152(4):1479–91.

119. Fan Y, Menon RK, Cohen P, et al. Liver-specific deletion of the growth hormone receptor reveals essential role of growth hormone signaling in hepatic lipid metabolism. J Biol Chem 2009;284(30):19937–44.

120. Mueller KM, Kornfeld JW, Friedbichler K, et al. Impairment of hepatic growth hormone and glucocorticoid receptor signaling causes steatosis and hepatocellular carcinoma in mice. Hepatology 2011;54(4):1398–409.

121. Ameen C, Linden D, Larsson BM, et al. Effects of gender and GH secretory pattern on sterol regulatory element-binding protein-1c and its target genes in rat liver. Am J Physiol Endocrinol Metab 2004;287(6):E1039–48.

122. Clemmons DR. The diagnosis and treatment of growth hormone deficiency in adults. Curr Opin Endocrinol Diabetes Obes 2010;17(4):377–83.

123. Liangpunsakul S, Chalasani N. Is hypothyroidism a risk factor for non-alcoholic steatohepatitis? J Clin Gastroenterol 2003;37(4):340–3.

124. Pagadala MR, Zein CO, Dasarathy S, et al. Prevalence of hypothyroidism in nonalcoholic fatty liver disease. Dig Dis Sci 2012;57(2):528–34.

125. Chung GE, Kim D, Kim W, et al. Non-alcoholic fatty liver disease across the spectrum of hypothyroidism. J Hepatol 2012. [Epub ahead of print].

126. Carulli L, Ballestri S, Lonardo A, et al. Is nonalcoholic steatohepatitis associated with a high-though-normal thyroid stimulating hormone level and lower cholesterol levels? Intern Emerg Med 2011. [Epub ahead of print].

127. Michalaki MA, Vagenakis AG, Leonardou AS, et al. Thyroid function in humans with morbid obesity. Thyroid 2006;16(1):73–8.

128. Dimitriadis G, Mitrou P, Lambadiari V, et al. Insulin action in adipose tissue and muscle in hypothyroidism. J Clin Endocrinol Metab 2006;91(12):4930–7.

129. Pucci E, Chiovato L, Pinchera A. Thyroid and lipid metabolism. Int J Obes Relat Metab Disord 2000;24(Suppl 2):S109–12.

130. Chicco AJ, Sparagna GC. Role of cardiolipin alterations in mitochondrial dysfunction and disease. Am J Physiol Cell Physiol 2007;292(1):C33–44.

131. Siciliano G, Monzani F, Manca ML, et al. Human mitochondrial transcription factor A reduction and mitochondrial dysfunction in Hashimoto's hypothyroid myopathy. Mol Med 2002;8(6):326–33.

132. Nanda N, Bobby Z, Hamide A, et al. Association between oxidative stress and coronary lipid risk factors in hypothyroid women is independent of body mass index. Metabolism 2007;56(10):1350–5.

133. Williams CD, Oxon BM, Lond H. Kwashiorkor: a nutritional disease of children associated with a maize diet. Lancet 1935;229:1151–2.

134. Fong DG, Nehra V, Lindor KD, et al. Metabolic and nutritional considerations in nonalcoholic fatty liver. Hepatology 2000;32(1):3–10.

135. Kwon DH, Kang W, Nam YS, et al. Dietary protein restriction induces steatohepatitis and alters leptin/signal transducers and activators of transcription 3 signaling in lactating rats. J Nutr Biochem 2011. [Epub ahead of print].

136. Milner RD. Insulin secretion in human protein-calorie deficiency. Proc Nutr Soc 1972;31(2):219–23.

137. Kim TS, Freake HC. High carbohydrate diet and starvation regulate lipogenic mRNA in rats in a tissue-specific manner. J Nutr 1996;126(3):611–7.

138. Tsukamoto M, Tanaka A, Arai M, et al. Hepatocellular injuries observed in patients with an eating disorder prior to nutritional treatment. Intern Med 2008; 47(16):1447–50.

139. Fong HF, Divasta AD, Difabio D, et al. Prevalence and predictors of abnormal liver enzymes in young women with anorexia nervosa. J Pediatr 2008;153(2): 247–53.

140. Narayanan V, Gaudiani JL, Harris RH, et al. Liver function test abnormalities in anorexia nervosa–cause or effect. Int J Eat Disord 2010;43(4):378–81.

141. Tajiri K, Shimizu Y, Tsuneyama K, et al. A case report of oxidative stress in a patient with anorexia nervosa. Int J Eat Disord 2006;39(7):616–8.

142. Sakada M, Tanaka A, Ohta D, et al. Severe steatosis resulted from anorexia nervosa leading to fatal hepatic failure. J Gastroenterol 2006;41(7):714–5.

143. Moller L, Stodkilde-Jorgensen H, Jensen FT, et al. Fasting in healthy subjects is associated with intrahepatic accumulation of lipids as assessed by 1H-magnetic resonance spectroscopy. Clin Sci 2008;114(8):547–52.

144. Evangeliou A, Vlassopoulos D. Carnitine metabolism and deficit–when supplementation is necessary? Curr Pharm Biotechnol 2003;4(3):211–9.

145. Flanagan JL, Simmons PA, Vehige J, et al. Role of carnitine in disease. Nutr Metab (Lond) 2010;7:30.

146. Scaglia F, Longo N. Primary and secondary alterations of neonatal carnitine metabolism. Semin Perinatol 1999;23(2):152–61.

147. Treem WR, Stanley CA. Massive hepatomegaly, steatosis, and secondary plasma carnitine deficiency in an infant with cystic fibrosis. Pediatrics 1989; 83(6):993–7.

148. Zeisel SH, Da Costa KA, Franklin PD, et al. Choline, an essential nutrient for humans. FASEB J 1991;5(7):2093–8.

149. Buchman AL, Dubin MD, Moukarzel AA, et al. Choline deficiency: a cause of hepatic steatosis during parenteral nutrition that can be reversed with intravenous choline supplementation. Hepatology 1995;22(5):1399–403.

150. Yao ZM, Vance DE. Head group specificity in the requirement of phosphatidyl-choline biosynthesis for very low density lipoprotein secretion from cultured hepatocytes. J Biol Chem 1989;264(19):11373–80.

151. Lombardi B, Pani P, Schlunk FF. Choline-deficiency fatty liver: impaired release of hepatic triglycerides. J Lipid Res 1968;9(4):437–46.

152. da Costa KA, Niculescu MD, Craciunescu CN, et al. Choline deficiency increases lymphocyte apoptosis and DNA damage in humans. Am J Clin Nutr 2006;84(1):88–94.

153. Albright CD, da Costa KA, Craciunescu CN, et al. Regulation of choline deficiency apoptosis by epidermal growth factor in CWSV-1 rat hepatocytes. Cell Physiol Biochem 2005;15(1–4):59–68.

154. Buchman AL, Moukarzel A, Jenden DJ, et al. Low plasma free choline is prevalent in patients receiving long term parenteral nutrition and is associated with hepatic aminotransferase abnormalities. Clin Nutr 1993;12(1):33–7.

155. Misra S, Ahn C, Ament ME, et al. Plasma choline concentrations in children requiring long-term home parenteral nutrition: a case control study. JPEN J Parenter Enteral Nutr 1999;23(5):305–8.

156. Compher CW, Kinosian BP, Stoner NE, et al. Choline and vitamin B12 deficiencies are interrelated in folate-replete long-term total parenteral nutrition patients. JPEN J Parenter Enteral Nutr 2002;26(1):57–62.

157. Buchman AL, Dubin M, Jenden D, et al. Lecithin increases plasma free choline and decreases hepatic steatosis in long-term total parenteral nutrition patients. Gastroenterology 1992;102(4 Pt 1):1363–70.

158. Buchman AL, Ament ME, Sohel M, et al. Choline deficiency causes reversible hepatic abnormalities in patients receiving parenteral nutrition: proof of a human

choline requirement: a placebo-controlled trial. JPEN J Parenter Enteral Nutr 2001;25(5):260–8.

159. D'Albuquerque LA, Gonzalez AM, Wahle RC, et al. Liver transplantation for subacute hepatocellular failure due to massive steatohepatitis after bariatric surgery. Liver Transpl 2008;14(6):881–5.

160. Castillo J, Fabrega E, Escalante CF, et al. Liver transplantation in a case of steatohepatitis and subacute hepatic failure after biliopancreatic diversion for morbid obesity. Obes Surg 2001;11(5):640–2.

161. Craig RM, Neumann T, Jeejeebhoy KN, et al. Severe hepatocellular reaction resembling alcoholic hepatitis with cirrhosis after massive small bowel resection and prolonged total parenteral nutrition. Gastroenterology 1980;79(1):131–7.

162. Drenick EJ, Fisler J, Johnson D. Hepatic steatosis after intestinal bypass–prevention and reversal by metronidazole, irrespective of protein-calorie malnutrition. Gastroenterology 1982;82(3):535–48.

163. Nazim M, Stamp G, Hodgson HJ. Non-alcoholic steatohepatitis associated with small intestinal diverticulosis and bacterial overgrowth. Hepatogastroenterology 1989;36(5):349–51.

164. Wigg AJ, Roberts-Thomson IC, Dymock RB, et al. The role of small intestinal bacterial overgrowth, intestinal permeability, endotoxaemia, and tumour necrosis factor alpha in the pathogenesis of non-alcoholic steatohepatitis. Gut 2001;48(2):206–11.

165. Miura K, Kodama Y, Inokuchi S, et al. Toll-like receptor 9 promotes steatohepatitis by induction of interleukin-1beta in mice. Gastroenterology 2010;139(1):323–34 e327.

166. Madrid AM, Poniachik J, Quera R, et al. Small intestinal clustered contractions and bacterial overgrowth: a frequent finding in obese patients. Dig Dis Sci 2011;56(1):155–60.

167. Sabate JM, Jouet P, Harnois F, et al. High prevalence of small intestinal bacterial overgrowth in patients with morbid obesity: a contributor to severe hepatic steatosis. Obes Surg 2008;18(4):371–7.

168. Turnbaugh PJ, Ley RE, Mahowald MA, et al. An obesity-associated gut microbiome with increased capacity for energy harvest. Nature 2006;444(7122):1027–31.

169. Frazier TH, DiBaise JK, McClain CJ. Gut microbiota, intestinal permeability, obesity-induced inflammation, and liver injury. J Parenter Enteral Nutr 2011;35(Suppl 5):14S–20S.

170. Mattila J, Aitola P, Matikainen M. Liver lesions found at colectomy in ulcerative colitis: correlation between histological findings and biochemical parameters. J Clin Pathol 1994;47(11):1019–21.

171. Eade MN, Cooke WT, Williams JA. Liver disease in Crohn's disease. A study of 100 consecutive patients. Scand J Gastroenterol 1971;6(3):199–204.

172. Riegler G, D'Inca R, Sturniolo GC, et al. Hepatobiliary alterations in patients with inflammatory bowel disease: a multicenter study. Caprilli & Gruppo Italiano Studio Colon-Retto. Scand J Gastroenterol 1998;33(1):93–8.

173. Bargiggia S, Maconi G, Elli M, et al. Sonographic prevalence of liver steatosis and biliary tract stones in patients with inflammatory bowel disease: study of 511 subjects at a single center. J Clin Gastroenterol 2003;36(5):417–20.

174. Bardella MT, Valenti L, Pagliari C, et al. Searching for coeliac disease in patients with non-alcoholic fatty liver disease. Dig Liver Dis 2004;36(5):333–6.

175. Valera JM, Hurtado C, Poniachik J, et al. Study of celiac disease in patients with non-alcoholic fatty liver and autoimmune hepatic diseases. Gastroenterol Hepatol 2008;31(1):8–11 [in Spanish].

176. Lo Iacono O, Petta S, Venezia G, et al. Anti-tissue transglutaminase antibodies in patients with abnormal liver tests: is it always coeliac disease? Am J Gastroenterol 2005;100(11):2472–7.
177. Grieco A, Miele L, Pignatoro G, et al. Is coeliac disease a confounding factor in the diagnosis of NASH? Gut 2001;49(4):596.
178. Miele L, Valenza V, La Torre G, et al. Increased intestinal permeability and tight junction alterations in nonalcoholic fatty liver disease. Hepatology 2009;49(6): 1877–87.
179. Nehra V, Angulo P, Buchman AL, et al. Nutritional and metabolic considerations in the etiology of nonalcoholic steatohepatitis. Dig Dis Sci 2001;46(11):2347–52.
180. Andresen BS, Dobrowolski SF, O'Reilly L, et al. Medium-chain acyl-CoA dehydrogenase (MCAD) mutations identified by MS/MS-based prospective screening of newborns differ from those observed in patients with clinical symptoms: identification and characterization of a new, prevalent mutation that results in mild MCAD deficiency. Am J Hum Genet 2001;68(6):1408–18.
181. Fishbein M, Smith M, Li BU. A rapid MRI technique for the assessment of hepatic steatosis in a subject with medium-chain acyl-coenzyme A dehydrogenase (MCAD) deficiency. J Pediatr Gastroenterol Nutr 1998;27(2):224–7.
182. Smith ET Jr, Davis GJ. Medium-chain acyl coenzyme-A dehydrogenase deficiency. Not just another Reye syndrome. Am J Forensic Med Pathol 1993; 14(4):313–8.
183. Perper JA, Ahdab-Barmada M. Fatty liver, encephalopathy, and sudden unexpected death in early childhood due to medium-chain acyl-coenzyme A dehydrogenase deficiency. Am J Forensic Med Pathol 1992;13(4):329–34.
184. Grabowski G, Charnas L, Du H. Lysosomal acid lipase deficiencies: the Wolman disease/cholesteryl ester storage disease spectrum. In: Valle D, Beaudet A, Vogelstein V, et al, editors. The online metabolic and molecular bases of inherited diseases (OMMBID). McGraw-Hill; 2012. Chapter 142.
185. Dalgic B, Sari S, Gunduz M, et al. Cholesteryl ester storage disease in a young child presenting as isolated hepatomegaly treated with simvastatin. Turk J Pediatr 2006;48(2):148–51.
186. Patrick AD, Lake BD. Deficiency of an acid lipase in Wolman's disease. Nature 1969;222(5198):1067–8.
187. Johncilla M, Mitchell KA. Pathology of the liver in copper overload. Semin Liver Dis 2011;31(3):239–44.
188. Muller T, Langner C, Fuchsbichler A, et al. Immunohistochemical analysis of Mallory bodies in Wilsonian and non-Wilsonian hepatic copper toxicosis. Hepatology 2004;39(4):963–9.
189. Jensen K, Gluud C. The Mallory body: morphological, clinical and experimental studies (part 1 of a literature survey). Hepatology 1994;20(4 Pt 1):1061–77.
190. Stromeyer FW, Ishak KG. Histology of the liver in Wilson's disease: a study of 34 cases. Am J Clin Pathol 1980;73(1):12–24.
191. Wasserman JM, Thung SN, Berman R, et al. Hepatic Weber-Christian disease. Semin Liver Dis 2001;21(1):115–8.
192. Kimura H, Kako M, Yo K, et al. Alcoholic hyalins (Mallory bodies) in a case of Weber-Christian disease: electron microscopic observations of liver involvement. Gastroenterology 1980;78(4):807–12.
193. Illingworth DR, Connor WE, Miller RG. Abetalipoproteinemia. Report of two cases and review of therapy. Arch Neurol 1980;37(10):659–62.
194. Sen D, Dagdelen S, Erbas T. Hepatosteatosis with hypobetalipoproteinemia. J Natl Med Assoc 2007;99(3):284–6.

195. Harada N, Soejima Y, Taketomi A, et al. Recurrent familial hypobetalipoproteinemia-induced nonalcoholic fatty liver disease after living donor liver transplantation. Liver Transpl 2009;15(7):806–9.

196. Chen Z, Fitzgerald RL, Averna MR, et al. A targeted apolipoprotein B-38.9-producing mutation causes fatty livers in mice due to the reduced ability of apolipoprotein B-38.9 to transport triglycerides. J Biol Chem 2000;275(42):32807–15.

197. Powell EE, Searle J, Mortimer R. Steatohepatitis associated with limb lipodystrophy. Gastroenterology 1989;97(4):1022–4.

198. Javor ED, Ghany MG, Cochran EK, et al. Leptin reverses nonalcoholic steatohepatitis in patients with severe lipodystrophy. Hepatology 2005;41(4):753–60.

199. Lemoine M, Barbu V, Girard PM, et al. Altered hepatic expression of SREBP-1 and PPARgamma is associated with liver injury in insulin-resistant lipodystrophic HIV-infected patients. AIDS 2006;20(3):387–95.

200. Haque WA, Shimomura I, Matsuzawa Y, et al. Serum adiponectin and leptin levels in patients with lipodystrophies. J Clin Endocrinol Metab 2002;87(5):2395.

201. Hall AM, Brunt EM, Chen Z, et al. Dynamic and differential regulation of proteins that coat lipid droplets in fatty liver dystrophic mice. J Lipid Res 2010;51(3):554–63.

202. Cortes VA, Curtis DE, Sukumaran S, et al. Molecular mechanisms of hepatic steatosis and insulin resistance in the AGPAT2-deficient mouse model of congenital generalized lipodystrophy. Cell Metab 2009;9(2):165–76.

203. Grimbert S, Fisch C, Deschamps D, et al. Effects of female sex hormones on mitochondria: possible role in acute fatty liver of pregnancy. Am J Phys 1995;268:G107–15.

Mechanisms of Disease Progression in NASH: New Paradigms

Brittany N. Bohinc, MD[a], Anna Mae Diehl, MD[b],*

KEYWORDS

- NASH • Nonalcoholic steatohepatitis • Hedgehog signaling pathway
- Hepatocellular carcinoma • Cirrhosis • Hepatic fibrosis

KEY POINTS

- Nonalcoholic steatohepatitis (NASH) is a significant health burden in the US population, with risk for progression to cirrhosis and hepatocellular carcinoma.
- Cell signaling pathways, notably Hedgehog (Hh), are important in the repair and regeneration of the liver in NASH and in other states of hepatic injury.
- Liver repair at the cellular level entails autocrine and paracrine signaling of the Hh ligand to promote the epithelial-to-mesenchymal transition of Hh-responsive cells and progenitors, stimulate fibrogenic repair, and trigger vascular remodeling.
- The fibrogenic response is highly dependent on the dose and duration of exposure of Hh-responsive cells to Hh ligand.
- When tissue injury is excessive, prolonged, or when there is aberrant Hh activation, the normal tissue repair response goes awry predisposing patients to end-stage liver complications, including cirrhosis and hepatocellular carcinoma.

NASH IN THE TWENTY-FIRST CENTURY: RISK FACTOR FOR LIVER FIBROSIS AND HEPATOCELLULAR CARCINOMA

Nonalcoholic fatty liver disease (NAFLD) and its more serious form, nonalcoholic steatohepatitis (NASH), are the hepatic manifestations of obesity and the metabolic syndrome.[1] NAFLD is currently the leading cause of chronic liver disease, with a prevalence estimated to affect nearly 30% of the US population.[2] According to the latest figures, NASH affects 2% to 5% of all Americans.[3] Interpatient variability in manifestations of the disease is apparent; some progress to fibrosis, cirrhosis, and, ultimately,

Financial disclosures: The authors have no financial disclosures to report.
[a] Department of Endocrinology, Diabetes and Metabolism, Duke University Hospital, 310 Baker House, 201 Trent Drive, Durham, NC 27710, USA; [b] Division of Gastroenterology, Duke Liver Center, Duke University, 595 LaSalle Street, Suite 1073, DUMC 3256, Durham, NC 27710, USA
* Corresponding author.
E-mail address: annamae.diehl@duke.edu

to hepatocellular carcinoma (HCC) or transplant.[4] Others have a more indolent disease course. Currently, NASH-related cirrhosis is expected to exceed viral hepatitis as the indication for liver transplantation by the year 2025.[5] Cirrhosis, a result of progressive liver injury and fibrosis, is also the most important risk factor in the development of HCC, a cancer that is currently the third leading cause of cancer death worldwide.[6,7] With such a daunting disease burden looming on the horizon, it is imperative that we better understand the risk factors and cellular signaling pathways that contribute to disease progression. Identifying an at-risk subpopulation among those with metabolic syndrome, understanding the mechanisms behind progressive liver injury, and considering future potential therapeutic targets are critical.

THE 2-HIT MODEL OF FIBROSIS

A 2-hit model has been proposed as an explanation for why some patients progress from NAFLD to NASH. Insulin resistance is at the forefront of the model,[8] contributing to enhanced adipose tissue triglyceride (TG) lipolysis, increased serum free fatty acids, and impaired hepatic TG export by very-low-density lipoprotein (VLDL). In this model, hepatic steatosis (hit 1) exposes the liver parenchyma to environmental and extracellular hepatic insults (hit 2), leading to inflammation, steatonecrosis, and fibrosis.[9] Described insults include diets high in fructose,[10] increased ingestion of saturated fatty acids and cholesterol,[11,12] a reduced ability of insulin to inhibit lipolysis (ie, insulin resistance),[13] and altered VLDL metabolism.[13–15] Insulin resistance and excess abdominal adiposity are associated with increased hepatic lipid accumulation and increased de novo hepatic lipogenesis.[16] Defects in lipid use via mitochondrial oxidation, and lipid export may also contribute to hepatic lipid accumulation. Aberrant adipocytokine signaling, lipotoxicity from saturated fatty acids, and exposure to high-fructose corn syrup have been all been implicated in causing hepatocyte injury through oxidative and endoplasmic reticulum stress.[17–19] Other potential contributors in progression to NASH include the following: (1) central hyperalimentation[20]; (2) rapid weight loss[21]; (3) lipid abnormalities, including hypertriglyceridemia and abetalipoproteinemia[22,23]; and (4) various drugs and environmental toxins.[24] Although these risk factors have been implicated in the development of NASH, there is a poor understanding of why some patients with NASH slowly progress, whereas others develop more insidious disease (ie, fibrosis or HCC). Our work in hedgehog (Hh) signaling suggests that aberrant/prolonged Hh signaling during hepatic tissue repair may be an integral component for disease progression in NASH.

OVERVIEW OF THE Hh SIGNALING PATHWAY

Hh is a morphogenic signaling pathway involved in cell fate decisions during embryogenesis. It is also involved in the repair and regeneration in many endodermal adult tissues. Hh signaling is critical in cellular proliferation, apoptosis, migration, differentiation, and the growth of progenitor cell populations. The pathway is highly conserved across species[25–27] and has been described in many tissues, including the liver, pancreas, and colon.[28–31]

Canonical Signaling

Hh signaling is activated by a family of Hh-specific ligands (ie, Sonic Hedgehog ([Shh], Indian Hedgehog [Ihh], Desert Hedgehog [Dhh]) that are preferentially expressed in various tissues. In the liver, Shh and Ihh are preferentially expressed by hepatocytes, bile ductular cells, and hepatic stellate cells (HSCs). The Hh ligand binds to its cell membrane surface receptor, Patched (Ptc), present on Hh-responsive target cells. After Hh binds to Ptc, there is a derepression on another cell membrane receptor, Smoothened (Smo), that is in a chronically inactivated state. The activation of Smo upon Hh ligand-Ptc binding results in the propagation of a host of intracellular signaling proteins, including the glioblastoma (Gli) family transcription factors Gli1, Gli2, and Gli3. Gli1 and Gli2 are generally reported to be transcriptional activators, whereas Gli3 can be either a repressor or activator depending on its posttranslational modification.[27] The increased production of Gli leads to the transcription of Gli target genes, including osteopontin (OPN), Hh interacting protein (Hhip), and SNAIL. Cellular signaling that uses the Hh ligand-Ptc-Smo interaction is referred to as canonical or classic Hh signaling and has been well described in the literature. The pathway is further complicated because the overexpression of Gli-associated target genes, Ptc or Hhip (a soluble antagonist of Hh ligand), can be present in excess of the Hh ligand and effectively silence Hh signaling.

When the Hh ligand is not present, unbound Ptc represses Smo to inhibit Hh signaling. Hh-regulated transcription factors are phosphorylated (ie, inactivated) by glycogen synthase kinase 3, protein kinase A, and casein kinase. Phosphorylated forms of Hh-responsive target genes are tagged for proteasome degradation and are prevented from translocating to the nucleus to bind with their respective nuclear receptors.[32]

Noncanonical Signaling

The activation of Gli-family transcription factors can also be triggered by noncanonical signals that do not involve the Hh ligand–Ptc-Smo interaction.[33] Potential activating factors include the following: (1) insulinlike growth factor with noncanonical activation of Gli1,[34] (2) transforming growth factor (TGF)-beta activation of Gli2,[35] and (3) epigenetic regulation of Hh target genes by changes in the methylation status.[36–39] In addition to noncanonical Hh signaling activation, the Hh pathway also influences alternate cell-fate regulating pathways. For example, the activation of Gli family members and other Hh-responsive gene products (by either Hh or by noncanonical mechanisms) regulates the transcription of pleiotropic TGF-beta target genes (ie, SNAIL) and influences the expression of activators/inhibitors in alternate cell signaling pathways, such as the Wingless (Wnt) ligand.

Hh LIGANDS: AUTOCRINE AND PARACRINE SIGNALING

Hh signaling can be activated by autocrine, paracrine, and endocrine mechanisms. Initially, Hh ligands are synthesized as propeptides. They then undergo autocatalyzed cleavage, generating an N-terminal fragment that is lipid modified before moving to the cellular membrane and then to the extracellular space. Hh propeptides can also undergo extracellular cleavage as seen in the proximal gastrointestinal tract.[40] Once cleaved and processed, Hh ligands then act on local Hh-responsive cells or move in an endocrine fashion to affect Hh-responsive cells in other tissues.[25,41,42] Exosomes containing the activated Hh ligand have been purified from the blood and bile of hepatically injured rodents, providing a mechanism for distant transport.[43] The release of Hh ligands from Hh-producing cells is facilitated by the cell membrane 12 transmembrane protein, Dispatched (Disp). Disp is similar to Ptc in that it has a sterol-sensing domain, which is a region found in proteins that regulates cholesterol trafficking.[44] Although Ptc and Disp are structurally similar, they perform seemingly opposite tasks in that the former sequesters the Hh ligand, whereas the latter releases it as a signaling molecule.

Hh ACTIVATION IN THE INJURED LIVER

Hh is virtually inactive in normal healthy livers.[45] Studies have shown that Hh is inactivated by resident quiescent HSCs (Q-HSCs) and endothelial cells that basally express high levels of Hhip, a protein that preferentially binds to the Hh ligand preventing it from interacting with Ptc.[45] In the acutely or chronically injured liver, however, the pathway is turned on and Hhip levels decrease.[46] The authors' group has demonstrated through a series of studies that ballooned hepatocytes (ie, injury-related hepatocyte enlargement characteristic of NASH) stain strongly for the Shh ligand.[47] The production of the Hh ligand by hepatocytes was further elicited by treating degenerating hepatocytes in vitro with tunicamycin, a drug that evokes endoplasmic reticulum stress. Although the treated cells were positive for the Hh ligand, stressed hepatocytes in vivo and in vitro were negative for Gli2, suggesting that, although they are Hh producing, they are not Hh responsive. Additional resident cells in the injured liver, including HSCs, cholangiocytes, progenitor cells, lymphocytes (ie, natural killer cells [NKTs]), reactive ductular cells, sinusoidal endothelial cells (SECs), and stromal cells, are capable of producing Hh ligands in states of liver injury.[28,43,47–51] Several growth factors, including platelet-derived growth factor BB, TGF-B1, and epidermal growth factor, can also stimulate immature ductular cells and HSCs to release the Hh ligand[43,52,53] and post-translationally stabilize Gli transcription factors via the PI3K/Akt pathway.[34] On enrichment of the hepatic microenvironment with the Hh ligand, Q-HSCs respond to the ligand via canonical signaling mechanisms and transition into myofibroblastic HSCs (MF-HSC) that contribute to fibrosis and cellular repair. Additional Hh-responsive cells include the following: (1) SECs, (2) ductular cells, (3) liver epithelial progenitors, (4) immature cholangiocytes, (5) T lymphocytes/NKTs, (6) HSCs, and (9) mature myofibroblasts. Active Hh ligand produced by injured hepatocytes and other cells act locally and in a paracrine/endocrine manner to influence Hh signaling activation in Hh-responsive cells. Experimental evidence suggests that once Hh is activated in diseased liver tissue, Hh-responsive signaling protein expression tends to auto-amplify as long as Hh ligands persist and become somewhat resistant to negative feedback from Ptc overexpression or Hhip.[54] However, when the insult abates and injury subsides, the Hh pathway turns off.

APOPTOSIS AND INFLAMMATION AS AMPLIFIERS OF Hh SIGNALING

Programmed cell death or apoptosis is a standard element of routine cellular turnover and maintenance. When appropriately regulated, cellular apoptotic mechanisms are highly controlled and limited to specific cells without the need to invoke an inflammatory reaction.[55,56] In the liver, programmed cell death is regulated intrinsically in the mitochondria or extrinsically by surface death receptors, including Fas (CD95),[57] that recruit caspase-8 and caspase-3 to complete the final apoptotic pathway.[58] Dysregulated apoptosis, as occurs in response to environmental toxins or noxious stimuli, is associated with both inflammatory and fibrotic responses.[59–61] Hepatocyte apoptosis in liver disease may directly or indirectly promote inflammation. Multiple studies have associated programmed cell death and caspase activation with the release of neutrophil chemoattractants, inflammatory cell recruitment (ie, neutrophils, monocytes, and T lymphocytes/NKTs), and proinflammatory chemokines (ie, CXC1 and MIP-2).[62–65] In addition, several studies have shown that engulfment of apoptotic bodies by monocytes or Kupffer cells (ie, hepatic macrophages) in states of liver damage promote the expression of death receptors, linking inflammation and apoptosis in states of hepatic tissue injury.[66,67]

One of the main differentiating factors between hepatosteatosis and NASH is the higher degree of hepatocyte injury and apoptosis in the latter.[68,69] Apoptotic bodies and degenerating hepatocytes are more numerous in NASH compared with NAFLD,[70] suggesting a role for apoptosis in worsening disease. In addition, hepatic accumulation of inflammatory cells is seen more often in NASH than in NAFLD, suggesting inflammatory and immune involvement in the former. Several studies have shown that patients with NASH have enhanced expression of nuclear factor kB, a transcription factor that promotes proinflammatory cytokines along with death receptors and proapoptotic ligands.[71,72]

The missing link between apoptosis in liver injury and aberrantly activated inflammation may be related to Hh activation. Indeed, recent data have shown that severely injured and dying liver epithelial cells produce and release Hh ligands to promote and activate Hh signaling. Once activated, Hh ligands stimulate immature ductular cells to produce CXCL16, the chemokine that recruits inflammatory NKT cells to the liver. On arrival, NKT cells respond to glycolipid antigens presented to them by CD1d molecules located on hepatocytes, bile ductular cells, and sinusoidal epithelial cells.[73,74] Once activated by these lipid antigens, NKT cells produce both T-helper 1 (Th1) cells and T-helper 2 (Th2) cells.[75] The production ratio of these cytokines can skew the hepatic microenvironment toward a proinflammatory/antifibrogenic setting (increased Th1 production) or an antiinflammatory/profibrogenic setting (Th2 overproduction).[76] NKT cells not only respond to Hh ligands to produce profibrogenic cytokines (ie, interleukin [IL] 13 and IL-4) but have also been shown to produce Hh ligands, which themselves promote Q-HSCs to convert to myofibroblasts.[50,77] In this way, inflammation and apoptosis may both contribute to the progression of disease in NASH.

The authors evaluated this hypothesis in the rodent model of NASH. In that experiment, wild-type (WT) mice fed a methionine choline–deficient (MCD) diet were compared with Ptc-deficient mice (Ptc±) with baseline upregulation of Hh pathway signaling because of the reduction in Smo repression for changes in NKT expression and fibrosis. The authors also evaluated CD1d-deficient mice with the absence of NKT cell expression. They found that both WT and Ptc ± mice had significant upregulation of Hh target genes after being fed the MCD diet to induce NASH but that Ptc ± mice had significantly worsened fibrosis as determined by fibrogenic markers and by histology. CD1d-deficient mice with the absence of NKT cells had significant attenuation of fibrosis compared with the WT animal. In the same study, the authors looked at liver specimens from human patients with NASH and stage 3 to 4 liver fibrosis. They found that the expression of the NKT cell cytokine, CXCL16, accompanied expression of Hh target genes, including Shh and Gli2, and that the highest expression was detected within fibrous septa.[77] Increased hepatic expression of CD1d has also been detected in human patients with severe NASH.[78] In all, both apoptosis and inflammation with immune regulatory cell recruitment seem to be associated with enhanced Hh signaling and disease progression in NASH.

THE Hh SIGNALING PATHWAY: ROLE IN REPAIR AND REGENERATION

Accumulating scientific evidence has demonstrated that Hh activation is not simply a by-product that simultaneously occurs with liver injury. Instead, it has been shown to be actively involved in liver repair and regeneration once exposed to insult. There are several areas of research that have shown that Hh is intricately involved in this regenerative process. Initial work showed that hepatic expression of both Shh and Ihh dramatically increase after 70% partial hepatectomy and on exposure to noxious stimuli.[79] Parallel work has described in detail how critical Hh activation is in the normal repair response.

Growth of a Progenitor Population of Cells and the Epithelial-to-Mesenchymal Transition Response

Healthy adult livers harbor small progenitor populations that concentrate along the Canals of Hering.[80] Because mature hepatocytes are not able to respond to Hh ligands and are unable to replicate during liver injury, the enrichment of the hepatic microenvironment with Hh ligand provides a selective survival advantage for cell types that are Hh responsive, leading to the outgrowth of Hh-responsive cells as long as injury persists. In this way, Hh ligands bind to Ptc on resident progenitor cells and activate proliferation while inhibiting progenitor cell apoptosis.[45,81] Progenitor populations in the rodent and human livers include oval cells, immature ductular cells, and young hepatocytic cells—all of which are Hh responsive.[48] Dying hepatocytes committed to apoptosis are unable to undergo regeneration and, therefore, stimulate progenitor cells (ie, oval cells) through the Hh ligand to proliferate and differentiate into ductular hepatocytes that then mature to hepatocytes. Likewise, progenitor cells can differentiate into cholangiocytes. In short, the progenitor cell population shrinks or grows in response to the Hh ligand, which is upregulated in injury.[45]

Support for this concept has been presented multiple times in the literature. In rodents, progenitor markers positively correlate with degree of Hh ligand production during liver injury and regress as injury abates.[49] A similar positive correlation between progenitor recruitment and growth and Hh activity has been reported in various human liver disease, including primary biliary cirrhosis,[51] chronic hepatitis B and C,[82] and in NAFLD.[83] The immunohistochemical analysis of healthy human and rodent livers has co-localized Hh ligand and Hh-responsive genes with progenitor cells located along the Canals of Hering.[45,49,51,84] Hh ligands are expressed by the primitive ventral endoderm, the tissue that ultimately gives rise to hepatic progenitor cells.[85] Further literature has shown that Hh regulates the growth of hepatoblastomas, which is a progenitor-derived liver tumor common in children.[86]

In addition to the recruitment of hepatic progenitors, plastic and immature cells are driven by Hh ligands to undergo another process common in embryogenesis: epithelial-to-mesenchymal transition (EMT) and reciprocal mesenchymal-to-epithelial transition (MET). In the epithelial phenotype (MET), cells become polarized and adherent to adjacent cells. On the contrary, mesenchymal cells (EMT) are mobile, migratory, and invasive.[87] In this complex process, epithelial cells gradually dissolve connections to adjacent cells, rearrange their cytoskeletons by activating Rac1 (a small cytoskeleton-associated GTPase important in the promotion of EMT),[88] remodel their matrix, and migrate out of epithelial sheets. Both Hh ligand and TGF beta are instrumental in EMT/MET in developing embryos.[89] Likewise, they are both important in adult liver repair and regeneration, inducing EMT among ductular progenitors and Q-HSC, and converting them into myofibroblasts that promote fibrous repair.[46,83,90]

Most of the published literature has focused on the EMT response in Q-HSCs and their role after liver injury. The authors' group, in particular, showed that freshly isolated Q-HSCs had a phenotype closely related to progenitor and immature epithelial cells. Specifically, these cells expressed peroxisome proliferator activating receptor, glial fibrillary acidic protein, E-cadherin, desmoplakin, and Ker-7 and -19. Although they did express desmin, a factor usually associated with a mesenchymal phenotype, they were lacking other typical myofibroblastic genes, including alpha smooth muscle actin (alpha-SMA) and collagen 1α1 (Col1α1). On activation of Hh signaling, Hhip, which is highly expressed in the Q-HSC, decreases dramatically, Shh and Gli are produced, and there is EMT (ie, downregulation of epithelial markers and upregulation of mesenchymal markers, including alpha-SMA, (Col1α1), vimentin, fibronectin, S100A4, SNAIL, and TGF beta-1). The process can conversely undergo MET after treatment of cells with an Smo antagonist, cyclopamine, to shut down Hh signaling and revert these cells to a less myofibroblastic and more quiescent phenotype.[46]

More recent data have confirmed the same finding in immature ductular cells using a model of biliary atresia and fibrosis.[90,91] The aggregate data from these studies suggested that activating Hh signaling in immature ductular cells (including adult liver-derived, small, immature, cholangiocytes) promotes EMT and represses MET. Consequently, in this model, immature ductular cells acquire a more mesenchymal phenotype capable of augmenting Hh ligand production and promoting fibrogenic repair.

Fibrogenesis and Fibrogenic Repair

Myofibroblasts are the main source of fibrosis in chronic liver injury. They are also involved in stromal remodeling, are major producers of matrix proteins, and are actively involved in matrix degradation. Therefore, they have a vital role in wound healing and repair.[92] The major source of these cells is the Hh-ligand mediated conversion of Q-HSC to MF-HSC during tissue/wound repair. Additional sources of myofibroblasts include bone marrow–derived monocytes, bone marrow–derived fibrocytes, and the EMT conversion of immature ductular cells to a more mesenchymal phenotype.[92] Bone marrow–derived monocytes/fibrocytes are recruited after the Hh ligand promotes the release of MCP-1, a known chemokine for these cells, from immature ductular cells.[65] Monocytes are also converted to fibrocytes after Hh ligands promote NKTs to upregulate Th2 cells that release profibrogenic cytokines, such as IL-13.[93] Alternate activation of Q-HSC conversion to MF-HSC has also been described. For example, leptin-activating leptin receptors (ObRb) activate downstream kinases, PI3K/Akt and JAK2/STAT3, which subsequently promote Hh signaling by stimulating HSC production of the Hh ligand.[94]

It has long been established that completely dead hepatocytes promote liver fibrosis by increasing fibrogenic activity in HSCs that have phagocytosed apoptotic hepatocytes.[68] Yet, more recent data have shown that dying epithelial cells can generate Hh ligands that promote the Q-HSC to MF-HSC conversion, progenitor growth, and inflammation/immune cell recruitment to liver parenchyma.[47,81,95] Another study showed that the way hepatocytes die (either via apoptosis, necrosis, necroptosis, autophagy, or other death mechanisms) may differently signal fibrogenic repair. In this study, diabetic db/db mice were fed MCD diets to induce NASH and liver fibrosis and then were treated with a pan-caspase inhibitor, VX-166, or vehicle. Treatment with VX-166 inhibited the activation of caspase-3 in the final apoptotic pathway and reduced the hepatic accumulation of cells expressing the myofibroblastic marker, alpha-SMA,[96] suggesting that apoptosis, in and of itself, is a robust signal for fibrogenic repair.

Multiple studies have supported the concept that the Hh ligand plays a major role in the hepatic accumulation of myofibroblasts. After partial hepatectomy in mice, myofibroblastic accumulation paralleled Hh signaling activation and was silenced on inhibition of Hh signaling.[79] A similar finding was seen after bile duct ligation and hepatic injury in rats, with upregulation of Hh signaling and the concurrent accumulation of collagen matrix and myofibroblastic cells.[84] In human patients, Hh-responsive proteins are positively correlated with the degree of fibrosis in several chronic liver diseases, including chronic viral hepatitis.[82,83]

OPN and Fibrogenesis

OPN is a proinflammatory cytokine and integrin-associated ligand that has been described in wound healing.[97–99] It is a Hh-target gene that is actively involved in fibrogenesis. In the liver, it is synthesized by fibroblasts, endothelial cells, and macrophages. It is upregulated in cirrhosis secondary to chronic hepatitis B infection and in obesity.[100–104] The authors' group recently reported that OPN may be an important glycoprotein in hepatic fibrosis. In this experiment, we fed an MCD diet to WT mice, Ptc ± mice (ie, mice that were overly responsive to the Hh ligand), and OPN −/− mice. It was found that although Ptc ± mice had increased liver fibrosis and overactivation of Hh compared with controls, OPN −/− mice had significantly reduced fibrosis (vs WT) despite similarly detected indices consistent with a similar degree of Hh pathway activation. At the cellular level, the incubation of HSCs with OPN increased the expression of fibrosis-associated markers, such as alpha-SMA and collagen. Treating HSCs with Hh agonists/antagonists similarly increased/decreased OPN expression. Increased serum OPN levels have also been associated with increased Gli2 expression in human models of NASH. In addition, OPN has been upregulated in other forms of human liver injury, including alcoholic and primary biliary cirrhosis.[105]

The Role of the Extracellular Matrix

Little is known about the 3-dimensional organization of the extracellular matrix during tissue repair. Recently, Hoehme and colleagues[106] developed a model (using immunostaining, fluorescent reporter mice, confocal microscopy, and computer modeling) that introduced the concept of hepatic sinusoidal alignment (HSA). In this study, mice underwent acute CCl4-induced liver damage. Mathematical modeling was performed, supporting a process of induced transient loss of polarity and enhanced migration in newly formed hepatocytes, allowing rapid cellular transit and alignment along hepatic sinusoids (ie, HSA). In their model, if HSA did not occur properly, normal hepatic microarchitecture and proper regeneration were not achieved. Thus, their findings suggest that if the correct cell-cell matrix interactions are not formed and the proper matrix 3-dimensional structure via cell polarization is not achieved, scar formation rather than liver regeneration will occur. The exact mechanisms by which HSA is regulated are unknown but several mediators have been proposed: (1) hepatocyte growth factor, (2) tumor necrosis factor alpha, (3) IL-6, (4) vascular endothelial growth factor (VEGF), (5) nitrous oxide, (6) Wnt ligand, and (7) Hh ligand.[107,108]

Vascular Remodeling

In addition to inflammation and fibrosis, cirrhosis is also often characterized by changes in hepatic sinusoidal architecture and perihepatic vascular remodeling.[92] Hh ligands have been shown to exert proangiogenic effects during embryogenesis and in adult wound healing.[109,110] Both Hh ligand and platelet-derived growth factor BB (which activates Hh signaling in liver progenitors and other Hh-responsive cells[43]) have been implicated in hepatic vascular remodeling.[84,111,112] Sinusoidal endothelial cells also respond to paracrine and endocrine Hh ligands to undergo phenotypic changes characteristic of that which happens during cirrhosis-related vascular remodeling.[43] Once activated, HSCs may also contribute to vascular revision by secreting angiogenic factors, notably angiopoietin 1.[113] In addition, myofibroblasts are known to produce several growth factors, including VEGF, that contribute to vascular repair in liver injury.[114]

NASH PROGRESSION: REPAIR GONE AWRY

It has not been well established why some hepatocytes and progenitors are successful in tissue repair and regeneration, whereas others undergo mis-repair with progression to cirrhosis. The level of Hh activation seems to be proportional to the severity and duration of liver injury in both rodents and humans.[49,115] In addition, the level of activation of Hh-responsive cells is directly related to Hh ligand production in both a time-dependent and concentration-dependent manner.[47] Taken together, this suggests that the degree and duration of Hh activation may play a role in whether injured hepatocytes regenerate normally or whether they form scar tissue in response to Hh overstimulation, which results in disorganized tissue repair that ultimately leads to cirrhosis.

Liver Fibrosis and the Stellate Cell

The transition of Q-HSC after Hh activation to myelofibroblastic hepatic stellate cells (MF-HSC) is important in liver repair and regeneration. Still, excess accumulation of MF-HSC out of proportion to hepatocyte regeneration is a key component to liver fibrosis and NASH progression. In vitro, HSCs require continued stimulation by Hh ligands to maintain their fibroblastic phenotype.[111] Variations in whether tissue regenerates or fibroses during liver injury likely reflects differences in the following: (1) local cytokine/growth factors, (2) the dose and duration of Hh ligand exposure, (3) the balance between Hh-responsive/unresponsive cell types, and (4) the presence/absence of poorly understood factors that contribute to fibrogenic repair mechanisms.[95]

Cirrhosis

In both hepatitis B and C infections and in NASH, the expression of Hh-responsive genes significantly correlates with the degree of fibrosis.[82,83,103] Ballooning degeneration, the presence of Mallory-Denk bodies (histologic findings characteristic of steatohepatitis), and hepatocyte apoptosis all independently predict the severity of liver fibrosis in NASH and indicate a greater risk for disease progression.[68,116,117] Early stages of NASH fibrosis are characterized by the deposition of fibrous matrix around hepatocytes and along sinusoids.[118] As the disease progresses, fibrosis involves the periportal area and involves bridging fibrosis between vascular structures. As more bridges form, hepatic architecture is further distorted because continued attempts at hepatocellular regeneration and contraction of fibrotic scars. When these changes diffusely involve the biopsy, the histopathologic diagnosis is classified as cirrhosis. Cirrhosis is, in fact, the result of suboptimal liver repair secondary to continued activation of Hh signaling that contributes to dysregulated fibrogenesis, inflammation, and vascular remodeling (ie, liver repair gone awry).

Dysregulation of Hh Signaling in HCC

It has been well established that cirrhosis predisposes to HCC. Multiple studies have suggested that the underlying mechanism progression to cancer may be related to Hh signaling.[7,37,82] Hh pathway activation has been detected in many forms of carcinoma, including cancer of the liver, colon, and pancreas.[119–122] Mechanisms for upregulation of Hh signaling include (1) upregulation of the Hh ligand, (2) activating mutations in Smo or the Gli family members, or (3) epigenetic silencing of Hhip via hypermethylation.[33,123–125] In the liver, enhanced Hh signaling has been described in both HCC and in cholangiocarcinoma,[122,126] with hypermethylation of Hhip described in as many as two-thirds of HCC.[127]

The development of various forms of liver carcinoma can be attributed, in part, to the enhanced survival of HSC, cholangiocytes, and epithelial progenitors by

Hh.[45,48,128] The growth and maintenance of HSCs, especially in states of MF-HSC excess as is seen in liver cirrhosis, play a large part in the development of HCC. After the activation of Hh signaling by dying hepatocytes, MF-HSCs are maintained by antiapoptotic mechanisms that appropriately wane after Hh pathway deactivation.[48] It is still unclear how Hh inhibits apoptosis in HSCs, but the mechanism may be similar to what has been reported in cholangiocarcinoma.

In cholangiocytes, apoptosis is normally triggered by the activation of death receptors, DR4 and DR5, and inhibited by Mcl-1, an antiapoptotic Bcl-2 family member.[129–131] Hh-responsive genes regulate the transcription of both apoptotic and antiapoptotic genes in these cells. For example, Gli3 has been shown to bind to the DR4 promoter to inhibit the transcription of the death receptor and protect the cell from apoptosis.[129] Likewise, Gli-family transcription factors have been shown to repress the transcription of miR29b, a factor in cholangiocarcinoma cells that represses the transcription of Mcl-1. Thus, Gli inhibition of this repressor of antiapoptosis promotes survival in the cell. Both mechanisms upregulated by Hh overactivation contribute to the development of cholangiocarcinoma.

After tissue injury, resident liver progenitor cells are instrumental in liver repair but can also contribute to carcinogenesis.[45,49,81] Multiple studies have established the role of Hh signaling in the growth and maintenance of this progenitor population.[49,81,109] One primary example of the interaction between progenitor growth and Hh signal activation is the hepatoblastoma, a common hepatic tumor in children derived from a pluripotent stem cell. Hh activity has been known to be upregulated in this tumor. In addition, the treatment of the hepatoblastoma cells in vitro with cyclopamine, a direct Smo inhibitor, prevented cell proliferation and induced cell death and apoptosis.[132] The same study also reported that the mechanism of action for Hh pathway overactivation may be hypermethylation of Hhip.[132] Progenitor cells have also been implicated in the development of HCC. In vitro studies using established HCC cells lines (including HepG2 and Hep3B cells) show that these cells are Hh responsive (via pharmacologic manipulation) and suggest that even mature malignant hepatocytes, which are normally Hh unresponsive, may maintain Hh sensitivity after arising from liver progenitors.[122]

Another recent work demonstrated that the extracellular matrix remodeling and EMT may also play a role in hepatocarcinogenesis and metastasis. Evidence suggests that EMT may correlate with tumor aggressiveness and metastasis in HCC.[133,134] As previously established, Hh signaling promotes EMT during adult liver repair and regeneration, inducing ductular progenitors and Q-HSC to convert into myofibroblasts that promote fibrosis. During hepatocarcinogenesis, genetic events that influence the migratory potential of these progenitors may occur. In fact, one recent article showed that the oncogene chromodomain helicase/ATPase DNA-binding protein 1-like gene (CDH1L) common in HCC, promotes the activation of Cdc42 and Rho kinases to induce EMT by modulating the assembly of the actin cytoskeleton, promotes filopodia formation and adherens junction disruption, and enhances cell migration.[135] Thus, liver progenitors or malignant hepatocytes become mobilized, permitting easy entry into the adjacent sinusoids and vasculature resulting in locoregional disease and distant metastasis.

FUTURE DIRECTIONS

Hh pathway overactivation has proven to be consistently present in NASH progression to liver cirrhosis and HCC. Recent articles suggest that there may be a role for Hh pharmacologic antagonists in the regression of liver fibrosis and primary liver cancer.[136] Novel drug therapy that inhibits Hh-responsive transcription factors, such as the Gli family, has also shown a possible therapeutic benefit in the cellular and animal models.[137,138] Future research will focus on continuing to search for new therapeutic and lifestyle interventions to prevent or slow the progression of NASH. Defining mechanisms of disease progression in NASH will continue to be a research priority as prevalence of disease burden increases.

REFERENCES

1. Boppidi H, Daram SR. Nonalcoholic fatty liver disease: hepatic manifestation of obesity and the metabolic syndrome. Postgrad Med 2008;120:E01–7.
2. Clark JM. The epidemiology of nonalcoholic fatty liver disease in adults. J Clin Gastroenterol 2006;40(Suppl 1):S5–10.
3. NIH Publication No. 07–4921The National Digestive Diseases Information Clearinghouse Web site, National Institute of Diabetes and Digestive and Kidney Diseases. National Institutes of Health; 2006. Available at: http://digestive.niddk.nih.gov/ddiseases/pubs/nash/. Accessed January 8, 2012.
4. Farrell GC, Larter CZ. Nonalcoholic fatty liver disease: from steatosis to cirrhosis. Hepatology 2006;43:S99–112.
5. Browning JD, Szczepaniak LS, Dobbins R, et al. Prevalence of hepatic steatosis in an urban population in the United States: impact of ethnicity. Hepatology 2004;40:1387–95.
6. Rahbari NN, Mehrabi A, Mollberg NM, et al. Hepatocellular carcinoma: current management and perspectives for the future. Ann Surg 2011;253:453–69.
7. Luedde T, Schwabe RF. NF-κB in the liver–linking injury, fibrosis and hepatocellular carcinoma. Nat Rev Gastroenterol Hepatol 2011;8:108–18.
8. McCullough AJ. Update on nonalcoholic fatty liver disease. J Clin Gastroenterol 2002;34(3):255–65.
9. Day C. Pathogenesis of steatohepatitis. Best practice and research. Clin Gastroenterol 2002;16(7):663.
10. Abdelmalek MF, Suzuki A, Guy C, et al. Increased fructose consumption is associated with fibrosis severity in patients with nonalcoholic fatty liver disease. Hepatology 2010;51(6):1961–71.
11. de Almeida IT, Cortez-Pinto H, Fidalgo G, et al. Plasma total and free fatty acids composition in human non-alcoholic steatohepatitis. Clin Nutr 2002;21(3):219–23.
12. Cassader M, Gambino R, Musso G, et al. Postprandial triglyceride-rich lipoprotein metabolism and insulin sensitivity in nonalcoholic steatohepatitis patients. Lipids 2001;36(10):1117–24.
13. Marchesini G, Forlani G. NASH: from liver diseases to metabolic disorders and back to clinical hepatology. Hepatology 2002;35(2):497–9.
14. Bernard S, Touzet S, Personne I, et al. Association between microsomal triglyceride transfer protein gene polymorphism and the biological features of liver steatosis in patients with type II diabetes. Diabetologia 2000;43(8):995–9.
15. Charlton M, Sreekumar R, Rasmussen D, et al. Apolipoprotein synthesis in nonalcoholic steatohepatitis. Hepatology 2002;35(4):898–904.
16. Tessari P, Coracina A, Cosma A. Hepatic lipid metabolism and non-alcoholic fatty liver disease. Nutr Metab Cardiovasc Dis 2009;19(4):291–302.
17. Yang S, Zhu H, Li Y, et al. Mitochondrial adaptations to obesity-related oxidant stress. Arch Biochem Biophys 2000;378:259–68.

18. Mantena SK, Vaughn DP, Andringa KK, et al. High fat diet induces dysregulation of hepatic oxygen gradients and mitochondrial function in vivo. Biochem J 2009; 417:183–93.

19. Collison KS, Saleh SM, Bakheet RH, et al. Diabetes of the liver: the link between nonalcoholic fatty liver disease and HFCS-55. Obesity (Silver Spring) 2009; 17(11):2003–13.

20. Allard JP. Other disease associations with non-alcoholic fatty liver disease (NAFLD). Best Pract Res Clin Gastroenterol 2001;16(5):783–95.

21. D'Albuquerque LA, Gonzalez AM, Wahle RC, et al. Liver transplantation for subacute hepatocellular failure due to massive steatohepatitis after bariatric surgery. Liver Transpl 2009;14(6):881–5.

22. Maruhama Y, Ohneda A, Tadaki H, et al. Hepatic steatosis and the elevated plasma insulin level in patients with endogenous hypertriglyceridemia. Metabolism 1975;24(5):653–64.

23. Sen D, Dagdelen S, Erbas T. Hepatosteatosis with hypobetalipoproteinemia. J Natl Med Assoc 2007;99(3):284–6.

24. Cave M, Deacluc I, Mendez C, et al. Nonalcoholic fatty liver disease: predisposing factors and the role of nutrition. J Nutr Biochem 2007;18(3): 184–95.

25. Hooper JE, Scott MP. Communicating with hedgehogs. Nat Rev Mol Cell Biol 2005;6:306–17.

26. Schuske K, Hooper JE, Scoot MP. Patched overexpression causes loss of wingless expression in Drosophila embryos. Dec Biol 1994;164:300–11.

27. Varjosalo M, Li SP, Taipale J. Divergence of hedgehog signal transduction mechanism between drosophila and mammals. Dev Cell 2006;10:177–86.

28. Sicklick JK, Li YX, Choi SS, et al. Role for hedgehog signaling in hepatic stellate cell activation and viability. Lab Invest 2005;85(11):1368–80.

29. Ramalho-Santos M, Melton DA, McMahon AP. Hedgehog signals regulate multiple aspects of gastrointestinal development. Dev 2000;127(12):2763–72.

30. Hebrok M, Kim SK, St Jacques B, et al. Regulation of pancreas development by hedgehog signaling. Dev 2000;127(22):4905–13.

31. Van den Brink GR. Hedgehog signaling in development and homeostasis of the gastrointestinal tract. Physiol Rev 2007;87:1343–75.

32. Pan Y, Wang C, Wang B. Phosphorylation of Gli2 by protein kinase A is required for Gli2 processing and degradation and the Sonic Hedgehog-regulated mouse development. Dev Biol 2009;326(1):177–89.

33. Lauth M, Toftgard R. Non-canonical activation of GLI transcription factors: implications for targeted anti-cancer therapy. Cell Cycle 2007;6:2458–63.

34. Riobo NA, Lu K, Ai X, et al. Phosphoinositide 3-kinase and Akt are essential for Sonic Hedgehog signaling. Proc Natl Acad Sci U S A 2006;103:4505–10.

35. Dennler S, Andre J, Alexaki I, et al. Induction of sonic hedgehog mediators by transforming growth factor-beta: Smad3-dependent activation of Gli2 and Gli1 expression in vitro and in vivo. Cancer Res 2007;67(14):6981–6.

36. Lauth M, Toftgård R. Non-canonical activation of Gli1 transcription factors: implications for targeted anti-cancer therapy. Cell Cycle 2007;6:2458–63.

37. Tada M, Kanai F, Tanaka Y, et al. Down-regulation of hedgehog-interacting protein through genetic and epigenetic alterations in human hepatocellular carcinoma. Clin Cancer Res 2008;14:3768–76.

38. Wolf I, Bose S, Desmond JC, et al. Unmasking of epigenetically silenced genes reveals DNA promoter methylation and reduced expression of PTCH in breast cancer. Breast Cancer Res Treat 2007;105:139–55.

39. Yakushiji N, Suzuki M, Satoh A, et al. Correlation between Shh expression and DNA methylation status of the limb-specific Shh enhancer region during limb regeneration in amphibians. Dev Biol 2007;312:171–82.

40. Zavros Y, Waghray M, Tessier A, et al. Reduced pepsin A processing of Sonic Hedgehog in parietal cells precedes gastric atrophy and transformation. J Biol Chem 2007;292:33265–74.

41. Porter JA, von Kessler DP, Ekker SC, et al. The product of hedgehog autoproteolytic cleavage active in local and long-range signaling. Nature 1995;374: 363–6.

42. Porter JA, Young KE, Beachy PA. Cholesterol modification of hedgehog signaling proteins in animal development. Science 1996;274:255–9.

43. Witek RP, Yang L, Liu R, et al. Liver cell-derived microparticles activate hedgehog signaling and alter gene expression in hepatic endothelial cells. Gastroenterology 2009;136:320–30.

44. Burke R, Nellen D, Bellotto M, et al. Dispatched, a novel sterol-sensing domain protein dedicated to the release of cholesterol-modified hedgehog from signaling cells. Cell 1999;99:803–15.

45. Sicklick JK, Li YX, Jayaraman A, et al. Hedgehog signaling maintains resident hepatic progenitors throughout life. Am J Physiol Gastrointest Liver Physiol 2006;290:G859–70.

46. Choi SS, Omenetti A, Witek RP, et al. Hedgehog pathway activation and epithelial-to-mesenchymal transitions during myofibroblastic transformation of rat hepatic cells in culture and cirrhosis. Am J Physiol Gastrointest Liver Physiol 2009;297:G1093–106.

47. Rangwala F, Guy CD, Lu J, et al. Increased production of Sonic Hedgehog by ballooned hepatocytes. J Pathol 2011;224:401–10.

48. Omenetti A, Yang L, Li YX, et al. Hedgehog-mediated mesenchymal-epithelial interactions modulate hepatic response to bile duct ligation. Lab Invest 2007; 87:499–514.

49. Fleig SV, Choi SS, Yang L, et al. Hepatic accumulation of hedgehog-reactive progenitors increases with severity of fatty liver damage in mice. Lab Invest 2007;87:1227–39.

50. Syn WK, Witek RP, Curbishley SM, et al. Role for hedgehog pathway in regulating growth and function of invariant NKT cells. Eur J Immunol 2009;39: 1879–92.

51. Jung Y, McCall SJ, Li YX, et al. Bile ductules and stromal cells express hedgehog ligands and/or hedgehog target genes in primary biliary cirrhosis. Hepatology 2007;45:1091–6.

52. Jung Y, Brown KD, Witek RP, et al. Accumulation of hedgehog-responsive progenitors parallels alcoholic liver disease severity in mice and humans. Gastroenterol 2008;134(5):1532–43.

53. Sanchez A, Fabregat I. Growth factor- and cytokine-driven pathways governing liver stemness and differentiation. World J Gastroenterol 2010;16(41):5148–61.

54. Omenetti A, Choi S, Michelotti G, et al. Hedgehog signaling in the liver. Journal of Hepatology 2011;54:366–73.

55. Kurosaka K, Takahashi M, Watanabe N, et al. Silent cleanup of very early apoptotic cells by macrophages. J Immunol 2003;171:4672–9.

56. Majno G, Joris I. Apoptosis, oncosis, and necrosis. An overview of cell death. Am J Pathol 1995;146:3–15.

57. Faubion WA, Gores GJ. Apoptosis: the nexus of liver injury and fibrosis. Hepatology 2004;39:273–8.

58. Elmore S. Apoptosis: a review of programmed cell death. Toxicol Pathol 2007; 35:495–516.

59. Canbay A, Friedman S, Gores GJ, et al. Apoptosis: the nexus of liver injury and fibrosis. Hepatology 2004;39:273–8.

60. Canbay A, Higuchi H, Bronk SF, et al. Fas enhances fibrogenesis in the bile duct ligated mouse: a link between apoptosis and fibrosis. Gastroenterology 2002; 123:1323–30.

61. Faouzi S, Burckhardt BE, Hanson JC, et al. Anti-Fas induces hepatic chemo-kines and promotes inflammation by an NF-kappa B-independent, caspase-3-dependent pathway. J Biol Chem 2001;276:49077–82.

62. Rogers HW, Callery MP, Deck B, et al. Listeria monoctogenes induces apoptosis of infected hepatocytes. J Immunol 1996;156:679–84.

63. Ebe Y, Hasegawa G, Takatsuka H, et al. The role of Kupffer cells and regulation of neutrophil migration into the liver by macrophage inflammatory protein-2 in primary listeriosis in mice. Pathol Int 1999;49:519–32.

64. Lawson JA, Fisher MA, Simmons CA, et al. Parenchymal cell apoptosis as a signal for sinusoidal sequestration and transendothelial migration of neutro-phils in murine models of endotoxin and Fas-antibody-induced liver injury. Hepatology 1998;28:761–7.

65. Omenetti A, Syn WK, Jung Y, et al. Repair-related activation of hedgehog signaling promotes cholangiocyte chemokine production. Hepatology 2009; 50:518–27.

66. Kiener PA, Davis PM, Rankin BM, et al. Human monocytic cells contain high levels of intracellular Fas ligand: rapid release following cellular activation. J Immunol 1997;159:1594–8.

67. Geske FJ, Monks J, Lehman L, et al. The role of the macrophage in apoptosis: hunter, gatherer, and regulator. Int J Hematol 2002;76:16–26.

68. Feldstein AE, Canbay A, Angulo P, et al. Hepatocyte apoptosis and fas expres-sion are prominent features of human nonalcoholic steatohepatitis. Gastroenter-ology 2003;125:437–43.

69. Wiechowska A, Zein NN, Yerian LM, et al. In vivo assessment of liver cell apoptosis as a novel biomarker of disease severity in nonalcoholic fatty liver disease. Hepatology 2006;44:27–33.

70. Puri P, Mirshahi F, Cheung O, et al. Activation and dysregulation of the unfolded protein response in non-alcoholic fatty liver disease. Gastroenterology 2008; 134:568–76.

71. Ghosh S, May MJ, Kopp EB. NF-kappaB and Rel proteins: evolutionarily conserved mediators of immune responses. Annu Rev Immunol 1998l;16:225–60.

72. Ribeiro PS, Cortez-Pinto H, Sola S, et al. Hepatocyte apoptosis, expression of death receptors, and activation of NF-kappaB in the liver of nonalcoholic and alcoholic steatohepatitis patients. Am J Gastroenterol 2004;99:1708–17.

73. De Lalla C, Galli G, Aldrighetti L, et al. Production of profibrotic cytokines by invariant NKT cells characterizes cirrhosis progression in chronic viral hepatitis. J Immunol 2004;173:1417–25.

74. Geissmann F, Cameron TO, Sidobre S, et al. Intravascular immune surveillance by CXCR6+ NKT cells patrolling liver sinusoids. PLoS Biol 2005;3:e113.

75. Kronenberg M. Toward an understanding of NKT: progress and paradoxes. Annu Rev Immunol 2005;23:877–900.

76. Mallevaey T, Fontaine J, Breuil L, et al. Invariant and noninvariant natural killer T cells exert opposite regulatory functions on the immune response during murine schistosomiasis. Infect Immun 2007;75:2171–80.

77. Syn WK, Oo YH, Pereira TA, et al. Accumulation of natural killer T cells in progressive nonalcoholic fatty liver disease. Hepatology 2010;51:1998–2007.
78. Tajiri K, Shimizu Y, Tsuneyama K, et al. Role of liver-infiltrating CD3+CD56+ natural killer T cells in the pathogenesis of nonalcoholic fatty liver disease. Eur J Gastroenterol Hepatol 2009;21:673–80.
79. Onchoa B, Syn WK, Delgado I, et al. Hedgehog signaling is critical for normal liver regeneration after partial hepatectomy in mice. Hepatology 2010;51:1712–23.
80. Zhang L, Theise N, Chua M, et al. The stem cell niche of human livers: symmetry between development and regeneration. Hepatology 2008;48:1598–607.
81. Jung Y, Witek RP, Syn WK, et al. Signals from dying hepatocytes trigger growth of liver progenitors. Gut 2010;59:655–65.
82. Pereira TA, Witek RP, Syn WK, et al. Viral factors induce hedgehog pathway activation in humans with viral hepatitis, cirrhosis, and hepatocellular carcinoma. Lab Invest 2010;90(12):1690–703.
83. Syn WK, Jung Y, Omenetti A, et al. Hedgehog-mediated epithelial-to-mesenchymal transition and fibrogenic repair in nonalcoholic fatty liver disease. Gastroenterology 2009;137:1478–88, e1478.
84. Omenetti A, Popov Y, Jung Y, et al. The hedgehog pathway regulates remodeling responses to biliary obstruction in rats. Gut 2008;57:1275–82.
85. Harmon EB, Ko AH, Kim SK. Hedgehog signaling in gastrointestinal development and disease. Curr Mol Med 2002;2:67–82.
86. Oue T, Yoneda A, Uehara S, et al. Increased expression of the hedgehog signaling pathway in pediatric solid malignancies. J Pediatr Surg 2010;45: 387–92.
87. Acloque H, Adams MS, Fishwick K, et al. Epithelial-mesenchymal transitions: the importance of changing cell state in development and disease. J Clin Invest 2009;119:1438–49.
88. Choi SS, Witek RP, Yang L, et al. Activation of Rac1 promotes hedgehog-mediated acquisition of the myofibroblastic phenotype in rat and human hepatic stellate cells. Hepatology 2010;52:278–90.
89. Baum B, Settleman J, Quinlan MP. Transitions between epithelial and mesenchymal states in development and disease. Semin Cell Dev Biol 2008;19: 294–308.
90. Omenetti A, Porrello A, Jung Y, et al. Hedgehog signaling regulates epithelial-mesenchymal transition during biliary fibrosis in rodents and humans. J Clin Invest 2008;118:3331–42.
91. Omenetti A, Bass LM, Anders RA, et al. Hedgehog activity, epithelial-mesenchymal transitions, and biliary dysmorphogenesis in biliary atresia. Hepatology 2011;53(4):1246–58.
92. Friedman SL. Mechanisms of hepatic fibrogenesis. Gastroenterology 2008;134: 1655–69.
93. Shao DO, Suresh R, Vakil V, et al. Pivotal advance: th-1 cytokines inhibit, and Th-2 cytokines promote fibrocyte differentiation. J Leukoc Biol 2008;83:1323–33.
94. Choi SS, Syn WK, Karaca GF, et al. Leptin promotes the myofibroblastic phenotype in hepatic stellate cells by activating the hedgehog pathway. J of Biol Chem 2010;285(47):36551–60.
95. Choi SS, Omenetti A, Syn WK, et al. The role of hedgehog signaling in fibrogenic liver repair. Int J Biochem Cell Biol 2011;43:238–44.
96. Witek RP, Stone WC, Karaca G, et al. Pan-caspase inhibitor VX-166 reduces fibrosis in an animal model of nonalcoholic steatohepatitis. Hepatology 2009; 50:1421–30.

97. Miyazaki K, Okada Y, Yamanaka O, et al. Corneal wound healing in an osteopontin-deficient mouse. Invest Ophthalmol Vis Sci 2008;49:1367–76.
98. Fujita N, Fujita S, Okada Y, et al. Impaired angiogenic response in the corneas of mice lacking osteopontin. Invest Ophthalmol Vis Sci 2010;51:790–4.
99. Lorena D, Darby IA, Gadeau AP, et al. Osteopontin expression in normal and fibrotic liver. Altered liver healing in osteopontin-deficient mice. J Hepatol 2006;44:383–90.
100. Gómez-Ambrosi J, Catalán V, Ramírez B, et al. Plasma osteopontin levels and expression in adipose tissue are increased in obesity. J Clin Endocrinol Metab 2007;92(9):3719–27.
101. Bertola A, Deveaux V, Bonnafous S, et al. Elevated expression of osteopontin may be related to tissue macrophage accumulation and liver steatosis in morbid obesity. Diabetes 2009;58(1):125–33.
102. Lee SH, Seo GS, Park YN, et al. Effects and regulation of osteopontin in rate hepatic stellate cells. Biochem Pharmacol 2004;68(12):2367–78.
103. Zhao L, Li T, Wang Y, et al. Elevated plasma osteopontin level is predictive of cirrhosis in patients with hepatitis B infection. Int J Clin Pract 2008;62(7): 1056–62.
104. Syn WK, Choi SS, Liaskou E, et al. Osteopontin is induced by hedgehog pathway activation and promotes fibrosis in nonalcoholic steatohepatitis. Hepatology 2011;53(1):106–15.
105. Harada K, Ozaki S, Sudo Y, et al. Osteopontin is involved in the formation of epithelioid granuloma and bile duct injury in primary biliary cirrhosis. Pathol Int 2003;53(1):8–17.
106. Hoehme S, Brulport M, Bauer A, et al. Prediction and validation of cell alignment along microvessels as order principle to restore tissue architecture in liver regeneration. Proc Natl Acad Sci U S A 2010;107:10371–6.
107. Rojkind M, Philips G, Diehl AM. Microarchitecture of the liver: a jigsaw puzzle. J of Hepatology 2011;54:187–8.
108. Rudolph KL, Trautwein C, Kubicks S, et al. Differential regulation of extracellular matrix synthesis during liver regeneration after partial hepatectomy in rates. Hepatology 1999;30:1159–66.
109. Asai J, Takenaka H, Kusano KF, et al. Topical Sonic Hedgehog gene therapy accelerates wound healing in diabetes by enhancing endothelial progenitor cell-mediated microvascular remodeling. Circulation 2006;113:2413–24.
110. Vokes SA, Yatskievch TA, Heimark RL, et al. Hedgehog signaling is essential for endothelial tube formation during vasculogenesis. Development 2004;131: 4371–80.
111. Yang L, Wang Y, Mao H, et al. Sonic Hedgehog is an autocrine viability factor for myofibroblastic hepatic stellate cells. J Hepatol 2008;48:98–106.
112. Semela D, Das A, Langer D, et al. Platelet-derived growth factor signaling through ephrin-b2 regulates hepatic vascular structure and function. Gastroenterology 2008;135:671–9.
113. Taura K, De Minicis S, Seki E, et al. Hepatic stellate cells secrete angiopoietin 1 that induces aniogenesis in liver fibrosis. Gastroenterology 2008;135:1729–38.
114. Ankoma-Sey V, Wang Y, Dai Z, et al. Hypoxic stimulation of vascular endothelial growth factor expression in activated rat hepatic stellate cells. Hepatology 2000; 31:141–8.
115. Guy CD, Suzuki A, Zdanowicz M, et al. Hedgehog pathway activation parallels histologic severity in nonalcoholic fatty liver disease. Hepatology 2011. DOI: 10.1002/hep.25559.

116. Gramlich T, Kleiner DE, McCullough AJ, et al. Pathologic features associated with fibrosis in non-alcoholic fatty liver disease. Hum Pathol 2004;35:196–9.

117. Matteoni CA, Younossi ZM, Gramlich T, et al. Non-alcoholic fatty liver disease: a spectrum of clinical and pathological severity. Gastroenterology 1999;116:1413–9.

118. Brunt EM. Histopathology of non-alcoholic fatty liver disease. Clin Liver Dis 2009;13:533–44.

119. Oniscu A, James RM, Morris RG, et al. Expression of Sonic Hedgehog pathway genes is altered in colonic neoplasia. J Pathol 2004;203(4):909–17.

120. Berman DM, Karhadkar SS, Maitra A, et al. Widespread requirement for hedgehog ligand stimulation in growth of digestive tract tumours. Nature 2003;425:846–51.

121. Thayer SP, Di Magliano MP, Heiser PW, et al. Hedgehog is an early and late mediator of pancreatic cancer tumorigenesis. Nature 2003;425:851–6.

122. Sicklick JK, Li YX, Jayaraman A, et al. Dysregulation of the hedgehog pathway in human hepatocarcinogenesis. Carcinogenesis 2006;27:748–57.

123. Toftgard R. Hedgehog signaling in cancer. Cell Mol Life Sci 2000;57:1720–31.

124. Saldanha G. The hedgehog signaling pathway in cancer. J Pathol 2001;193:427–32.

125. Freeman JW, Wang Y, Glies FJ. Epigenetic modulation and attacking the hedgehog pathway: potentially synergistic therapeutic targets for pancreatic cancer. Cancer Biol Ther 2009;8:1227–39.

126. Beachy PA, Karhadkar SS, Berman DM. Tissue repair and stem cell renewal in carcinogenesis. Nature 2004;432:324–31.

127. Villanueva A, Newell P, Chiang DY, et al. Genomics and signaling pathways in hepatocellular carcinoma. Semin Liver Dis 2007;27:55–76.

128. Harnois DM, Que FG, Celli A, et al. Bcl-2 is overexpressed and alters the threshold for apoptosis in a cholangiocarcinoma cell line. Hepatology 1997;26:884–90.

129. Kurita S, Mott JL, Almada LL, et al. GLI3-dependent repression of DR4 mediates hedgehog antagonism of TRAIL-induced apoptosis. Oncogene 2010;29:4848–58.

130. Takeda K, Kojima Y, Ikejima K, et al. Death receptor 5 mediated-apoptosis contributes to cholestatic liver disease. Proc Natl Acad Sci U S A 2008;105:10895–900.

131. Mott JL, Kobayashi S, Bronk SF, et al. Mir-29 regulated Mcl-1 protein expression and apoptosis. Oncogene 2007;26:6133–40.

132. Eichenmuller M, Gruner I, Hagl B, et al. Blocking the hedgehog pathway inhibits hepatoblastoma growth. Hepatology 2009;49:482–90.

133. Yang MH, Chen CL, Chau GY, et al. Comprehensive analysis of the independent effect of twist and snail in promoting metastasis of hepatocellular carcinoma. Hepatology 2009;50(5):1464–74.

134. Matsuo N, Shiraha H, Fujikawa T, et al. Twist expression promotes migration and invasion in hepatocellular carcinoma. BMC Cancer 2009;9:240.

135. Chen L, Chan TH, Yuan YF, et al. CHD1L promotes hepatocellular carcinoma progression and metastasis in mice and is associated with these processes in human patients. J Clin Invest 2010;120(4):1178–91.

136. Philips GM, Chan IS, Swiderska M, et al. Hedgehog signaling antagonist promotes regression of both liver fibrosis and hepatocellular carcinoma in a murine model of primary liver cancer. PLoS ONE 2011;6(9):e23943.

137. Xu Y, Chenna V, Hu C, et al. A polymeric nanoparticle encapsulated hedgehog pathway inhibitor HPI-1 inhibits systemic metastases in an orthotopic model of human hepatocellular carcinoma. Clin Cancer Res 2012;18(5):1291–302.

138. Kim Y, Yoon JW, Xiao X, et al. Selective down-regulation of glioma-associated oncogene 2 inhibits the proliferation of hepatocellular carcinoma cells. Cancer Res 2007;67(8):3583–93.

Can Nash Be Diagnosed, Graded, and Staged Noninvasively?

Garfield A. Grandison, MD, Paul Angulo, MD*

KEYWORDS

- Nonalcoholic fatty liver disease • Nonalcoholic steatohepatitis • Noninvasive
- CK-18 • Fibrosis • Fibrogenesis • FibroScan • Magnetic resonance elastography

KEY POINTS

- Nonalcolohic fatty liver disease (NAFLD) affects a substantial proportion of the population worldwide.
- Few subjects who have the condition develop liver-related complications.
- Predicting which patients will develop progressive disease is problematic.
- Currently, there is no available noninvasive test demonstrated to be simple, reproducible, and valid for disease staging in patients with NAFLD.
- Liver biopsy remains the gold standard investigation to distinguish between patients with nonalcoholic steatohepatitis and those without NASH or bland steatosis, and to determine disease prognosis based on fibrosis staging.

BACKGROUND

Nonalcoholic fatty liver disease (NAFLD) refers to the accumulation of fat (mainly triglycerides) in hepatocytes that results from insulin resistance.[1] It is the most common chronic liver disease in the Western world. Data from the National Health and Nutrition Survey from 1988 to 2008 show that the prevalence of common chronic liver diseases has remained stable, except for NAFLD, as defined by idiopathic elevation of liver enzymes, which is increasing.[2] The clinicopathologic spectrum of NAFLD ranges from bland hepatic steatosis, which is clinically associated with a similar long-term prognosis as compared to the general population, to nonalcoholic steatohepatitis (NASH), which when associated with increased liver fibrosis, may progress to cirrhosis and liver failure. As such, distinguishing between steatosis and NASH with and without fibrosis has important implications for management and patient counseling.

Conflict of interest: Nothing to disclose.
Division of Digestive Diseases & Nutrition, Department of Medicine, University of Kentucky Medical Center, 800 Rose Street, Lexington, KY 40536-0298, USA
* Corresponding author.
E-mail address: paul.angulo@uky.edu

NAFLD is a growing medical problem affecting any age range, with a reported prevalence of 9.6% among adolescents and preadolescents,[3] and 34% among patients aged 30 to 65 years.[4] However, the reported prevalence of this condition varies based on the study population studied and the diagnostic modality used. For instance, liver biopsies performed in otherwise healthy potential liver donors revealed a prevalence of NAFLD (as defined by greater than 30% of steatosis) of 20%,[5] whereas studies using magnetic resonance (MR) spectroscopy reported a prevalence of 34% in the general adult population in Dallas County, Texas.[4] Studies using idiopathic elevations in liver enzymes as a case definition yielded a wide NAFLD prevalence of 8% to 75%.[6–8]

ROLE OF LIVER BIOPSY IN DIAGNOSING AND STAGING NASH

The decision regarding whom and when to biopsy should take into account whether the information likely to be obtained would affect the patient's care. There are 2 general indications for performing a liver biopsy in patients with suspected NAFLD:

1. Confirming the diagnosis and staging the disease. Establishing the diagnosis, activity grade (degree of inflammation and cellular injury), and stage of fibrosis of NAFLD requires a liver biopsy. Given the high prevalence in the population, the invasive nature of liver biopsy, and the paucity of effective therapies, however, there is often an understandable reluctance to perform liver biopsy for the sole purpose of confirming the diagnosis. In most patients, therefore, the diagnosis of suspected NAFLD is based on clinical and laboratory data, and imaging studies with appropriate exclusion of other liver conditions.

2. Determining prognosis based on the severity of liver injury and fibrosis. Liver biopsy is the only investigation that can reliably distinguish between simple steatosis and NASH, as well as stage the extent of fibrosis. The prognosis of NAFLD depends on the severity of liver injury and fibrosis. While most studies suggest that there is no increased mortality associated with simple steatosis, mortality in patients with NASH, particularly those with advanced fibrosis and cirrhosis, is increased as compared to the general population of same age and gender. For instance, the prevalence of cirrhosis and liver-related mortality within the first 15 years of diagnosis is less than 1% (0.7% and 0.9% respectively) in patients with bland steatosis, but this increases to 11% and 7%, respectively, in patients with NASH.[9] The highest liver-related morbidity and mortality are undoubtedly among those patients with advanced (stage 3 or 4) fibrosis.[10–12] Additionally, the identification of early cirrhosis or advanced (bridging) fibrosis may alter management, as such patients should undergo upper endoscopies to screen for gastroesophageal varices and periodic liver ultrasound imaging to screen for hepatocellular carcinoma.[12]

Hence, in the absence of clinical and radiologic features of cirrhosis, liver biopsy remains the only way to reliably assess prognosis.

Over the last decade, several simple laboratory tests (in isolation or in combination), serum markers of fibrogenesis, and imaging studies (ultrasound, computed tomography [CT] and magnetic resonance imaging [MRI]) have been evaluated as a substitute for liver biopsy in NAFLD and had showed varying degrees of accuracy when compared to liver biopsy. There remains a high degree of interest in accurately diagnosing, grading, and staging this disease noninvasively.

LIMITATIONS OF LIVER BIOPSY

The potential drawbacks of liver biopsy are well documented. These include sampling error, problems with inadequate biopsy size, variability in pathologist interpretation, cost, and associated morbidity. Liver biopsy samples only a tiny portion, roughly 1/50,000, of the liver. Sampling error is therefore common, with 30% to 40% of patients with NAFLD undergoing simultaneous paired liver biopsies having samples differing by at least 1 fibrosis stage.[13,14] Larger biopsy samples are more likely to demonstrate features supporting a diagnosis of NASH with or without fibrosis, so that small samples are more likely to be associated with diagnostic and fibrosis staging error.[13,15] Interobserver variability between pathologists is reasonable, although imperfect, adding to the inaccuracy of liver biopsy for staging purposes.[16,17] Finally, percutaneous liver biopsy is associated with serious complications in 0.3% of cases and a mortality rate of 0.01%.[18] These drawbacks of liver biopsy have led investigators to examine noninvasive markers as potential substitutes in the diagnosis and staging of NASH. The ideal noninvasive test should be simple, reproducible, readily available, less expensive than liver biopsy, able to predict the full spectrum of liver fibrosis stages, and reflect changes occurring with therapy.

NONINVASIVE DIAGNOSIS OF STEATOSIS
Clinical and Laboratory Variables

Three indices have been developed to make the diagnosis of steatosis; among them is the (SteatoTest, Biopredictive, Paris, France), a proprietary formula based on the 6 variables of FibroTest-ActiTest plus body mass index (BMI), cholesterol, triglycerides, and glucose adjusted by age and gender.[19] A cutoff of 0.3 has a sensitivity of 85% or more to make the diagnosis of fatty liver, and a cutoff of 0.7 has a specificity of 80%.[19] The fatty liver index or FLI includes 4 variables: BMI, waist circumference, triglycerides, and gamma-glutamyl-transpeptidase.[20] The FLI can be calculated using a specific formula, with a score of 30 or less having a sensitivity of 87%, and a score of 60 or more having a specificity of 86% in the diagnosis of steatosis.[20] The lipid accumulation product or LAP includes 3 variables, waist circumference, triglycerides, and gender.[21] These indices,[19–21] however, did not gain much popularity, and they may not add much to the information provided by clinical, laboratory, and imaging studies done routinely in patients with suspected NAFLD.

Routine Imaging Studies

Ultrasound, CT, and MRI can noninvasively diagnose fatty infiltration of the liver. Hepatic steatosis causes increased echogenicity on ultrasound, which can be contrasted against the lower echogenicity of the spleen or renal cortex. A similar pattern can be seen with diffuse fibrosis, giving rise to the term fatty–fibrotic pattern, although the echo shadows tend to be coarser in the presence of pure fibrosis. The sensitivity and specificity of ultrasound for detecting hepatic steatosis vary from 60% to 94% and 88% to 95%, respectively. However, the sensitivity of ultrasound decreases with lower degrees of fatty infiltration. In the presence of a 30% or more fatty infiltration, the sensitivity of ultrasound is 80% compared with a sensitivity of 55% when hepatic fat content is 10% to 19%.[22] In addition, the ultrasonography sensitivity for the detection of steatosis progressively decreases as the BMI increases, with a sensitivity as low as 39% in individuals with BMI of 35 kg/m^2 or higher.[23]

On noncontrast CT scan images, hepatic steatosis has a low attenuation and appears darker than the spleen. On contrast images, CT scan has a sensitivity between 50% and 86%, and a specificity between 75% and 87%, for the detection of steatosis.[24,25] Confounding factors such as iron, copper, or fibrous tissue that alter the Hounsfield density of liver and differences in the rate of contrast injection and the timing of the scanning may explain the differences in diagnostic accuracy reported in several studies.[24,25] Overall, the sensitivity of CT at detecting greater than 33% hepatic steatosis is up to 93%, with a positive predictive value of 76%.[26] CT, however, is not sensitive in detecting mild-to-moderate amounts of steatosis between 5% and 30%.[26]

Both MRI and MR spectroscopy are reliable at detecting steatosis and offer good correlation with hepatic fat volume.[27,28] The sensitivity and specificity of MRI in detecting as low as 5% of liver fat infiltration are 85% and 100%, respectively.[27] MR spectroscopy studies of the human liver have been based on the ubiquitous protons hydrogen (1H) and phosphorus (31P). More than 5% of hepatic fat content on MR spectroscopy indicates presence of steatosis.[28] However, the routine application of MR images is limited by cost and lack of availability.

NONINVASIVE DIAGNOSIS OF NASH
Clinical and Laboratory Variables

Different indices have been proposed to make the diagnosis of NASH (**Table 1**). One is the (NashTest, Biopredictive, Paris, France), another proprietary formula that includes 12 variables and has an area under the receiving characteristic (AUROC) curve of 0.79.[29] The indices described by Palekar and colleagues[30] as well as Shimada and colleagues[31] include a combination of several other variables described in **Table 1**. The reported accuracy of these indices seems fair, but the number of patients included was too small; further validation of these indices is needed.

Markers of Apoptosis

Cytokeratin (CK) 18 is the serum marker of NASH that has been most validated to date. CK-18 fragments come from apoptosis of hepatocytes accomplished by the enzyme caspase 3. CK-18 fragments can be investigated in liver tissue using immunostaining, or measured in plasma using monoclonal antibodies. In the original study,[32] 39 patients with suspected NAFLD were included, and CK-18 plasma values of 395 U/L had a petty high AUROC curve, with high sensitivity and specificity to differentiate between patients with NASH and non-NASH. Subsequently, a validation study was conducted and included 139 patients with liver biopsy-confirmed NAFLD.[33] The AUROC curve was estimated to be 0.83, with 95% confidence interval (CI) 0.75, 0.91. A CK-18 plasma value of about 250 U/L had a sensitivity of 0.75 (95% CI 0.64, 0.83) and a specificity of 0.81 (95% CI 0.61, 0.93). Subsequently, several validation studies have been reported in the literature, essentially reproducing the same results.[34] These studies suggest plasma CK-18 levels may help in distinguishing between simple steatosis from NASH, but the test is far from perfect, as indicated by the lower 95% CI in the 0.60 range for sensitivity and specificity. CK-18 assay is commercially available, but still has not been cleared by the US Food and Drug Administration (FDA).

Routine Imaging Studies

Ultrasonography, CT, and MRI are insensitive in differentiating hepatic steatosis from NASH, and they cannot be used to stage fibrosis.[26] A small CT study of patients with NAFLD found that patients with NASH had increased liver size and increased caudate lobe-to-right lobe size ratio, compared with those with steatosis only.[35] The caudate-to-right lobe size ratio was statistically higher in NASH (mean, 0.43; range, 0.31–0.55) compared with steatosis only (mean, 0.36; range, 0.22–0.47). However, measurements showed considerable overlap in both categories, and it is unlikely that these measurements will be useful in individual patients.

Table 1
Noninvasive diagnosis of NASH

Author (Reference)	n	Variables	Cutoff	AUROC	Sensitivity (%)	Specificity (%)	PPV (%)	NPV (%)
Poynard et al,[29] 2006	257, 97, 383	Age, gender, BMI, triglycerides, cholesterol, α-2 macroglobulin, gamma-GT, AST, ALT, haptoglobin, apolipoprotein A1, total bilirubin	ND	0.79	29	98	91	71
Palekar et al,[30] 2006	80	Age $\geq$50, female, AST $\geq$45, AST/ALT ratio $\geq$0.8, BMI $\geq$30, hyaluronate $\geq$55 μg/L	$\geq$3	0.76	74	66	68	71
Shimada et al,[31] 2007	85	Serum adiponectin, type 4 collagen 7s level, HOMA-IR	ND	ND	94	74	94	74
Wieckowska et al,[32] 2006; Feldstein et al,[33] 2009	39 139 (validation)	CK-18 levels	395 U/L 250 U/L	0.93 0.83 (95% CI 0.75, 0.91)	87 0.75 (95% CI 0.64, 0.83)	100 0.81 (95% CI 0.61, 0.93)	100	86

Abbreviations: GT, glutamyl-transpeptidase; HOMA-IR, homeostatic model assessment of insulin resistance; ND, not determined.

SERUM MARKERS OF LIVER FIBROSIS IN NASH
Simple Laboratory Tests as Markers of Fibrosis

Several routinely available laboratory tests may be abnormal in the presence of advanced liver fibrosis. Markers of synthetic liver function, such as albumin and prothrombin time, often are altered in the presence of cirrhosis, and serum bilirubin may be increased. A low platelet count in the setting of advanced liver disease is usually a sign of hypersplenism related to portal hypertension. Advanced liver disease is often already clinically and radiologically apparent, however, when these laboratory markers become abnormal. Although these markers may assist in assessing the severity of liver decompensation, they are insensitive at detecting noncirrhotic stages of fibrosis.

Elevated aminotransferase levels are found to correlate with liver fibrosis in certain select populations of patients with NAFLD, such as those undergoing bariatric surgery. Among nearly 1000 morbidly obese subjects undergoing gastrointestinal bariatric surgery in Italy, an aspartate aminotransferase (AST) or alanine aminotransferase (ALT) level greater than twice the upper limit of normal had a positive predictive value (PPV) for bridging fibrosis of 21% and a negative predictive value (NPV) of 93%.[36] An AST greater than twice the upper limit of normal was also independently predictive of portal or bridging fibrosis in an Asian study of 60 patients with NAFLD.[37] However, other studies have failed to confirm an association between simple aminotransferase levels and degree of fibrosis in patients who have NAFLD.[38–40] Furthermore, studies comparing NAFLD patients who had persistently raised ALT levels to those who had persistently normal ALT levels found no difference in the prevalence of advanced fibrosis and cirrhosis between the groups.[41,42] The association between aminotransferase levels and fibrosis is therefore inconsistent and cannot sufficiently predict fibrosis stage in individual patients.

An association between an elevated AST/ALT ratio and fibrosis has been recognized in chronic liver disease and may reflect impaired AST clearance by sinusoidal cells in the liver.[43] Among patients who have NAFLD without advanced fibrosis, the AST/ALT ratio is typically less than 1, but it tends to reverse as the degree of fibrosis progresses to bridging fibrosis or cirrhosis.[38] Consequently, several studies have found an association between advanced fibrosis on liver biopsy and an AST/ALT ratio greater than 1. An early study examining 144 biopsy-proven cases of NASH found that an AST/ALT ratio greater than 1 remained significantly associated with advanced fibrosis when adjusted for multiple factors.[38] In that study, 82% of patients who had an AST/ALT ratio of up to 1 did not have fibrosis, whereas 47% of those who had a ratio of greater than 1 had advanced fibrosis, indicating that the AST/ALT ratio may be a useful clinical adjunct for predicting or excluding advanced fibrosis in patients with NASH.

Another simple laboratory ratio proposed as a marker of advanced fibrosis is the AST-to-platelet ratio index (APRI). While it was initially proposed as a marker of fibrosis in chronic hepatitis C infection, it has been validated in a cohort of 111 patients with NAFLD.[44] In this validation study, the APRI was significantly higher in NASH patients who had advanced fibrosis. The AUROC curve for APRI was 0.85, with an optimal cutoff of 0.98, leading to a sensitivity and specificity of 75% and 86% respectively. The PPV of the APRI was only 54%, with an NPV of 93%. The APRI may therefore be useful in identifying patients unlikely to have advanced fibrosis, but it is less useful in predicting the presence of advanced fibrosis.

Serum ferritin levels are elevated in 21%–40% of patients who have NAFLD and seem related to insulin resistance and liver damage rather than reflecting increased hepatic iron stores.[40,45] Ferritin has been found to be a significant independent predictor of severe fibrosis in 167 subjects from Italy who had NAFLD.[45] While several studies have failed to replicate this, a large recent study showed a serum ferritin greater than 1.5 times the upper limit of normal was associated with advanced hepatic fibrosis in a cohort of 628 patients with NAFLD.[46] The precise role for isolated serum ferritin as a marker of fibrosis is unsettled. Manousou and colleagues[47] have recently found that serum ferritin, particularly when combined with an elevated BMI, is a useful discriminant marker for liver fibrosis in patients with NAFLD. This combination may therefore prompt consideration for obtaining a liver biopsy to identify the severity of fibrosis.

Combination of Simple Laboratory Tests and Clinical Markers of Liver Fibrosis

In an effort to increase the predictive value of simple laboratory parameters for liver fibrosis, several routine laboratory tests and clinical variables have been identified by multivariate analyses (**Table 2**).[38,48–53] As insulin resistance is a driving force behind the pathogenesis of NAFLD and is associated with stimulating fibrogenic hepatic growth factors,[54,55] it is not surprising that the clinical correlates of insulin resistance (obesity, diabetes mellitus, and hypertriglyceridemia) are associated with advanced fibrosis and are incorporated with laboratory tests to predict liver fibrosis.

Among 144 patients who had biopsy-proven NASH, 66% of those who had the combination of obesity, diabetes, age 45 years or older, and AST/ALT ratio greater than 1 had bridging fibrosis or cirrhosis.[38] In contrast, no patient had severe fibrosis in the absence of all of these factors. Another study found age, 50 years or older; BMI, 28 kg/m^2 or more; elevated serum triglyceride; and ALT levels to be associated with septal fibrosis in a French cohort of 93 obese subjects who had abnormal liver tests.[48] No patient in this cohort who had 1 or fewer of these factors had septal fibrosis, whereas all 4patients who had all 4 factors had septal fibrosis. Additionally, an Australian algorithm involving systemic hypertension, elevated ALT, and insulin resistance (the HAIR index) provided a sensitivity and specificity of 80% and 89%, respectively, for detecting NASH in patients who were morbidly obese and undergoing bariatric surgery.[49] In the presence of at least 2 of the 3 predictive factors in the HAIR index, 10 of 11 patients who had bridging fibrosis or cirrhosis were identified. Unfortunately, the specificity of the index was low, with at least 11 other patients who had a score of 2 or more not having advanced fibrosis.

Based on the results of multivariate analyses, several predictive scores for advanced fibrosis have been developed based on a combination of clinical and routine laboratory parameters. They are the NAFLD fibrosis score, the BARD score, and the FIB-4 index (**Table 3**).[51,52,56] These score formulas may assist in deciding when to perform a liver biopsy for fibrosis staging.

In an international multicenter study, data from 733 patients with liver-biopsy confirmed NAFLD were analyzed to create (480 patients) and validate (253 patients) a scoring system to distinguish between patients with (stage 3–4) and without (stage 0–2) advanced fibrosis using Kleiner's staging system.[51] The NAFLD fibrosis score was created using 6 variables (as shown in **Table 3**) that were significant by multivariate analysis. The AUROC curve for this score to distinguish between patients with and without advanced fibrosis was high, 0.88 in the estimation group and 0.82 in the validation group. A score less than −1.455 had high accuracy in excluding advanced fibrosis, with an NPV of 93% and 88% in the training and validation groups, respectively; a score greater than 0.676 had high accuracy in identifying advanced fibrosis, with a PPV of 90% and 92% respectively, in the training and validation groups. If the NAFLD fibrosis score had been applied to the entire cohort of 733 patients, the

Table 2
Routine laboratory and clinical predictors of advanced fibrosis in patients with NAFLD

Author (Reference)	n	Patient Population	Risk Factors	Odds Ratio (95% Confidence Interval)
Angulo et al,[38] 1999	144	NASH	Age ≥45 years	5.6 (1.5, 21.7)
			Obesity (BMI >30 kg/m²)	4.3 (1.4, 13.8)
			Diabetes	3.5 (1.2, 9.8)
			AST/ALT ratio >1	4.3 (1.5, 12)
Marceau et al,[50] 1999	551	Bariatric surgery patients	Age	NA
			Diabetes	NA
			Waist-hip ratio	NA
			BMI	NA
Ratziu et al,[48] 2000	93	Overweight, raised liver tests	Age ≥50 years	14.1 (3.7, 54.0)
			BMI ≥28 kg/m²	5.7 (1.6, 20.0)
			Triglyceride ≥1.7 mmol/L	5.0 (1.4, 17.0)
			ALT ≥2 × ULN	4.6 (1.3, 16.0)
Dixon et al,[49] 2001	105	Bariatric surgery patients	Hypertension	NA
			ALT >40 IU/L	NA
			Insulin resistance >5.0	NA
Angulo et al,[51] 2007	733	NAFLD	Age (years)	1.04 (1.01, 1.07)
			BMI (kg/m²)	1.10 (1.04, 1.16)
			IFG/diabetes	3.12 (1.77, 5.51)
			AST/ALT ratio	2.70 (1.33, 5.62)
			Platelet count ($\times 10^9$/L)	0.987 (0.98, 0.99)
			Albumin (g/dl)	0.51 (0.25, 1.05)
Harrison et al,[52] 2008	827	NAFLD	BMI ≥28 kg/m²	2.4 (1.2, 4.8)
			AST/ALT ratio ≥0.8	9.3 (6.3, 13.6)
			Diabetes	4.0 (2.8, 5.7)
Miyaaaki et al,[53] 2008	182	NAFLD	Female gender	4.60 (1.68, 12.58)
			Age ≥60	2.73 (1.23, 5.94)
			Type 2 diabetes	3.43 (1.48, 7.92)
			Hypertension	3.58 (1.63, 7.90)

Abbreviations: IFG, impaired fasting glucose; NA, not available; ULN, upper limit of normal.

liver biopsy for fibrosis staging could have been avoided in 75% of patients, that is those correctly identified, and performed in only the 25% of patients that fell in the indeterminate range. Several studies of independent populations have since reproduced the high accuracy of the NAFLD fibrosis score in distinguishing patients with and without advanced fibrosis.[57,58] In 1 study of 162 Chinese patients (low prevalence of NAFLD), the lower cutoff value of less than −1.455 was used and had an NPV of 91% in excluding advanced fibrosis.[57] Qureshi and colleagues[58] evaluated 331 morbidly obese patients with NAFLD who underwent bariatric surgery. The lower cut-off score had an NPV of 98% in ruling out advanced fibrosis.

The BARD score was created by analyzing data collected retrospectively from a group of 827 patients with NAFLD.[52] Based on logistic regression analysis, the BARD score included a combination of 3 variables as shown in **Table 3**. The authors reported a score of 2 to 4 associated with an odds ratio of 17 for advanced fibrosis. It was unclear how many of the 827 retrospectively evaluated patients had the 3 variables measured and were in fact included in the evaluation of the BARD score. A BARD score of 2 to 4 was associated with an odds ratio for advanced fibrosis of 17.3 and an NPV of 97%. The BARD score has since been cross-validated in a Polish population of 104 patients with NAFLD.[59]

Table 3
Predicting advanced fibrosis (F3-4) using routine clinical and laboratory variables in NAFLD

Predictive Score (Reference)	n	Variables/Formula	AUROC (95% Confidence Interval)	Cut-off Points	PPV (%)	NPV (%)
NAFLD fibrosis score[51]	733	$-1.675 + 0.037$ × age (years) + 0.094 × BMI (kg/m^2) + 1.13 × IFG/diabetes (yes = 1, no = 0) + 0.99 × AST/ALT ratio -0.013 × platelet count (×10^9/L) -0.66 × albumin (g/dL)	0.88 (0.85, 0.92)	≤-1.455 ≥ 0.676	56 90	93 85
BARD score[52]	827	BMI $\geq 28 = 1$ AST/ALT ratio $\geq 0.8 = 2$ Diabetes = 1 Score ≥ 2, odds ratio for advanced fibrosis = 17	ND	<2 points		96
FIB-4 score[56]	541	Age (years) × AST (U/L)/ platelet (×10^9/L) × ALT [U/L]	0.80 (0.76, 0.85)	≤ 1.30 ≥ 2.67	43 80	90 83

Abbreviation: IFG, impaired fasting glucose.

The FIB-4 score was originally developed to predict advanced fibrosis in patients coinfected with hepatitis C and human immunodeficiency virus (HIV). The FIB-4 score was validated in a database of 541 patients with NAFLD to calculate jackknife-validated AUROC curves based on 4 variables as shown in **Table 3**.[56] The AUROC curve was 0.80. Using a cut-off of :2.67 or more, the PPV was 80%, and the NPV was 83%. Using a cut-off of less than 1.30, the PPV was only 43%, but the NPV was 90%, suggesting that the FIB-4 index may be useful in excluding patients without advanced fibrosis. The FIB-4 score has been cross-validated in a cohort of 576 Japanese patients with biopsy-proven NAFLD.[60] However, the cut-off values used were different from those used in the original study.[56] In the Japanese study,[60] the lower cut-off used was less than 1.45. Only 6 of 308 patients with a FIB-4 index below the proposed low cut-off point (<1.45) were understaged, giving a high NPV of 98%. Twenty-eight of 59 patients with an FIB-4 index above the high cut-off point (>3.25) were overstaged, giving a low PPV of 53%. Using these cutoffs, 91% of the 395 patients with FIB-4 values outside 1.45 to 3.25 would be correctly classified, and implementation of the FIB4 index in the Japanese population would be estimated to avoid 58% of liver biopsies.

The performance characteristics of the NAFLD fibrosis score, BARD score, FIB-4 score, as well as the AST/ALT ratio and APRI have been compared in an independent population of 145 patients from the United Kingdom.[61] The AUROC curve to distinguish between patients with and without advanced (stage 3–4) fibrosis was 0.86 for the FIB-4 score, 0.83 for the AST/ALT ratio, 0.81 for the NAFLD fibrosis score, 0.77 for the BARD score, and 0.67 for the AST-to-platelet ratio index. The AST/ALT ratio, BARD score, FIB-4 score, and NAFLD fibrosis score all had NPVs between 92% and 95% to rule out advanced fibrosis, although PPVs were modest for all of them. Based on the data from this study, in order to exclude advanced fibrosis, liver biopsy could potentially be avoided in 69% of patients with AST/ALT ratio, 62% with FIB-4,

52% with NAFLD fibrosis score, and 38% with BARD. Adams and colleagues[62] calculated simple (APRI, BARD) and complex (eg, hepascore, Fibrotest, FIB-4) fibrosis models in 242 NAFLD subjects undergoing liver biopsy. For significant fibrosis (stage 2–4), noninvasive fibrosis models had modest accuracy (AUC 0.707–0.743) with BARD being least accurate (area under the curve [AUC] 0.609, $P<.05$ vs others). For advanced fibrosis (stage 3–4), complex models were more accurate than BARD (AUC 0.802–0.858 vs 0.701, $P<.05$). The authors concluded that in NAFLD subjects, noninvasive models have modest accuracy for determining significant fibrosis and have predictive values less than 90% in the majority of subjects, although complex models are more accurate than simple models across a range of fibrosis.

While these combined clinical and laboratory models may be useful in identifying a subset of patients at low risk of advanced liver fibrosis who may therefore avoid liver biopsy for staging and prognostic purposes, they are not sufficiently accurate to replace liver biopsy for staging and prognostic purposes if advanced fibrosis is suspected.

Direct Serum Markers of Liver Fibrogenesis

Hepatic fibrosis is a dynamic process involving complex interaction between enzymes involved in extracellular matrix synthesis and degradation. Extracellular matrix components, such as hyaluronic acid, collagen components (type 4 collagen and type 3 procollagen peptide, P3NP), and laminin circulate in the serum at low levels and have been examined in isolation and in combination as potential predictors of liver fibrosis in NAFLD (**Table 4**).[30,63–69]

Serum levels of hyaluronic acid are increased in liver fibrosis reflecting increased deposition of collagen and decreased clearance by sinusoidal endothelial cells.[63] Several studies have determined that hyaluronic acid predicts bridging fibrosis or cirrhosis in patients who have NAFLD, with accuracy between 80% and 89%.[30,63,64] Hyaluronic acid, however, is less accurate for detecting lesser degrees of fibrosis, with an AUC for any degree of fibrosis varying between 0.67 and 0.73.[63,65] In addition, hyaluronic acid increases in systemic inflammatory conditions, which may produce falsely positive predictive results.

Type 4 collagen is a product of collagen degradation and a marker of fibrolysis. Serum levels of the 7S domain are increased in the presence of severe fibrosis in patients who have NAFLD. Among 112 Japanese patients who had NAFLD, a cutoff point of 5.0 ng/mL provided a PPV and an NPV of 68% and 84%, respectively, for the presence of severe fibrosis.[64] Laminin is a component of extracellular matrix cleared by hepatic endothelial cells. A small study found levels >282 ng/mL reasonably predictive for the presence of any fibrosis in 30 patients who had NAFLD.[65] Serum YKL-40 is glycoprotein secreted by several different cell types, including hepatic stellate cells. Elevated serum YKL-40 levels have been proposed as a marker of fibrosis in NAFLD,[70] based on a small study that lacked a validation group. However, other studies have failed to show an association between YKL-40 and fibrosis in NAFLD.[71]

Proprietary Predictive Panels

To increase the accuracy of noninvasive markers of liver fibrosis, multiple serum markers have been combined into mathematic models to produce predictive scores. The Fibrotest is one algorithm, consisting of a combination of age, gender, bilirubin, g-glutamyltransferase, apolipoprotein A1, haptoglobin, and a2-macroglobulin. It has been validated in a variety of chronic liver conditions and was examined in a cohort of 267 patients, 85% of whom had NAFLD.[66] A score of less than 0.3 (range 0.0–1.0) provided an NPV of 98% for the presence of bridging fibrosis or cirrhosis,

Table 4
Serum markers of fibrogenesis and clinical predictors of advanced fibrosis (F3-4) in patients with NAFLD

Author (Reference)	n	Serum Marker	AUROC	Sensitivity (%)	Specificity (%)
Suzuki et al,[63] 2005	79	Hyaluronic acid >46.1 ng/mL	0.89	85.0	79.7
Sukugaya et al,[64] 2005	112	Hyaluronic acid ≥50 ng/mL	0.80	68.8	82.8
		Type 4 collagen 7S ≥5 ng/mL	0.82	81.3	71.4
Palekar et al,[30] 2006	80	Hyaluronic acid >45.3 ng/mL	0.88	85.7	80.3
Kaneda et al,[69] 2006	148	Hyaluronic acid >42 ng/mL		100.0	89.0
Santos et al,[65,a] 2005	30	Hyaluronic acid >24.6 ng/mL	0.73	82.0	68.0
		Type 4 collagen >145 ng/mL	0.80	64.0	89.0
		Laminin >282 ng/mL	0.87	82.0	89.0
Ratziu et al,[66] 2006	267	Fibrotest 0.30	0.88	92.0	71.0
		Fibrotest 0.70	0.88	25.0	97.0
Guha et al,[67] 2008	192	ELF score = −7.412 + (ln(HA)*0.681) + (ln(P3NP)*0.775) + (ln(TIMP1)*0.494) ELF = 0.3576[b]	0.93	80	90
Nobili et al,[68] 2009	112	ELF (different cut-of values)	0.90–0.99	88–100	76–98

Abbreviations: AUROC, area under the receiver operating characteristics curve. The AUROC is used to distinguish between patients with and without advanced fibrosis; ELF, enhanced liver fibrosis panel; TIMP1, tissue inhibitor of metalloproteinase 1.

[a] Predicting the presence of fibrosis versus the absence of fibrosis.

[b] An ELF score of 0.3576 has a sensitivity of 80% in detecting advanced fibrosis and a specificity of 90% in ruling out advanced fibrosis.

whereas a score of greater than 0.7 provided a 60% PPV for bridging fibrosis or cirrhosis. However, 33% of individuals had a score between 0.3 and 0.7, indicating that the Fibrotest cannot predict severity of liver fibrosis in one-third of patients with NAFLD.

The European Liver Fibrosis Group assessed the combination of age and serum levels of hyaluronic acid, aminoterminal propeptide of type III collagen, and tissue inhibitor of matrix metalloproteinase 1 in predicting advanced fibrosis in patients who had a wide range of liver diseases.[72] The proposed algorithm had an acceptable accuracy overall, but only 61 out of the 912 patients studied had NAFLD—a number too small to derive meaningful conclusions about the NAFLD population. The same group therefore evaluated the same 3 serum markers: hyaluronic acid, aminoterminal propeptide of type III collagen, and tissue inhibitor of matrix metalloproteinase 1 (named Enhanced Liver Fibrosis panel, ELF, iQur Ltd, Southampton, United Kingdom) in predicting fibrosis in 192 patients with NAFLD.[67] An ELF score of 0.3576 had an area under the ROC curve of 0.93, and a sensitivity of 80% for detecting advanced fibrosis and a specificity of 90% in ruling out advanced fibrosis. ELF was also evaluated in 112 children with NAFLD[68]; the AUROC curve to distinguish among the stages of fibrosis varied from 0.90 to 0.99. In that study, values of ELF from 9.28 to 10.51 had a sensitivity of 88%–100% and a specificity of 76%–98% to distinguish among the stages.

IMAGING ASSESSMENT OF FIBROSIS IN NASH

Conventional ultrasound, CT, and MRI can noninvasively detect hepatic steatosis, and have a good level of accuracy in detecting cirrhosis with portal hypertension. However, they are far less reliable at detecting NASH and the associated stages of fibrosis. The radiologic features of splenomegaly, reversal of hepatic blood flow, change in caudate to right lobe ratio, and hepatic vein narrowing aid the sensitivity of detecting cirrhosis with portal hypertension, but they are less useful in earlier stages of disease. However, new imaging technologies, such as the ultrasonography-based transient elastography (FibroScan, Echosens, Paris, France) and MRI-based elastography offer promise in determining severity of liver fibrosis associated with NASH.

Ultrasound-Based Elastography (FibroScan)

Transient elastography (FibroScan) is a technique whereby shear waves, at a low frequency of 50 Hz, are created by a vibrating probe and transducer applied to the skin overlying the liver. The velocity of the propagated wave is correlated with the stiffness or elasticity of the underlying liver; simplistically, the propagated wave travels faster with increasing fibrosis. A pulse–echo ultrasound allows measurement of the wave velocity, and the results are presented as kilopascals (kPa). At least 10 validated measures must be obtained. The validity of measurement is assessed by the interquartile range and ratio of successful measurements to unsuccessful measurements, which should be over 60%.

The transient elastography technique measures the liver stiffness within a cylinder of 1 cm in width and 4 cm in length, producing an estimated sampling area that is 100 times greater than biopsy, although the portion of liver sampled is still small. The reproducibility of the technique has been evaluated in a large study including 800 examinations in 200 patients who had heterogeneous liver disease; the intraclass correlation coefficient was 0.98 by 2 operators.[73] The test is inexpensive, and the equipment has a capital cost. The threshold for detecting significant fibrosis varied from 4 to 9 kPa in 4 selected studies that have included patients with mixed causes of chronic liver disease including NAFLD.[73–76] Good diagnostic performance occurs above these critical thresholds. The AUROC curve varied from 0.74 to 0.86, with a sensitivity and specificity of the selected kPa threshold from 68% to 94% and 33 to 85%, respectively. Similar to laboratory tests, FibroScan shows better performance in detecting cirrhotic stage disease.

Few studies have evaluated the performance of FibroScan in staging fibrosis in patients with NAFLD. In the largest study on NAFLD reported to date, 274 patients with NAFLD underwent transient elastography to measure liver stiffness with liver biopsy as the gold standard; the AUROC curve was 0.84 for significant fibrosis (F$\geq$2), 0.93 for advanced fibrosis (F$\geq$3), and 0.95 for cirrhosis (F = 4).[77] A cutoff value of 7.9 kPa was accurate in identifying late-stage fibrosis with an associated sensitivity, specificity, PPV, and NPV of 91%, 75%, 52%, and 97% in identifying fibrosis stage F$\geq$3.[77] However, FibroScan failed to achieve the 10 validated measures required to assess liver stiffness in 28 of the 274 (10.2%) patients. The AUROC curve for FibroScan to distinguish between advanced (stage 3–4) and nonadvanced (stage 0–2) fibrosis nevertheless compared favorably to the AUROC curve for AST/ALT ratio, APRI, FIB-4 score, NAFLD fibrosis score, and BARD score in the 246 patients with reliable FibroScan examinations. After intention-to-treat (or to diagnose) analysis, however, a cut-off of 8.7 kPa had an NPV of 89% to exclude advanced fibrosis, which did not differ from the NPV for the other previously mentioned simple indices. Furthermore, the PPV to predict the presence of advanced fibrosis was only 48.5% with FibroScan, lower than the NAFLD fibrosis score (61.1%) and the FIB-4 score (59.1%).

Castera and colleagues[78] investigated the frequency and causes of failure and unreliable results in measuring liver stiffness by FibroScan over a 5-year period, based on more than 13,000 examinations. Failure of FibroScan occurred in 3.1% of all examinations and was independently associated at first examination with BMI greater than 30 kg/m^2; operator experience of fewer than 500 examinations; age, older than 52 years; and type 2 diabetes. Unreliable results were obtained in an additional 15.8% of cases and were independently associated with BMI greater than 30 kg/m^2, operator experience fewer than 500 examinations, age older than 52 years, female sex, hypertension, and type 2 diabetes. The authors concluded that liver stiffness measurements were uninterpretable in nearly 1 in 5 cases (19%).

Due to the poor accuracy of the standard M probe of FibroScan in detecting liver fibrosis in overweight/obese patients,[78,79] a new XL probe has been developed and recently evaluated in 2 large studies.[80,81] In a group of 274 patients with chronic liver disease of different etiology who had a BMI of 28 kg/m^2 or higher, the XL probe provided reliable measurements of liver stiffness in 73% of patients as compared to only 50% of patients with the M probe.[80] Despite the better performance of the XL probe in overweight/obese patients, the XL probe did not provide reliable measurements of liver stiffness in 27% of the patients, and thus, the XL probe was unsuccessful in 1 out 4 overweight/obese patients.[80] Further studies are needed to determine the role of the XL probe in overweight/obese patients with NAFLD.

Transient elastography has been evaluated in children with NAFLD.[82] Nobili and colleagues[82] evaluated the accuracy of the FibroScan in 52 consecutive children with biopsy-proven NAFLD and showed that cutoff values between 7 and 9 kPa predict fibrosis stages 1 or 2, and cutoff values of 9 kPa or more are associated with the presence of advanced fibrosis. These similarities in the cutoff values suggest that the diagnostic accuracy of FibroScan is independent of the patient's age.

Magnetic Resonance Elastography

In contrast to FibroScan, which estimates liver stiffness of a small fraction of the liver, magnetic resonance elastography (MRE) estimates the average degree of liver fibrosis throughout most of the liver parenchyma by assessing the propagation of mechanical waves through the tissue. First, shear waves are generated in the liver tissue by a driver (pneumatic or electromechanical) attached to the abdominal wall. Magnetic resonance images are then obtained depicting the propagated shear waves, and finally, images of the shear waves are analyzed and used to generate quantitative maps of tissue stiffness, referred to as elastograms.[83] As the entire liver can be sequenced, the area of sampling is greatly increased, and the heterogeneous distribution of fibrosis is more commonly appreciated. In a study by Huwart and colleagues,[84] MRE performed better than FibroScan and AST-to-platelet ratio index (APRI) in 141 patients with chronic liver disease of various etiologies. The AUROC curves were significantly greater for distinguishing any stage of fibrosis using MRE. The technical success rate of MRE was significantly higher than that of FibroScan (94% vs 84%). The AUROC curve of MRE (0.994 for F≥2; 0.985 for F≥3; 0.998 for F = 4) were significantly higher than those of FibroScan, APRI, and the combination of FibroScan and APRI. The study demonstrated that MRE has a higher technical success rate than FibroScan and better diagnostic accuracy than FibroScan and APRI for staging liver fibrosis. In a tertiary center in Asia, MRE was shown to increase systematically along with fibrosis stage in a cohort of 60 patients—55 with chronic hepatobiliary diseases and 5 living related liver donors.[85] With a shear stiffness cut-off of 3.05 kPa, the predicted sensitivity and specificity for differentiating liver fibrosis (F ≥2) from mild fibrosis (F1) were 89.7% and 87.1%, respectively. Impressively, MRE was able to discriminate between patients with severe fibrosis (F3) and those with liver cirrhosis (sensitivity 100%, specificity 92.2%), with a shear stiffness cut-off value of 5.32 kPa.

Rather intriguing are the recent findings showing that MRE is useful in helping to identify patients with steatohepatitis, even prior to the onset of fibrosis.[86] In this retrospective study of 58 NAFLD patients, hepatic stiffness had high accuracy in discriminating patients with NASH from those with simple steatosis (AUROC =0.93, sensitivity 94%, specificity 73% by using a threshold of 2.74 kPa). NAFLD patients with inflammation (NASH) but no fibrosis have greater liver stiffness than those with simple steatosis and lower mean stiffness than those with fibrosis.[86]

Despite these encouraging results, there are still issues of concern with MRE techniques. These include the increased acquisition time of scanning, the costs of the equipment, the expertise in analysis, and standardized thresholds of measurement. Nevertheless, it holds great promise as a noninvasive alternative to liver biopsy in staging fibrosis in NASH, but more studies are needed to determine the role of MRE to distinguish between simple steatosis and NASH.

Other Imaging Modalities

Other modalities that are still being evaluated and may be more widely utilized in the future include acoustic radiation force impulse imaging to assess liver fibrosis,[87,88] optical analysis of CT-generated images to predict fibrosis stage and distribution,[89] and diffusion-weighted MRI for the diagnosis of liver fibrosis and cirrhosis.[90] These imaging modalities need to be evaluated in patients with NAFLD to determine their accuracy in diagnosing and staging this disease.

SUMMARY

NAFLD affects a substantial proportion of the population worldwide. Few subjects who have the condition develop liver-related complications. Predicting which patients will develop progressive disease is problematic. Currently, there is no available noninvasive test demonstrated to be simple, reproducible, and valid for disease staging in patients with NAFLD. Liver biopsy remains the gold standard investigation to distinguish between patients with NASH and those without NASH or bland steatosis, and to determine disease prognosis based on fibrosis staging. Measuring plasma levels of cytokeratin-18 is the most promising but imperfect noninvasive test to distinguish NASH from bland steatosis. Several simple scoring formulas that combine routinely measured clinical and laboratory variables as well as some proprietary serum panels are currently available to predict severity of liver fibrosis. Both the proprietary panels and simple indices seem equally accurate. Liver stiffness measured by ultrasound-based elastography or FibroScan may detect occult cirrhosis, but the technique is often unreliable in patients with NAFLD and obesity. In addition, FibroScan is not superior to simple indices in predicting severity of liver fibrosis in NAFLD. Magnetic resonance-based elastography or MRE has a high sensitivity and specificity for diagnosing and staging liver fibrosis in patients with chronic liver disease of various etiologies. However, further work is needed to determine the accuracy of MRE in diagnosing and staging liver fibrosis in patients with NAFLD and in distinguishing between patients with bland steatosis and those with NASH. MRE is not yet widely available, and cost and expertise in interpretation are likely to be limiting factors to its use. In the future, indirect and direct serum markers of NASH and liver fibrosis alone or in combination with imaging modalities will likely be increasingly translated into simple diagnostic kits and algorithms for viable, noninvasive alternatives to liver biopsy.

REFERENCES

1. Cusi K. Role of obesity and lipotoxicity in the development of nonalcoholic steatohepatitis: pathophysiology and clinical implications. Gastroenterology 2012;142:711–25.
2. Younossi ZM, Stepanova M, Afendy M, et al. Changes in the prevalence of the most common causes of chronic liver diseases in the United States from 1988 to 2008. Clin Gastroenterol Hepatol 2011;9(6):524–530.e1 [quiz: e60].
3. Schwimmer JB, Deutsch R, Kahen T, et al. Prevalence of fatty liver in children and adolescents. Pediatrics 2006;118(4):1388–93.
4. Browning JD, Szczepaniak LS, Dobbins R, et al. Prevalence of hepatic steatosis in an urban population in the United States: impact of ethnicity. Hepatology 2004; 40(6):1387–95.
5. Marcos A, Fisher RA, Ham JM, et al. Selection and outcome of living donors for adult-to-adult right lobe transplantation. Transplantation 2000;69(11):2410–5.
6. Patt CH, Yoo HY, Dibadj K, et al. Prevalence of transaminase abnormalities in asymptomatic, healthy subjects participating in an executive health-screening program. Dig Dis Sci 2003;48(4):797–801.
7. Clark JM, Brancati FL, Diehl AM. The prevalence and etiology of elevated aminotransferase levels in the United States. Am J Gastroenterol 2003;98(5):960–7.
8. Ioannou GN, Boyko EJ, Lee SP. The prevalence and predictors of elevated serum aminotransferase activity in the United States in 1999–2002. Am J Gastroenterol 2006;101(1):76–82.
9. Angulo P. Long-term mortality in nonalcoholic fatty liver disease: is liver histology of any prognostic significance? Hepatology 2010;51(2):373–5.
10. Younossi ZM, Stepanova M, Rafiq N, et al. Pathologic criteria for nonalcoholic steatohepatitis: interprotocol agreement and ability to predict liver-related mortality. Hepatology 2011;53:1874–82.
11. Sanyal AJ, Banas C, Sargeant C, et al. Similarities and differences in outcomes of cirrhosis due to nonalcoholic steatohepatitis and hepatitis C. Hepatology 2006;43: 682–9.
12. Bhala N, Angulo P, van der Poorten D, et al. The natural history of nonalcoholic fatty liver disease with advanced fibrosis or cirrhosis: an international collaborative study. Hepatology 2011;54:1208–16.
13. Ratziu V, Charlotte F, Heurtier A, et al. Sampling variability of liver biopsy in nonalcoholic fatty liver disease. Gastroenterology 2005;128(7):1898–906.
14. Janiec DJ, Jacobson ER, Freeth A, et al. Histologic variation of grade and stage of non-alcoholic fatty liver disease in liver biopsies. Obes Surg 2005;15(4): 497–501.
15. Vuppalanchi R, Unalp A, Van Natta ML, et al. Effects of liver biopsy sample length and number of readings on sampling variability in nonalcoholic fatty liver disease. Clin Gastroenterol Hepatol 2009;7:481–6.
16. Kleiner DE, Brunt EM, Van Natta M, et al. Design and validation of a histological scoring system for nonalcoholic fatty liver disease. Hepatology 2005;41(6):1313–21.
17. Fukusato T, Fukushima J, Shiga J, et al. Liver Disease Working Group-Kanto. Interobserver variation in the histopathological assessment of nonalcoholic steatohepatitis. Hepatol Res 2005;33:122–7.
18. Piccinino F, Sagnelli E, Pasquale G, et al. Complications following percutaneous liver biopsy. A multicentre retrospective study on 68,276 biopsies. J Hepatol 1986;2(2):165–73.
19. Poynard T, Ratziu V, Naveau S, et al. The diagnostic value of biomarkers (SteatoTest) for the prediction of liver steatosis. Comp Hepatol 2005;4:10.

20. Bedogni G, Bellentani S, Miglioli L, et al. The Fatty Liver Index: a simple and accurate predictor of hepatic steatosis in the general population. BMC Gastroenterol 2006;6:33.
21. Bedogni G, Kahn HS, Bellentani S, et al. A simple index of lipid overaccumulation is a good marker of liver steatosis. BMC Gastroenterol 2010;10:98.
22. Ryan CK, Johnson LA, Germin BI, et al. One hundred consecutive hepatic biopsies in the workup of living donors for right lobe liver transplantation. Liver Transpl 2002;8:1114–22.
23. Mottin CC, Moretto M, Padoin AV, et al. The role of ultrasound in the diagnosis of hepatic steatosis in morbidly obese patients. Obes Surg 2004;14:635–7.
24. Jacobs JE, Birnbaum BA, Shapiro MA, et al. Diagnostic criteria for fatty infiltration of the liver on contrast-enhanced helical CT. AJR Am J Roentgenol 1998;171: 659–64.
25. Johnston RJ, Stamm ER, Lewin JM, et al. Diagnosis of fatty infiltration of the liver on contrast enhanced CT: limitations of liver-minus-spleen attenuation difference measurements. Abdom Imaging 1998;23:409–15.
26. Saadeh S, Younossi ZM, Remer EM, et al. The utility of radiological imaging in nonalcoholic fatty liver disease. Gastroenterology 2002;123:745–50.
27. Mazhar SM, Shiehmorteza M, Sirlin CB. Noninvasive assessment of hepatic steatosis. Clin Gastroenterol Hepatol 2009;7:135–40.
28. Reeder SB, Cruite I, Hamilton G, et al. Quantitative assessment of liver fat with magnetic resonance imaging and spectroscopy. J Magn Reson Imaging 2011; 34:729–49.
29. Poynard T, Ratziu V, Charlotte F, et al. LIDO Study Group; CYTOL study group. Diagnostic value of biochemical markers (NashTest) for the prediction of nonalcoholic steatohepatitis in patients with non-alcoholic fatty liver disease. BMC Gastroenterol 2006;6:34.
30. Palekar NA, Naus R, Larson SP, et al. Clinical model for distinguishing nonalcoholic steatohepatitis from simple steatosis in patients with nonalcoholic fatty liver disease. Liver Int 2006;26:151–6.
31. Shimada M, Kawahara H, Ozaki K, et al. Usefulness of a combined evaluation of the serum adiponectin level, HOMA-IR, and serum type IV collagen 7S level to predict the early stage of nonalcoholic steatohepatitis. Am J Gastroenterol 2007;102:1931–8.
32. Wieckowska A, Zein NN, Yerian LM, et al. In vivo assessment of liver cell apoptosis as a novel biomarker of disease severity in nonalcoholic fatty liver disease. Hepatology 2006;44(1):27–33.
33. Feldstein AE, Wieckowska A, Lopez AR, et al. Cytokeratin-18 fragment levels as noninvasive biomarkers for nonalcoholic steatohepatitis: a multicenter validation study. Hepatology 2009;50(4):1072–8.
34. Alkhouri N, Carter-Kent C, Feldstein AE. Apoptosis in nonalcoholic fatty liver disease: diagnostic and therapeutic implications. Expert Rev Gastroenterol Hepatol 2011;5:201–12.
35. Oliva MR, Mortele KJ, Segatto E, et al. Computed tomography features of nonalcoholic steatohepatitis with histopathologic correlation. J Comput Assist Tomogr 2006;30:37–43.
36. Papadia FS, Marinari GM, Camerini G, et al. Liver damage in severely obese patients: a clinical-biochemical-morphologic study on 1,000 liver biopsies. Obes Surg 2004;14(7):952–8.
37. Tsang SW, Ng WF, Wu BP, et al. Predictors of fibrosis in Asian patients with non-alcoholic steatohepatitis. J Gastroenterol Hepatol 2006;21(1 Pt 1):116–21.

38. Angulo P, Keach JC, Batts KP, et al. Independent predictors of liver fibrosis in patients with nonalcoholic steatohepatitis. Hepatology 1999;30:1356–62.

39. Brunt EM, Neuschwander-Tetri BA, Oliver D, et al. Nonalcoholic steatohepatitis: histologic features and clinical correlations with 30 blinded biopsy specimens. Hum Pathol 2004;35(9):1070–82.

40. Chitturi S, Weltman M, Farrell GC, et al. HFE mutations, hepatic iron, and fibrosis: ethnic-specific association of NASH with C282Y but not with fibrotic severity. Hepatology 2002;36(1):142–9.

41. Mofrad P, Contos MJ, Haque M, et al. Clinical and histologic spectrum of nonalcoholic fatty liver disease associated with normal ALT values. Hepatology 2003; 37(6):1286–92.

42. Sorrentino P, Tarantino G, Conca P, et al. Silent non-alcoholic fatty liver disease—a clinical–histological study. J Hepatol 2004;41(5):751–7.

43. Sheth SG, Flamm SL, Gordon FD, et al. AST/ALT ratio predicts cirrhosis in patients with chronic hepatitis C virus infection. Am J Gastroenterol 1998;93(1): 44–8.

44. Kruger FC, Daniels CR, Kidd M, et al. APRI: a simple bedside marker for advanced fibrosis that can avoid liver biopsy in patients with NAFLD/NASH. S Afr Med J 2011;101(7):477–80.

45. Bugianesi E, Manzini P, D'Antico S, et al. Relative contribution of iron burden, HFE mutations, and insulin resistance to fibrosis in nonalcoholic fatty liver. Hepatology 2004;39(1):179–87.

46. Kowdley KV, Belt P, Wilson LA, et al. Serum ferritin is an independent predictor of histologic severity and advanced fibrosis in patients with nonalcoholic fatty liver disease. Hepatology 2012;55(1):77–85.

47. Manousou P, Kalambokis G, Grillo F, et al. Serum ferritin is a discriminant marker for both fibrosis and inflammation in histologically proven non-alcoholic fatty liver disease patients. Liver Int 2011;31(5):730–9.

48. Ratziu V, Giral P, Charlotte F, et al. Liver fibrosis in overweight patients. Gastroenterology 2000;118(6):1117–23.

49. Dixon JB, Bhathal PS, O'Brien PE. Nonalcoholic fatty liver disease: predictors of nonalcoholic steatohepatitis and liver fibrosis in the severely obese. Gastroenterology 2001;121(1):91–100.

50. Marceau P, Biron S, Hould FS, et al. Liver pathology and the metabolic syndrome X in severe obesity. J Clin Endocrinol Metab 1999;84(5):1513–7.

51. Angulo P, Hui JM, Marchesini G, et al. The NAFLD fibrosis score: a noninvasive system that identifies liver fibrosis in patients with NAFLD. Hepatology 2007; 45(4):846–54.

52. Harrison SA, Oliver D, Arnold HL, et al. Development and validation of a simple NAFLD clinical scoring system for identifying patients without advanced disease. Gut 2008;57(10):1441–7.

53. Miyaaki H, Ichikawa T, Nakao K, et al. Clinicopathological study of nonalcoholic fatty liver disease in Japan: the risk factors for fibrosis. Liver Int 2008;28(4): 519–24.

54. Paradis V, Perlemuter G, Bonvoust F, et al. High glucose and hyperinsulinemia stimulate connective tissue growth factor expression: a potential mechanism involved in progression to fibrosis in nonalcoholic steatohepatitis. Hepatology 2001;34(4 Pt 1):738–44.

55. Sugimoto R, Enjoji M, Kohjima M, et al. High glucose stimulates hepatic stellate cells to proliferate and to produce collagen through free radical production and activation of mitogen-activated protein kinase. Liver Int 2005;25(5):1018–26.

56. Shah AG, Lydecker A, Murray K, et al. Nash Clinical Research Network. Comparison of noninvasive markers of fibrosis in patients with nonalcoholic fatty liver disease. Clin Gastroenterol Hepatol 2009;7(10):1104–12.

57. Wong VW, Wong GL, Chim AM, et al. Validation of the NAFLD fibrosis score in a Chinese population with low prevalence of advanced fibrosis. Am J Gastroenterol 2008;103(7):1682–8.

58. Qureshi K, Clements RH, Abrams GA. The utility of the "NAFLD fibrosis score" in morbidly obese subjects with NAFLD. Obes Surg 2008;18(3):264–70.

59. Raszeja-Wyszomirska J, Szymanik B, Ławniczak M, et al. Validation of the BARD scoring system in Polish patients with nonalcoholic fatty liver disease (NAFLD). BMC Gastroenterol 2010;10:67.

60. Sumida Y, Yoneda M, Hyogo H, et al. Validation of the FIB4 index in a Japanese nonalcoholic fatty liver disease population. BMC Gastroenterol 2012;12(1):2.

61. McPherson S, Stewart SF, Henderson E, et al. Simple non-invasive fibrosis scoring systems can reliably exclude advanced fibrosis in patients with nonalcoholic fatty liver disease. Gut 2010;59(9):1265–9.

62. Adams LA, George J, Bugianesi E, et al. Complex non-invasive fibrosis models are more accurate than simple models in non-alcoholic fatty liver disease. J Gastroenterol Hepatol 2011;26(10):1536–43.

63. Suzuki A, Angulo P, Lymp J, et al. Hyaluronic acid, an accurate serum marker for severe hepatic fibrosis in patients with non-alcoholic fatty liver disease. Liver Int 2005;25(4):779–86.

64. Sakugawa H, Nakayoshi T, Kobashigawa K, et al. Clinical usefulness of biochemical markers of liver fibrosis in patients with nonalcoholic fatty liver disease. World J Gastroenterol 2005;11(2):255–9.

65. Santos VN, Leite-Mór MM, Kondo M, et al. Serum laminin, type IV collagen and hyaluronan as fibrosis markers in non-alcoholic fatty liver disease. Braz J Med Biol Res 2005;38(5):747–53.

66. Ratziu V, Massard J, Charlotte F, et al. Diagnostic value of biochemical markers (FibroTest-FibroSURE) for the prediction of liver fibrosis in patients with non-alcoholic fatty liver disease. BMC Gastroenterol 2006;6:6.

67. Guha IN, Parkes J, Roderick P, et al. Noninvasive markers of fibrosis in nonalcoholic fatty liver disease: validating the European Liver Fibrosis Panel and exploring simple markers. Hepatology 2008;47(2):455–60.

68. Nobili V, et al. Performance of ELF serum markers in predicting fibrosis stage in pediatric non-alcoholic fatty liver disease. Gastroenterology 2009;136(1):160–7.

69. Kaneda H, Hashimoto E, Yatsuji S, et al. Hyaluronic acid levels can predict severe fibrosis and platelet counts can predict cirrhosis in patients with nonalcoholic fatty liver disease. J Gastroenterol Hepatol 2006;21(9):1459–65.

70. Johansen JS, Christoffersen P, Møller S, et al. Serum YKL-40 is increased in patients with hepatic fibrosis. J Hepatol 2000;32(6):911–20.

71. Malik R, Chang M, Bhaskar K, et al. The clinical utility of biomarkers and the nonalcoholic steatohepatitis CRN liver biopsy scoring system in patients with nonalcoholic fatty liver disease. J Gastroenterol Hepatol 2009;24(4):564–8.

72. Rosenberg WM, Voelker M, Thiel R, et al. Serum markers detect the presence of liver fibrosis: a cohort study. Gastroenterology 2004;127(6):1704–13.

73. Fraquelli M, Rigamonti C, Casazza G, et al. Reproducibility of transient elastography in the evaluation of liver fibrosis in patients with chronic liver disease. Gut 2007;56(7):968–73.

74. Gomez-Dominguez E, Mendoza J, Rubio S, et al. Transient elastography: a valid alternative to biopsy in patients with chronic liver disease. Aliment Pharmacol Ther 2006;24(3):513–8.
75. Chang PE, Lui HF, Chau YP, et al. Prospective evaluation of transient elastography for the diagnosis of hepatic fibrosis in Asians: comparison with liver biopsy and aspartate transaminase platelet ratio index. Aliment Pharmacol Ther 2008; 28(1):51–61.
76. Myers RP, Elkashab M, Ma M, et al. Transient elastography for the noninvasive assessment of liver fibrosis: a multicentre Canadian study. Can J Gastroenterol 2010;24(11):661–70.
77. Wong VW, Vergniol J, Wong GL, et al. Diagnosis of fibrosis and cirrhosis using liver stiffness measurement in nonalcoholic fatty liver disease. Hepatology 2010;51(2):454–62.
78. Castéra L, Foucher J, Bernard PH, et al. Pitfalls of liver stiffness measurement: a 5-year prospective study of 13,369 examinations. Hepatology 2010;51: 828–35.
79. Foucher J, Castéra L, Bernard PH, et al. Prevalence and factors associated with failure of liver stiffness measurement using FibroScan in a prospective study of 2114 examinations. Eur J Gastroenterol Hepatol 2006;18(4):411–2.
80. Myers RP, Pomier-Layrargues G, Kirsch R, et al. Feasibility and diagnostic performance of the FibroScan XL probe for liver stiffness measurement in overweight and obese patients. Hepatology 2012;55(1):199–208.
81. de Ledinghen V, Wong VW, Vergniol J, et al. Diagnosis of liver fibrosis and cirrhosis using liver stiffness measurement: comparison between M and XL probe of FibroScan. J Hepatol 2012;56:833–9.
82. Nobili V, Vizzutti F, Arena U, et al. Accuracy and reproducibility of transient elastography for the diagnosis of fibrosis in pediatric nonalcoholic steatohepatitis. Hepatology 2008;48(2):442–8.
83. Mariappan YK, Glaser KJ, Ehman RL. Magnetic resonance elastography: a review. Clin Anat 2010;23(5):497–511.
84. Huwart L, Sempoux C, Vicaut E, et al. Magnetic resonance elastography for the noninvasive staging of liver fibrosis. Gastroenterology 2008;135(1):32–40.
85. Kim BH, Lee JM, Lee YJ, et al. MR elastography for noninvasive assessment of hepatic fibrosis: experience from a tertiary center in Asia. J Magn Reson Imaging 2011;34(5):1110–6.
86. Chen J, Talwalkar JA, Yin M, et al. Early detection of nonalcoholic steatohepatitis in patients with nonalcoholic fatty liver disease by using MR elastography. Radiology 2011;259(3):749–56.
87. Friedrich-Rust M, Wunder K, Kriener S, et al. Liver fibrosis in viral hepatitis: noninvasive assessment with acoustic radiation force impulse imaging versus transient elastography. Radiology 2009;252(2):595–604.
88. Castera L. Acoustic radiation force impulse imaging: a new technology for the noninvasive assessment of liver fibrosis? J Gastrointestin Liver Dis 2009;18(4): 411–2.
89. Romero-Gomez M, Gómez-González E, Madrazo A, et al. Optical analysis of computed tomography images of the liver predicts fibrosis stage and distribution in chronic hepatitis C. Hepatology 2008;47(3):810–6.
90. Do RK, Chandarana H, Felker E, et al. Diagnosis of liver fibrosis and cirrhosis with diffusion-weighted imaging: value of normalized apparent diffusion coefficient using the spleen as reference organ. AJR Am J Roentgenol 2010;195(3): 671–6.

Is Nonalcoholic Fatty Liver Disease in Children the Same Disease as in Adults?

Evelyn Hsu, MD*, Karen Murray, MD

KEYWORDS

- Adolescents • Children • Nonalcoholic fatty liver disease
- Nonalcoholic steatohepatitis

KEY POINTS

- Nonalcoholic fatty liver disease (NAFLD) is the leading cause of chronic liver disease in children, and can present as early as toddlerhood.
- There is a differential distribution of NAFLD in children based on race and gender.
- The gold standard for diagnosis and classification of pediatric NAFLD is liver biopsy although ongoing studies aim to identify and define noninvasive investigations for pediatric NAFLD.
- Pediatric NAFLD can have a different histologic presentation than adult NAFLD.
- Treatments that have been shown to be successful in adult NAFLD, such as insulin sensitizers and Vitamin E, have not been proven to be as definitively successful in children with NAFLD.

Before the late twentieth century, hepatic steatosis was largely associated with alcoholic liver disease. In 1980, physicians at the Mayo Clinic described nonalcoholic steatohepatitis (NASH), giving this disease a name.[1] NASH was first reported in the pediatric population 3 years later,[2] when a case series described 3 Caucasian children, aged 10 to 15 years, who presented with a persistent elevation in the levels of liver-associated enzymes. Infectious, anatomic, and metabolic work-up was found to be negative, and liver biopsy results showed varying degrees of macrovesicular steatosis, inflammation, and fibrosis. All 3 children were overweight, and with diet and exercise, the levels of liver-associated enzymes improved over the short-term. Pediatric nonalcoholic fatty liver disease (NAFLD)/NASH is now known to be the leading cause of chronic liver disease in children.

The prevalence of obesity and overweight for adults and children in most Westernized countries has increased markedly over the last half century, particularly in the 1980s and 1990s. The most recent data from the National Health and Nutrition

Division of Pediatric Gastroenterology and Hepatology, Seattle Children's Hospital, 4800 Sand Point Way Northeast, Mailstop W7830, Seattle, WA 98115, USA
* Corresponding author.
E-mail address: evelyn.hsu@seattlechildrens.org

Clin Liver Dis 16 (2012) 587–598
doi:10.1016/j.cld.2012.05.004
1089-3261/12/$ – see front matter © 2012 Elsevier Inc. All rights reserved.

Examination Survey (NHANES), 2009 to 2010, show that 16.9% of American children aged from 2 to 19 years are considered obese,[3] which is defined as body mass index (BMI, calculated as the weight in kilograms divided by height in meters squared) greater than the 97th percentile for age. This prevalence is consistent overall with percentages reported over the past decade although there may be a trend toward increasing rates in adolescent men. By comparison, the most recent NHANES data on the adults of the United States found more than 30% prevalence of BMI-defined obesity (>30) in most sex-age groups, a significant increase over the past decade.[4]

Given the high incidence of obesity and the association of NAFLD with obesity, several minimally invasive markers have been used in an attempt to describe the prevalence of NAFLD in the pediatric population, including elevated serum alanine aminotransferase (ALT) level, ultrasonography (US), and fast gradient echo magnetic resonance imaging (MRI). Data from the NHANES III (1988–1994) focused on the association between elevated ALT levels and obesity and found that 16% of obese (10%) and overweight (6%) adolescents had elevated ALT level, defined as ALT level greater than 40 IU/L.[5] A retrospective study of a cohort of 119 obese children with type 2 diabetes mellitus (T2DM) found that elevated ALT level was present in 48% of children.[6] ALT level has not, however, been well correlated with the presence and degree of histologic inflammation and fibrosis in NASH.[7]

Ultrasonography (US) was initially used as a tool to assess steatosis in adults, with sensitivity of 94% and specificity of 84% when correlated with liver biopsy, it was less reliably a predictor of fibrosis, however.[8] US has been valued in the pediatric population because of low cost and noninvasive nature. In an early study of 75 consecutive obese patients, defined as 160% of ideal body weight, 52.8% were found to have abnormalities on US thought to be secondary to steatosis, and only 25% had abnormalities in the level of ALT.[9] In 810 northern Japanese school children aged 4 to 12 years, US was used to assess steatosis by ascertaining the liver-kidney echo discrepancy, ultrasonic penetration into the deepest portion of the liver, and clarity of the liver blood vessel structures. Overall prevalence of hepatic steatosis in this group was 2.6%. In those patients who were defined as obese (BMI >20) there was a prevalence of hepatic steatosis in 22.5% in girls and 25% in boys. There was a strong linear relationship between the thickness of abdominal subcutaneous fat and the prevalence of fatty liver.[10] US and ALT levels were used to study a similar cohort of 84 obese (average BMI 39.3) Chinese children aged 7 to 18 years. In this population, 77% had hepatic steatosis by established ultrasonographic criteria as described above, compared with 24% who had elevated ALT levels.[11]

Because of the established lack of concordance between the elevated ALT levels and US findings of steatosis, hepatic fast gradient echo MRI has also been investigated as an imaging modality. The benefit of MRI is that the presence of fatty liver can be determined by signal differences between fat and water and is absolute rather than subject to interpretation. Most scans can be completed within a single breath hold, increasing its practicality in the pediatric population. In a population of 22 obese pediatric patients aged 6 to 18 years, hepatic steatosis was present in 21 of 22 subjects, and showed a strong correlation with abnormal ALT level when calculated fat fraction is greater than 18%.[12]

Only 1 pediatric epidemiologic study has incorporated liver histology, the gold standard of diagnosing NAFLD. The Study of Child and Adolescent Liver Epidemiology (SCALE) was a retrospective autopsy-based study of liver histology in 742 subjects aged 2 years to 19 years who had died a sudden unexpected death in San Diego county.[13] When controlled for age, race, gender, and ethnicity, the overall prevalence of fatty liver (defined by >5% steatosis) was 9.6%. Prevalence rates were lowest in those aged 2 to 4 years (0.7%) and highest in those aged 15 to 19 years (17.3%). Fatty liver was present in 38% of obese children (defined by BMI >95th percentile for age). In comparison, an adult autopsy study was done in 1990 that had described an overall prevalence of steatosis of 19% in obese adults.[14]

In the pediatric population, race, ethnicity, and gender can predict the presence of NAFLD. Elevated ALT level was used as a surrogate for suspected NAFLD after excluding other causes of abnormalities (hepatitis B, C, α_1-antitrypsin deficiency, auto-immune hepatitis, and Wilson disease) in obese (mean BMI = 35.2) 12th-grade partic-ipants in the Child and Adolescent Trial for Cardiovascular Health (CATCH). After controlling for gender and BMI, this study found that Hispanic ethnicity significantly pre-dicted greater ALT level than those of black race, and boys were 6 times more likely than girls to have unexplained elevated ALT level.[15] The autopsy-based prevalence study revealed similar findings, with fatty liver more prevalent in boys than girls (11.1% vs 7.9%), most prevalent in children and adolescents of Hispanic ethnicity, and least prev-alent in those of black race. Children and adolescents of Asian race were of interme-diate prevalence, with major variability within the subgroups of Asian race.[13] A study of adults in the Nonalcoholic Steatohepatitis Clinical Research Network (NASH CRN) has shown an under-representation of Black individuals and an adequate representa-tion of Hispanic individuals with respect to the general adult population of the United States. Hispanic individuals with NASH were younger with less physical activity.[16]

PATHOPHYSIOLOGY

The most accepted paradigm of NASH pathogenesis in both children and adults is the two-hit hypothesis in which a primarily abnormality in the liver (ie, the accumulation of triglyceride droplets within the hepatocytes, or steatosis) is a result of peripheral insulin resistance leading to hyperinsulinemia, which then potentiates hepatic lipogen-esis, increasing the flow of free fatty acids to the liver. The steatotic liver is then made more vulnerable to additional damage from free oxygen radicals.[17]

Dyslipidemia, hypertriglyceridemia, and insulin resistance are common in children with NAFLD. Steatosis often precedes the development of insulin resistance and metabolic syndrome, with fat overpowering the storage capacity of the adipocyte and accumulating in the liver and skeletal muscle. Fatty liver can potentiate the devel-opment of type DM by causing acquired insulin signaling defects, insulin resistance, and T2DM. Adipose tissue is a hormonally active organ, releasing adipokines (leptin, tumor necrosis factor α, and adiponectin) that affect and may add to liver toxicity.[18]

Metabolic syndrome (MetS), defined as central obesity, dyslipidemia, impaired fast-ing glucose, and hypertension, is strongly associated with pediatric NAFLD. The National Institute of Diabetes and Digestive and Kidney Diseases, with additional support from the National Institute of Childhood Health and Human Development, funded the NASH CRN beginning in 2002 to assess the etiology, natural history, and therapy for NAFLD/NASH.[19] In a study of 254 children aged 6 to 17 years enrolled in the NASH CRN, 26% met the criteria for MetS, with a majority (77.2%) having 1 to 3 features present.[17] Risk of MetS was greatest among those with severe steatosis and advanced fibrosis, and severity of insulin resistance was most consistently associated with the histologic features of pediatric NASH. Achieving greater insight into the asso-ciation between MetS and NASH will provide potential targets for therapeutic interven-tion and prognostic markers to predict disease severity.

GENETICS

Identifying genetic variants that predispose toward hepatic damage can open insights toward the molecular mechanisms underlying NASH, allowing clinicians to identify high-risk individuals and provide targeted therapy. A single nucleotide polymorphism (SNP), rs738509, in the patatin-like phospholipase 3 gene (PNPLA3) has been associated with hepatic steatosis in adults.[20–23] It is a common missense variant, characterized by a C-to-G substitution encoding an isoleucine-to-methionine substitution at amino acid position 148 (I148M) in the PNPLA3 gene. The PNPLA3 gene product is adiponutrin, which is a member of the calcium-independent phospholipase A2 family and has hydrolyzing capability. In humans, adiponutrin is primarily expressed in white adipose tissue and liver. Adiponutrin may have a role in generating adipocytes and has been shown to increase in incidence with obesity.

To investigate the role of this polymorphism in the pediatric population, a multiethnic group of 85 children was recruited from a pediatric obesity clinic. Fast MRI was performed in all the participants, subcutaneous fat biopsy in 18 children, and liver biopsy in 6 children. The common variant (the G allele) did confer an increased susceptibility to hepatic steatosis in obese patients without increasing the level of insulin resistance.[24] Analysis of 149 consecutive children and adolescents of Caucasian-Italian descent for the same I148M SNP of PNPLA3 was done. In this study, the G allele was strongly associated with hepatocellular ballooning, lobular inflammation, and presence of fibrosis. In particular, individuals who were homozygous for the G allele were at risk for severe steatosis, heterozygotes were at intermediate risk, and individuals with negative G allele had milder form of steatosis.[25] Body mass, dyslipidemia, and insulin resistance were unaffected by the presence of this SNP. A study of 475 overweight or obese children found that the PNPLA3 I148M was associated with elevated ALT level and hepatic steatosis as determined by US. As with previous studies, there was no positive association with measures of insulin resistance.[26]

Another SNP of interest is the rs1260326 glucokinase regulatory protein (GCKR). The rs1260326 is a functionally relevant SNP consisting of a C-to-T substitution that codes for a proline-to-leucine substitution at position 446 (P446L). This SNP may influence the ability of GCKR to inhibit glucokinase in response to fructose-6-phosphate. This process increases glucose uptake by the liver, which can increase levels of malonyl CoA, favoring hepatic fat accumulation by inhibiting carnitine-palmitoyltransferase-1 (CPT-1) through blocking the oxidation of fatty acids.[27]

Studying the genomic DNA of 455 obese children recruited through the Yale Pediatric Obesity Clinic, it was found that the GCKR SNP was associated with high triglycerides, elevated very low-density lipoprotein levels, and increased hepatic fat fraction. The PNPLA3 SNP, as demonstrated previously, was associated with increased hepatic fat fraction, but not with triglyceride levels. There was a joint effect between PNPLA3 and GCKR SNPs, accounting for nearly one-third of the variance. Analysis of an SNP associated with apolipoprotein C3 promoter (APOC3) did not have a predictive association in this population; however, as previously described in sedentary Asian Indian adult men, a population known to have an increased prevalence of NAFLD and insulin resistance.[28,29]

NATURAL HISTORY AND QUALITY OF LIFE

In adults, severe liver disease and fibrosis with progression to cirrhosis is common, with cirrhosis occurring in as many as 17% of adults at time of diagnosis.[30] Progression to cirrhosis in pediatric NAFLD is possible and cases have been reported in the literature.[31,32] Alarmingly, there are 4 reported cases of liver transplantation for NAFLD in childhood.[33–35] Reported cases of liver transplantation for pediatric NAFLD are associated with hepatopulmonary syndrome, a finding not described in the adult

NAFLD/NASH literature. Early recurrence of NASH within the graft with progressive disease is common and concerning, especially if there is a need for re-transplant.

In a hospital-based cohort study of 66 patients with up to 20 years of follow-up at the Mayo Clinic, children with NAFLD had a nearly 14 times increased risk of mortality or liver transplantation relative to the general population.[35]

In addition, adult NAFLD has been linked to the development of hepatocellular carcinoma (HCC) and may be contributing to the increase in age-adjusted incidence in the United States.[36] The occurrence of HCC in noncirrhotic NASH is a recent finding.[37] By extrapolation, in addition to being at increased risk of progression to end-stage liver disease with potential need for liver transplantation, pediatric patients with NASH are at risk for HCC in adulthood.

The establishment of the NASH CRN has enabled studies for characterizing quality of life (QOL) in children with NAFLD/NASH, which is a crucial part of understanding the disease-related morbidity in these individuals.[38] A study of 239 individuals with NAFLD/NASH was conducted using the Pediatric Quality of Life Inventory version 4.0 (PedsQL 4.0, Mapi Research Trust, Lyon, France), and compared with age-matched healthy controls. Children with NAFLD/NASH were found to have significantly lower QOL (40% of children with NAFLD had impaired QOL), physical health, and psychosocial health. There were no significant differences in QOL based on histologic severity or classification. Females more commonly than males had impaired QOL, and non-Hispanic children had more impairment of QOL than did Hispanic children. Persistent fatigue was very common in children with NAFLD, a finding not shown to be independently associated with obesity. Life-threatening depression and attempted suicide have been reported in children with NAFLD.[39]

DIAGNOSIS AND HISTOLOGY

Despite the use of new noninvasive radiologic imaging techniques, discrimination between NASH and hepatic steatosis, an important distinction for managing and determining prognosis, remains elusive without histologic analysis. Liver biopsy, when the specimen is of adequate length and diameter, remains the best way to characterize NAFLD/NASH. The drawback of live biopsy is its invasiveness with risk of complications, but it is beneficial in excluding other causes of liver disease. In a review of 354 adult liver biopsies for suspected NAFLD, 66% of patients were confirmed to have NAFLD with 50% of those patients having NASH with fibrosis. Fully one-third of these adult patients had something other than NAFLD on histologic review.[40] Furthermore, in children as well as in adults elevated ALT levels are not predictive of degree of fibrosis or steatohepatitis.[41]

In adults, the histopathology of NAFLD is well described, with established criteria for classification and characterization of injury and parenchymal changes.[42] The primary components of steatosis and steatohepatitis occur in the perivenular (zone 3) portions of the hepatic acinus, an area that is not well oxygenated because it is farthest from hepatic artery and portal vein inflow. Triglyceride accumulation can be described as macrovesicular (single large droplets that displace nucleus) or microvesicular, called small droplet steatosis (smaller droplets mixed in with cytoplasmic contents). Steatohepatitis is defined as inflammation and hepatocyte injury usually characterized as a lymphocytic lobular inflammation. In adults, ballooning is described as enlarged hepatocytes that have a fluffy flocculent appearance to the cytoplasm. Cytoplasmic aggregates called Mallory-Denk Bodies or Mallory hyaline can be present. Other histologic features of NASH include apoptotic hepatocytes (acidophil bodies), glycogen-filled hepatocyte nuclei, and megamitochondria. The NAFLD Activity Score (NAS) was developed by the NASH CRN and enables scoring the severity once the diagnosis of NAFLD/NASH has been established. The NAS score totals the sum of scores for steatosis, lobular inflammation, and ballooning, and ranges from 0 to 8.[43]

Pediatric studies of NAFLD/NASH have described significantly different histopathological findings, suggesting that this may be a distinct entity from the adult disease. In the first large biopsy series of pediatric NAFLD, Schwimmer and colleagues[41] characterized the liver biopsy results of 106 consecutive pediatric patients with NAFLD and established a histologic definition of pediatric NASH. Two distinct histologic patterns of steatohepatitis were demonstrated. Type 1 NASH was more common in adults and Caucasian children, with the presence of steatosis, ballooning degeneration, and perisinusoidal fibrosis. Type 1 NASH represented only 17% of the cases described in this series. Type 2 NASH was more common in Asian, Native American and Hispanic children; has typical features of steatosis, but portal inflammation and portal fibrosis; and represented 51% of pediatric NAFLD. Type 2 NASH was characterized by moderate-to-marked steatosis, but was distinguished from type 1 NASH by the absence of ballooning degeneration, a predominance of lymphocytic portal inflammation, and fibrosis in the portal region that spares the central veins. In addition, children were younger and had a greater severity of obesity, and advanced fibrosis was more common in type 2 compared with type 1 NASH. Sixteen percent of the pediatric patients with NAFLD in this series did not meet criteria for simple steatosis and had overlapping features of both type 1 and type 2 NASH. These biopsy results had a higher prevalence of megamitochondria and less macrovesicular steatosis. Of note, about half of the cases clustered with type 2 and the other half with type 1.

There is a subset of adults with NAFLD who also exhibit a pattern consistent with type 2 NASH. In a case control study of morbidly obese adults (definition BMI >40) undergoing liver biopsies and gastric bypass surgery, 33% of the biopsy results showed isolated portal fibrosis fitting the criteria of type 2 NASH. In this subset of patients, the mean age was slightly lower (38.6 years vs 40.8 years), and greater than 80% of the subjects were non-Hispanic women.[44] Furthermore, in a recent investigation of 1101 subjects who underwent liver biopsies enrolled in the NASH CRN studies, portal inflammation was described in 25% of subjects who had the presence of definite NASH.[7]

Using the same criteria for classification of NASH as either type 1 or type 2, a multicenter retrospective cohort study was completed taking into account the liver biopsies of 130 children with NAFLD.[45] The mean age in this cohort was 12 years, and liver biopsy samples were classified based on the following criteria: (1) type 1 NASH: zone 3 dominance of steatosis, ballooning, and zone 3 perisinusoidal fibrosis, (2) type 2 NASH: steatosis with portal inflammation in the absence of ballooning and portal fibrosis, and (3) overlap, with characteristics from both types 1 and 2. This series described that overlapping features of both type 1 and type 2 NASH were present in a majority of biopsies (82%), and 20% had bridging fibrosis. In this same series, the presence of lobular and portal inflammation correlated with the presence and severity of fibrosis.

By examining the liver biopsies from 149 children enrolled in the NASH CRN, 110 biopsies were determined to be definite NASH, with 42.7% showing features of both types 1 and 2, 32.5% as type 2, and 24.5% as type 1. Subjects classified as type 2 NASH were more likely to be boys (86.1%).[46] A subset of patients with more severe obesity and increased insulin resistance may progress to cirrhosis without zone 3 injuries because increased inflammation does seem to correlate with increased hepatocellular injury and fibrosis. It does not seem clear, however, that type 2 NASH, or what is sometimes described as pediatric NASH, is an entity unto itself. Type 2 NASH may simply be a predictor of a subset of patients who have more severe disease on the spectrum of NASH. Please refer to **Figs. 1–4** for further demonstration of NASH histology.

TREATMENT/MANAGEMENT

In the past decade, largely through the collaborative efforts of the NASH CRN, tremendous gains have been made toward achieving clarity and insight on the treatment of NAFLD in adults, children, and adolescents. Based on the supporting evidence of several small pilot studies for the use of insulin sensitizers and vitamin E in adults to improve the features of NASH,[47–50] the NASH CRN conducted a phase 3, multicenter, randomized, placebo-controlled, double-blind clinical trial of pioglitazone or vitamin E for the treatment of 247 adults without diabetes who had NASH.[51] There were 3 treatment arms; pioglitazone at a dosage of 30 mg daily, vitamin E at a dosage of 800 IU daily, and placebo. Length of treatment was 96 weeks, and primary outcome was improvement in the histologic features of NASH with secondary outcome comprising change in overall NASH activity score, ALT levels, insulin resistance, and lipid profiles. The investigators found that vitamin E compared with placebo was associated with a significantly higher rate of improvement in the ALT level (43% vs 19%), whereas pioglitazone did not reach significance (34% vs 19%). Improvements in hepatic steatosis and lobular inflammation were also seen in both of the treatment groups although neither treatment had an effect on the level of fibrosis.

Initial small pilot studies in children supported the use of metformin and vitamin E to improve outcome in children with NAFLD.[52,53] The NASH CRN conducted a randomized, double-blind, double-dummy, placebo-controlled clinical trial of vitamin E and metformin in 173 patients aged 8 to 17 years and who were confirmed by biopsy to have NAFLD.[39] Patients were randomized into 3 treatment groups: (1) vitamin E 800 IU daily + placebo (2) metformin 1000 mg daily + placebo (3) 2 placebo medications. Primary outcome was sustained reduction in ALT level, defined as 50% reduction from baseline. Secondary outcome measures were improvements in histologic features of NASH. Patients in the 3 treatment groups were given standard of care advice on diet and exercise throughout the treatment duration of 96 weeks. Neither vitamin E nor

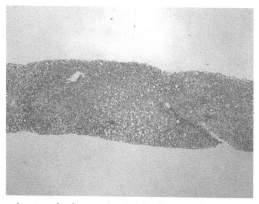

Fig. 1. Low power micrograph shows classic histology of pediatric NASH with steatosis surrounding the portal tract and sparing the zone 3 region. Ballooning degeneration is not obvious. (Hematoxylin-eosin, original magnification ×40). (*Courtesy of* Matthew M. Yeh, MD, PhD, Department of Pathology, University of Washington, Seattle, WA.)

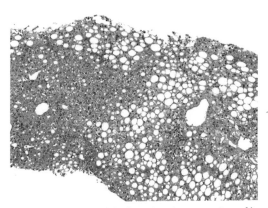

Fig. 2. Biopsy typical of type 1 NASH with ballooning degeneration of hepatocytes and peri-sinusoidal fibrosis. (Hematoxylin-eosin, original magnification ×100). (*Courtesy of* Matthew M. Yeh, MD, PhD, Department of Pathology, University of Washington, Seattle, WA.)

metformin resulted in a sustained reduction in ALT level. Among the 121 patients with NASH at the commencement of the trial, vitamin E reduced the degree of NASH when compared with placebo (58% vs 28%), with a significant improvement in hepatocellular ballooning (44% vs 21%), but no improvement in steatosis, inflammation, or fibrosis. In the patients treated with metformin, there were improvements in hepatocellular ballooning (44% vs 21%) but not in steatosis, inflammation, or NAS. In all subjects there was a mean increase in weight, BMI, and waist circumference despite standard of care recommendations provided on diet and exercise.

Sustained weight loss reliably improves NASH histologic activity. A randomized controlled trial using lifestyle modification as an active treatment intervention was completed in 33 adult patients with well-characterized NASH.[54] This study showed that it was possible for patients who are overweight and obese with NASH to successfully achieve a weight reduction of 7% to 10%. With this weight reduction, improvements were seen in overall NASH histologic activity, degree of steatosis, and ALT levels. Increased degree of weight loss was associated with increased improvement. The degree of hepatic fibrosis, however, did not change, suggesting that either the

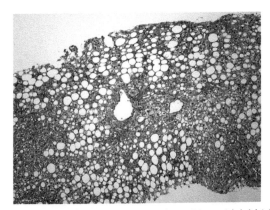

Fig. 3. Typical fibrosis pattern of type 1 NASH with perisinusoidal (chicken wire) fibrosis. (Masson trichrome stain, original magnification ×100). (*Courtesy of* Matthew M. Yeh, MD, PhD, Department of Pathology, University of Washington, Seattle, WA.)

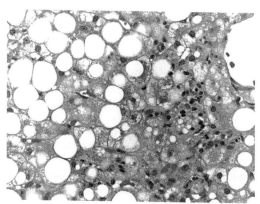

Fig. 4. High-power micrograph showing typical appearance of ballooning degeneration of hepatocytes. (Hematoxylin-eosin, original magnification ×400). (*Courtesy of* Matthew M. Yeh, MD, PhD, Department of Pathology, University of Washington, Seattle, WA.)

sample size was too small or the finding of hepatic fibrosis is less likely to reverse, particularly in adults.

Weight reduction through lifestyle interventions, such as dietary change and physical activity, is a primary part of counseling pediatric patients with NAFLD. In 1994, a case series of 9 obese children with elevated ALT levels who experienced 10% weight loss had sustained improvement of ALT levels.[55] Subsequently, a trial of 53 pediatric patients (mean age 12 years) underwent 2 years of lifestyle intervention with a diet modified toward individual calorie requirement and prescribed increased physical activity. The intervention was associated with a significant improvement in the severity of steatosis, inflammation, and hepatocyte ballooning,[56] whereas BMI remained stable or decreased. Secondary end points such as insulin resistance and levels of lipids as well as ALT also improved significantly. Although this is the first moderately sized study to examine liver histology as a primary endpoint, there was no control group for lifestyle intervention.

SUMMARY

NAFLD is the leading cause of chronic liver disease in children, with some patients progressing to severe fibrosis, cirrhosis, and end-stage liver disease. Although there are significant areas of concordance between adults and children regarding genetics and associations with obesity and insulin resistance, there is also alarming evidence that the histopathologic presentation of NAFLD/NASH in children is distinct from that of adults and may be associated with a worse prognosis. Also of concern is the large multi-center trials of medical therapy such as insulin sensitizers and anti-oxidant therapy that have shown improvement in liver histology in adults have not produced similar results when performed in the pediatric population. Considerable resources have been invested in the study of pediatric NAFLD to date and must continue to help characterize, treat, and eradicate this disease.

REFERENCES

1. Ludwig J, Viggiano TR, McGill DB, et al. Nonalcoholic steatohepatitis: Mayo Clinic experiences with a hitherto unnamed disease. Mayo Clin Proc 1980; 55(7):434–8.

2. Moran JR, Ghishan FK, Halter SA, et al. Steatohepatitis in obese children: a cause of chronic liver dysfunction. Am J Gastroenterol 1983;78(6):374–7.

3. Ogden CL, Carroll MD, Kit BK, et al. Prevalence of obesity and trends in body mass index among US children and adolescents, 1999-2010. JAMA 2012; 307(5):483–90.

4. Flegal KM, Carroll MD, Kit BK, et al. Prevalence of obesity and trends in the distribution of body mass index among US adults, 1999-2010. JAMA 2012;307(5): 491–7.

5. Strauss RS, Barlow SE, Dietz WH. Prevalence of abnormal serum aminotransferase values in overweight and obese adolescents. J Pediatr 2000;136(6): 727–33.

6. Nadeau KJ, Klingensmith G, Zeitler P. Type 2 diabetes in children is frequently associated with elevated alanine aminotransferase. J Pediatr Gastroenterol Nutr 2005;41(1):94–8.

7. Neuschwander-Tetri BA, Clark JM, Bass NM, et al. Clinical, laboratory and histological associations in adults with nonalcoholic fatty liver disease. Hepatology 2010;52(3):913–24.

8. Saverymuttu SH, Joseph AE, Maxwell JD. Ultrasound scanning in the detection of hepatic fibrosis and steatosis. Br Med J (Clin Res Ed) 1986;292(6512):13–5.

9. Franzese A, Vajro P, Argenziano A, et al. Liver involvement in obese children. Ultrasonography and liver enzyme levels at diagnosis and during follow-up in an Italian population. Dig Dis Sci 1997;42(7):1428–32.

10. Tominaga K, Kurata JH, Chen YK, et al. Prevalence of fatty liver in Japanese children and relationship to obesity. An epidemiological ultrasonographic survey. Dig Dis Sci 1995;40(9):2002–9.

11. Chan DF, Li AM, Chu WC, et al. Hepatic steatosis in obese Chinese children. Int J Obes Relat Metab Disord 2004;28(10):1257–63.

12. Fishbein M, Castro F, Cheruku S, et al. Hepatic MRI for fat quantitation: its relationship to fat morphology, diagnosis, and ultrasound. J Clin Gastroenterol 2005;39(7):619–25.

13. Schwimmer JB, Deutsch R, Kahen T, et al. Prevalence of fatty liver in children and adolescents. Pediatrics 2006;118(4):1388–93.

14. Wanless IR, Lentz JS. Fatty liver hepatitis (steatohepatitis) and obesity: an autopsy study with analysis of risk factors. Hepatology 1990;12(5):1106–10.

15. Schwimmer JB, McGreal N, Deutsch R, et al. Influence of gender, race, and ethnicity on suspected fatty liver in obese adolescents. Pediatrics 2005;115(5):e561–5.

16. Bambha K, Belt P, Abraham M, et al. Ethnicity and nonalcoholic fatty liver disease. Hepatology 2012;55(3):769–80.

17. Patton HM, Yates K, Unalp-Arida A, et al. Association between metabolic syndrome and liver histology among children with nonalcoholic fatty liver disease. Am J Gastroenterol 2010;105(9):2093–102.

18. Schwimmer J. Non-alcoholic fatty liver disease. In: Suchy F Sr, Balistreri W, editors. Liver disease in children. 3rd edition, Cambridge University Press; 2007. p. 830–9.

19. Lavine JE, Schwimmer JB. Pediatric initiatives within the Nonalcoholic Steatohepatitis-Clinical Research Network (NASH CRN). J Pediatr Gastroenterol Nutr 2003;37(3):220–1.

20. Romeo S, Kozlitina J, Xing C, et al. Genetic variation in PNPLA3 confers susceptibility to nonalcoholic fatty liver disease. Nat Genet 2008;40(12):1461–5.

21. Kotronen A, Johansson LE, Johansson LM, et al. A common variant in PNPLA3, which encodes adiponutrin, is associated with liver fat content in humans. Diabetologia 2009;52(6):1056–60.

22. Romeo S, Sentinelli F, Dash S, et al. Morbid obesity exposes the association between PNPLA3 I148M (rs738409) and indices of hepatic injury in individuals of European descent. Int J Obes (Lond) 2010;34(1):190–4.
23. Speliotes EK, Butler JL, Palmer CD, et al. PNPLA3 variants specifically confer increased risk for histologic nonalcoholic fatty liver disease but not metabolic disease. Hepatology 2010;52(3):904–12.
24. Santoro N, Kursawe R, D'Adamo E, et al. A common variant in the patatin-like phospholipase 3 gene (PNPLA3) is associated with fatty liver disease in obese children and adolescents. Hepatology 2010;52(4):1281–90.
25. Valenti L, Alisi A, Galmozzi E, et al. I148M patatin-like phospholipase domain-containing 3 gene variant and severity of pediatric nonalcoholic fatty liver disease. Hepatology 2010;52(4):1274–80.
26. Romeo S, Sentinelli F, Cambuli VM, et al. The 148M allele of the PNPLA3 gene is associated with indices of liver damage early in life. J Hepatol 2010;53(2):335–8.
27. Valenti L, Alisi A, Nobili V. Unraveling the genetics of fatty liver in obese children: additive effect of P446L GCKR and I148M PNPLA3 polymorphisms. Hepatology 2012;55(3):661–3.
28. Santoro N, Zhang CK, Zhao H, et al. Variant in the glucokinase regulatory protein (GCKR) gene is associated with fatty liver in obese children and adolescents. Hepatology 2012;55(3):781–9.
29. Petersen KF, Dufour S, Hariri A, et al. Apolipoprotein C3 gene variants in nonalcoholic fatty liver disease. N Engl J Med 2010;362(12):1082–9.
30. Lee RG. Nonalcoholic steatohepatitis: a study of 49 patients. Hum Pathol 1989;20(6):594–8.
31. Molleston JP, White F, Teckman J, et al. Obese children with steatohepatitis can develop cirrhosis in childhood. Am J Gastroenterol 2002;97(9):2460–2.
32. Rashid M, Roberts EA. Nonalcoholic steatohepatitis in children. J Pediatr Gastroenterol Nutr 2000;30(1):48–53.
33. Jonas MM, Krawczuk LE, Kim HB, et al. Rapid recurrence of nonalcoholic fatty liver disease after transplantation in a child with hypopituitarism and hepatopulmonary syndrome. Liver Transpl 2005;11(1):108–10.
34. Jankowska I, Socha P, Pawlowska J, et al. Recurrence of non-alcoholic steatohepatitis after liver transplantation in a 13-yr-old boy. Pediatr Transplant 2007;11(7):796–8.
35. Feldstein AE, Charatcharoenwitthaya P, Treeprasertsuk S, et al. The natural history of non-alcoholic fatty liver disease in children: a follow-up study for up to 20 years. Gut 2009;58(11):1538–44.
36. Baffy G, Brunt EM, Caldwell SH. Hepatocellular carcinoma in nonalcoholic fatty liver disease: an emerging menace. J Hepatol 2012;56(6):1384–91.
37. Cuadrado A, Orive A, Garcia-Suarez C, et al. Non-alcoholic steatohepatitis (NASH) and hepatocellular carcinoma. Obes Surg 2005;15(3):442–6.
38. Kistler KD, Molleston J, Unalp A, et al. Symptoms and quality of life in obese children and adolescents with non-alcoholic fatty liver disease. Aliment Pharmacol Ther 2010;31(3):396–406.
39. Lavine JE, Schwimmer JB, Van Natta ML, et al. Effect of vitamin E or metformin for treatment of nonalcoholic fatty liver disease in children and adolescents: the TONIC randomized controlled trial. JAMA 2011;305(16):1659–68.
40. Skelly MM, James PD, Ryder SD. Findings on liver biopsy to investigate abnormal liver function tests in the absence of diagnostic serology. J Hepatol 2001;35(2):195–9.

41. Schwimmer JB, Behling C, Newbury R, et al. Histopathology of pediatric nonalcoholic fatty liver disease. Hepatology 2005;42(3):641–9.
42. Brunt EM. Pathology of nonalcoholic fatty liver disease. Nat Rev Gastroenterol Hepatol 2010;7(4):195–203.
43. Kleiner DE, Brunt EM, Van Natta M, et al. Design and validation of a histological scoring system for nonalcoholic fatty liver disease. Hepatology 2005;41(6): 1313–21.
44. Abrams GA, Kunde SS, Lazenby AJ, et al. Portal fibrosis and hepatic steatosis in morbidly obese subjects: a spectrum of nonalcoholic fatty liver disease. Hepatology 2004;40(2):475–83.
45. Carter-Kent C, Yerian LM, Brunt EM, et al. Nonalcoholic steatohepatitis in children: a multicenter clinicopathological study. Hepatology 2009;50(4):1113–20.
46. Vos MB, Colvin R, Belt P, et al. Correlation of vitamin E, uric acid, and diet composition with histologic features of pediatric NAFLD. J Pediatr Gastroenterol Nutr 2012;54(1):90–6.
47. Belfort R, Harrison SA, Brown K, et al. A placebo-controlled trial of pioglitazone in subjects with nonalcoholic steatohepatitis. N Engl J Med 2006;355(22):2297–307.
48. Promrat K, Lutchman G, Uwaifo GI, et al. A pilot study of pioglitazone treatment for nonalcoholic steatohepatitis. Hepatology 2004;39(1):188–96.
49. Sanyal AJ, Mofrad PS, Contos MJ, et al. A pilot study of vitamin E versus vitamin E and pioglitazone for the treatment of nonalcoholic steatohepatitis. Clin Gastroenterol Hepatol 2004;2(12):1107–15.
50. Harrison SA, Torgerson S, Hayashi P, et al. Vitamin E and vitamin C treatment improves fibrosis in patients with nonalcoholic steatohepatitis. Am J Gastroenterol 2003;98(11):2485–90.
51. Sanyal AJ, Chalasani N, Kowdley KV, et al. Pioglitazone, vitamin E, or placebo for nonalcoholic steatohepatitis. N Engl J Med 2010;362(18):1675–85.
52. Lavine JE. Vitamin E treatment of nonalcoholic steatohepatitis in children: a pilot study. J Pediatr 2000;136(6):734–8.
53. Schwimmer JB, Middleton MS, Deutsch R, et al. A phase 2 clinical trial of metformin as a treatment for non-diabetic paediatric non-alcoholic steatohepatitis. Aliment Pharmacol Ther 2005;21(7):871–9.
54. Promrat K, Kleiner DE, Niemeier HM, et al. Randomized controlled trial testing the effects of weight loss on nonalcoholic steatohepatitis. Hepatology 2010;51(1): 121–9.
55. Vajro P, Fontanella A, Perna C, et al. Persistent hyperaminotransferasemia resolving after weight reduction in obese children. J Pediatr 1994;125(2):239–41.
56. Nobili V, Manco M, Devito R, et al. Lifestyle intervention and antioxidant therapy in children with nonalcoholic fatty liver disease: a randomized, controlled trial. Hepatology 2008;48(1):119–28.

The Cardiovascular Link to Nonalcoholic Fatty Liver Disease
A Critical Analysis

Tommy Pacana, MD*, Michael Fuchs, MD, PhD, FEBG, AGAF*

KEYWORDS

- Nonalcoholic fatty liver disease • Nonalcoholic steatohepatitis
- Subclinical atherosclerosis • Cardiovascular disease

KEY POINTS

- Nonalcoholic fatty liver disease (NAFLD), the most common chronic liver disease in Western countries that can progress from simple steatosis to liver cirrhosis, is increasing because of the epidemics in obesity and diabetes and is becoming a serious public health burden.
- The overall mortality in patients with NAFLD is higher compared with the general population, with cardiovascular disease rather than liver cirrhosis as the leading cause of death.
- NAFLD and the metabolic syndrome share common features, such as insulin resistance, systemic inflammation, and atherogenic dyslipidemia, implicating a role of NAFLD in the development and progression of cardiovascular disease.
- A growing body of evidence suggests that NAFLD is independent of traditional risk factors and features of the metabolic syndrome associated with markers of subclinical atherosclerosis and strongly associated with incident cardiovascular disease.
- Being at a high risk for future cardiovascular events, patients with NAFLD deserve special attention for cardiovascular risk screening and surveillance strategies to allow early targeted intervention.

INTRODUCTION

Nonalcoholic fatty liver disease (NAFLD), the most common cause of chronic liver disease in the United States and other Western countries, encompasses a histologic spectrum of liver disease ranging from simple steatosis to nonalcoholic steatohepatitis (NASH), which may progress to cirrhosis and liver cancer.[1-4] Although the true prevalence of NAFLD is unknown, NAFLD affects approximately 20% to 30% of adults

Division of Gastroenterology, Hepatology and Nutrition, Virginia Commonwealth University School of Medicine, MCV Box 980341, Richmond, VA 23298-0341, USA
* Corresponding author.
E-mail addresses: typacana@mcvh-vcu.edu; mfuchs@vcu.edu

Clin Liver Dis 16 (2012) 599–613
doi:10.1016/j.cld.2012.05.008
1089-3261/12/$ – see front matter © 2012 Elsevier Inc. All rights reserved.

liver.theclinics.com

in Western countries of which 10% develop NASH.[5,6] Up to 20% of patients with NASH will progress to liver cirrhosis and 30% to 40% may suffer liver-related deaths.[7] Epidemiologic studies suggest that 75% of obese individuals have NAFLD and up to 20% may have NASH.[8] Furthermore, with the increase of obesity in children, NAFLD is now recognized as the most common cause of liver disease in the pediatric population.[9] NAFLD is closely associated with the metabolic syndrome and its individual components, such as obesity, insulin resistance, hyperlipidemia, diabetes, and hypertension.[10,11] This association has led to the concept that NAFLD represents the hepatic manifestation of the metabolic syndrome. Moreover, the presence of multiple features of the metabolic syndrome is associated with the underlying severity of NAFLD.[12] It is not surprising that the epidemics in obesity, diabetes, and metabolic syndrome will increase the prevalence of NAFLD and threaten to become one of the most serious public health burdens.[13,14]

Metabolic syndrome features are established risk factors for cardiovascular disease (CVD),[15] and the syndrome per se predicts incident CVD and diabetes mellitus.[16] A meta-analysis further showed that the metabolic syndrome is associated with a twofold increased risk for CVD, CVD mortality, and stroke. It is important to mention that the metabolic syndrome remains associated with a high risk for CVD even in the absence of diabetes mellitus.[17] A growing body of evidence suggests that NAFLD is associated with an increased risk for CVD independent of classical and metabolic syndrome risk factors.[18] Studies by Targher and colleagues[19] in patients with diabetes mellitus have demonstrated a higher prevalence of CVD among patients with NAFLD.[20] The outcomes are independent of traditional risk factors, metabolic syndrome features, and medications. Furthermore, recent prospective studies link NAFLD to markers of subclinical cardiovascular risk.[21] Survival among patients with NAFLD is worse than expected in comparison with the general population,[22,23] and those with NASH have a poorer prognosis.[24,25] In addition, several but not all population-based cohort studies have pointed out CVD as the leading cause of death in patients with NAFLD.[24–27]

Therefore, it is important to address the role of NAFLD as a potential independent risk factor for the development and progression of CVD. The aim of this review is to provide insights into the relationships between NAFLD and subclinical markers of atherosclerosis and incidence of CVD. Potential biologic mechanisms linking NAFLD to CVD are also discussed.

NAFLD AND SUBCLINICAL CVD MARKER

Noninvasive and inexpensive tests to enhance risk stratification and improve cardiovascular risk prediction, especially in individuals at lower risk, are of considerable interest lately. Subclinical atherosclerosis may be assessed with measurements of carotid intima-media thickness, ankle-arm index, aortic pulse-wave velocity, or the detection of carotid plaques and coronary artery calcifications. It has been shown that a negative test result conveys a lower risk for CVD.[28] Therefore, screening for early atherosclerosis by subclinical marker testing may be useful in patients with NAFLD. Choosing vascular imaging as a surrogate marker for CVD is particularly appealing because it assesses the atherosclerotic disease process itself, whereas soluble surrogate markers would only partially reflect the complex pathobiology of atherosclerosis.

Ultrasonography of the Carotid Artery

Thickness of the intima-media layer or the total plaque area of the carotid artery may serve as marker of subclinical CVD and can be measured with ultrasonography.

Studies have demonstrated that carotid intima-media thickness and carotid plaques predict CVD and stroke.[29–31] In the Diabetes Heart Study, no correlation was observed between carotid intima-media thickness and NAFLD diagnosed by computed tomography.[32] These findings were in agreement with data obtained in obese children and adolescents whereby NAFLD was confirmed histologically.[33] In contrast, a study in adult patients with biopsy-proven NAFLD showed a smaller carotid intima-media thickness in controls. Furthermore, patients with NASH had a greater carotid intima-media thickness than those with steatosis alone, independent of traditional risk factors and the metabolic syndrome.[34] A meta-analysis of 3497 individuals recruited from 7 studies examining the relationship between carotid intima-media thickness and NAFLD suggests that patients with hepatic steatosis have a carotid intima-media thickness that is increased by 13%.[35]

Carotid artery plaques are more prevalent in patients with NAFLD compared with controls.[35] A Norwegian comparative study involving 6226 participants followed for 6 years illustrated that carotid artery plaques rather than carotid intima-media thickness represents a stronger predictor of first-ever myocardial infarction.[36] This finding has been corroborated further by a French study of 5895 healthy older adults indicating that an increasing number of carotid artery plaques, not intima-media thickness of the carotid artery, independently predicted greater risk of first coronary heart disease over 6 years of follow-up.[37] To resolve some of the discrepancies, large prospective studies are needed to compare the independent value of both tests in predicting CVD in patients with NAFLD. One also has to consider that ultrasonography measurements have their limitations in the imaging of atherosclerosis, inherent to its physical properties. Although ultrasonography provides a 2-dimensional image of the vessel wall, atherosclerosis is a 3-dimensional disease. Measurement variability also depends to a large extent on the ability to find the same anatomic location for repeat examinations and the ability to reproduce the same angle of insonation.

Computed Tomography of Coronary Artery Calcifications

After adjusting for risk factors and imaging-derived measures, the Multi-Ethnic Study of Atherosclerosis suggests that coronary artery calcification judged by computed tomography is a better predictor of coronary heart disease and events compared with carotid artery intima-media thickness.[38] The significance of this test with regard to NAFLD is that the prevalence of NAFLD increases with the severity of coronary artery calcification.[39] In individuals with a low to intermediate risk for coronary artery disease, there is a higher frequency of coronary plaques by cardiac computed tomography in patients with NAFLD independent of metabolic syndrome features.[40] Moreover, patients with both hepatic steatosis and alanine aminotransferase (ALT) greater than 30 U/L have a coronary calcium score greater than 100 as assessed by computed tomography.[41] Arad and colleagues[42] previously demonstrated that a coronary calcium score greater than 100 is associated with a higher rate of CVD events compared with patients with a score less than 100.

Future studies, however, should be performed with magnetic resonance imaging because this technology enables more accurate visualization of plaque composition and vulnerability. In addition, this technique will also allow the assessment of functional properties of the artery wall.

Brachial Artery Flow-Mediated Vasodilation

Brachial artery flow-mediated vasodilation is a test of endothelial dysfunction that is associated with the early stages of atherosclerosis. The measurement is done by assessing end-diastolic brachial artery diameters continually before and after a short period of forearm ischemia. The superimposed blood flow and increased shear stress after ischemia stimulates local nitric oxide release from the endothelium resulting in vasodilation. NAFLD is inversely correlated with percent brachial flow-mediated vasodilation independent of components of the metabolic syndrome.[43] Although this test of endothelial dysfunction does not provide additional predictive value to the Framingham risk score, the test independently predicts incident cardiovascular events in adults without known CVD.[44] Aside from the difficulty in reproducibility and nonexisting cutoff levels between normal and abnormal test results, variability of the vasodilation can be ascribed to inconsistency of the endothelial response and environmental factors.

Pulse-Wave Velocity

Pulse-wave velocity is the proposed gold standard of arterial stiffness and an indicator for early atherosclerosis.[45] This method calculates pulse-wave propagation velocity between 2 sites. Following the documentation of the distance between the 2 recording sites, the determination of the pulse transit time allows calculation of the pulse-wave velocity. Studies have suggested that aortic pulse-wave velocity predicts cardiovascular mortality, coronary heart disease, and stroke regardless of cardiovascular risk factors.[46,47] Increased pulse-wave velocity is observed in patients with NAFLD independent of age, sex, and features of the metabolic syndrome.[48] These findings are supported by the fact that biopsy-proven NAFLD is an independent determinant of pulse-wave velocity.[49]

NAFLD AND CVD INCIDENCE

Given the strong association between NAFLD and markers of subclinical CVD, it is important to investigate if this also results in an increased incidence of cardiovascular event.

Liver Enzymes as Surrogate Marker for the Diagnosis of NAFLD

Several prospective studies have shown that elevated gamma-glutamyl transferase (GGT), as a surrogate marker of NAFLD, is independently associated with the incidence of CVD. In a study of 163,944 Austrian adults followed for up to 17 years, elevated GGT was significantly associated with total CVD mortality.[50] In addition, a longitudinal increase in GGT from baseline normal levels in another Austrian study suggests an increased risk of CVD mortality.[51] Albeit the confounding effect of alcohol consumption to GGT elevation, a recent meta-analysis analyzing 10 prospective studies indicated that, even in the subgroup of nondrinkers, an increase of 1 U/L of natural logged GGT is associated with an increased risk of coronary heart disease, stroke, or both.[52] In patients with no history of coronary heart disease, stroke, or diabetes, an increase in GGT not only predicts 24-year fatal coronary heart disease and stroke regardless of other cardiovascular risk factors but also provides prognostic information beyond that of the Framingham risk score for coronary heart disease and CVD mortality.[53] Thus, GGT may be a promising prognostic index in cardiovascular risk stratification.

The potential role of ALT, another surrogate marker of NAFLD, in predicting cardiovascular events has been controversial. The Hoorn study has reported a positive association between ALT and 10-year coronary heart disease events independent of traditional risk factors and features of the metabolic syndrome.[54] Ioannou and colleagues[55] suggested that patients with elevated ALT, in the absence of viral hepatitis or excessive alcohol consumption, have a higher calculated risk of coronary heart disease based on the Framingham risk score. On the contrary, a meta-analysis of 2 studies by Fraser and colleagues[52] indicated a negative association of ALT with coronary heart disease, stroke, or both. This finding is supported in multivariate-adjusted analyses in the Framingham Offspring Heart Study and an Australian study by Olynyk and colleagues that observed no significant association between ALT and incident CVD events over a 20-year and 10-year follow-up period, respectively.[56,57] The incongruity in the findings may be attributed to age difference, length of follow-up, or underestimation of incident CVD because of various methodological definitions of incident CVD.

The mechanism behind the stronger association of GGT than ALT with CVD risk remains largely unknown. GGT may be involved directly in the pathogenesis of atherosclerosis by participating in extracellular catabolism of glutathione and contributing to atherosclerotic plaque formation.[58] In retrospect, caution should be exercised when correlating surrogate markers of NAFLD with CVD incidents because liver enzymes can be normal in patients with NAFLD and normal liver enzymes do not exclude significant underlying liver damage. Thus, large-scale prospective studies in patients with biopsy-proven NAFLD with incremental GGT or ALT values are necessary in an ideal setting to provide evidence as to whether an increase of GGT reflects the association between the progression of NAFLD and CVD events, above and beyond the established CVD risk factors, and whether NAFLD or elevated GGT can add additional information in CVD risk prediction.

Ultrasonography as Surrogate Marker for the Diagnosis of NAFLD

Few prospective studies have been performed to assess the relationship of the incidence of both fatal and nonfatal CVD events with NAFLD as judged by ultrasonography (**Table 1**). In the Valpolicella Heart Diabetes Study, with a follow-up of 5 years, findings have initially demonstrated that NAFLD is associated with an increased incidence of CVD among patients with diabetes after controlling for sex, age, smoking, diabetes duration, hemoglobin A1C, low-density lipoprotein cholesterol, medications, and metabolic syndrome.[59] Subsequently, the same cohort complements the previous outcomes during a follow-up of 6.5 years.[60] This study, however, constitutes a high-risk group to develop CVD because of the presence of diabetes. Hamaguchi and colleagues[61] have reported that, among healthy male and female Japanese patients, NAFLD retains an independent correlation with CVD events in multivariate analyses.

With regard to fatal CVD outcomes only, 2 studies with different follow-up periods have conflicting findings. Haring and colleagues[62] demonstrated that a hyperechogenic ultrasound in correlation with elevated GGT has a higher all-cause and CVD mortality in men during a mean duration of 7.2 years of follow-up than elevated GGT only. Their study stresses the importance of performing liver ultrasound in patients with increased GGT levels for further CVD risk stratification. In contrast, a recent study by Lazo and colleagues[27] from the Third National Health and Nutrition Examination Survey cohort dismissed the association between NAFLD, with or without increased liver enzyme levels, and the increased risk of death from all-causes and CVD mortality in the US general population. Because of chronicity of the disease, additional prospective studies in the general population with a longer follow-up and inclusion of a complete panel of established risk factors are needed to correlate NAFLD with all-cause and specific-cause mortality.

To the authors' knowledge, there are no population-based studies that prospectively assess the association between histologically proven NAFLD and major cardiovascular events. The difficulty in performing liver biopsy in a population study

Table 1
Prospective studies linking ultrasound-diagnosed NAFLD to fatal or nonfatal CVD incidence

Authors	Study Population	Participants	Follow-Up Duration (y)	Cardiovascular Outcomes	Findings
Targher et al,[59] 2005	2103 patients with type 2 diabetes (aged 40–79 y) in the Valpolicella Heart Diabetes Study without CVD or secondary causes of chronic liver disease at baseline	248 with CVD events (94 NAFLD) and 496 without CVD events (56 NAFLD)	5	Cardiovascular death, nonfatal CHD (MI and coronary revascularization) and ischemic stroke	Increased risk of fatal and nonfatal CVD events independent of age, sex, smoking, diabetes duration, glycated hemoglobin, LDL-C, GGT, use of medications, and MS
Targher et al,[60] 2007	2103 patients with type 2 diabetes (aged 40–79 y) in the Valpolicella Heart Diabetes Study without CVD or secondary causes of chronic liver disease at baseline	384 with CVD events (96 NAFLD) and 1719 without CVD (61 NAFLD)	6.5	Cardiovascular death, nonfatal CHD (MI and coronary revascularization) and ischemic stroke	Increased risk of fatal and nonfatal CVD events independent of age, sex, smoking, diabetes duration, glycated hemoglobin, LDL-C, GGT, use of medications, and MS
Hamaguchi et al,[61] 2007	1637 healthy adults (aged 22–83 y) in Japan	231 with NAFD and 990 without NAFLD	5	Nonfatal CHD (unstable angina, acute MI, silent MI), ischemic stroke and cerebral hemorrhage	Increased risk of nonfatal CVD events independent of age, smoking, systolic blood pressure, LDL-C, and MS

| Haring et al,[62] 2009 | 4160 adults (aged 20–79 y) in the Study of Health in Pomerania without hepatitis B and C or liver cirrhosis at baseline | 1249 with hyperechogenic ultrasound pattern (779 in men and 470 in women) and 2911 with normal ultrasound (1265 in men and 1646 in women) | 7.2 | CVD mortality | Increased risk of CVD mortality among men with NAFLD and elevated GGT independent of age, waist circumference, alcohol consumption, physical activity, education level, civil status, equalized income, Functional Comorbidity Index, and multiplicative interaction term of continuous GGT with liver ultrasound |
| Lazo et al,[27] 2011 | 11,371 adults (aged 20–74 y) in the Third National Health and Nutrition Examination Survey of the US general population without viral hepatitis and iron overload | 426 with hepatic steatosis and increased liver enzyme levels, 2089 with hepatic steatosis only, and 8856 with no hepatic steatosis | 18 | CVD mortality | No increased risk of CVD mortality among patients with NAFLD, with or without increased liver enzyme levels, independent of sex, race, education, smoking, alcohol consumption, physical activity, body mass index, hypertension, hypercholesterolemia, and diabetes |

Abbreviations: CHD, coronary heart disease; LDL-C, low-density lipoprotein cholesterol; MI, myocardial infarction; MS, metabolic syndrome.

precludes not only the accurate diagnoses of hepatic steatosis and NASH but also the identification of progression of hepatic steatosis over time. This difficulty results in a potential nondifferential misclassification of NAFLD solely by liver ultrasound, which partially limits study findings because of its poor sensitivity when hepatic infiltration is less than 33%.[63] But because ultrasonography is accessible, safe, and cheap, it may be reasonable to consider it as the imaging of choice for screening fatty liver in clinical and population settings.

CVD: LEADING CAUSE OF DEATH IN NAFLD

Although CVD is close to malignancy as the leading cause of death in patients with biopsy-proven NAFLD,[64] several published studies have linked CVD as the primary cause of mortality (**Table 2**). In a 14-year follow-up, Ekstedt and colleagues[24] reported that patients with NASH die mainly of CVD, followed by extrahepatic malignancy and liver-related causes. Soderberg and colleagues[25] and Rafiq and colleagues[26] concur with the previous study that CVD is the main cause of death in patients with NAFLD who were followed for a mean period of 21 and 13 years, respectively. Sanyal and colleagues[65] indicated that cardiovascular mortality is higher in patients with cirrhosis caused by NASH than cirrhosis caused by hepatitis C over a 10-year follow-up. Given the relative small sample size of these studies, drawing a firm generalized conclusion will be premature at this point. Nevertheless, these studies further supplement the existing literature that mortality is higher in patients with NAFLD than in the general population.

BIOLOGIC MECHANISMS LINKING NAFLD TO CVD: ROLE OF HIGH-DENSITY LIPOPROTEIN

It is currently not entirely clear if NAFLD associated with CVD is a consequence of the common shared risk factors or whether NAFLD contributes to CVD independently of shared factors. As reviewed elsewhere,[18,66] expanded and inflamed visceral fat, especially in the steatotic and inflamed liver (NASH), releases inflammatory cytokines and adipokines and promotes insulin resistance. This release not only further aggravates liver disease but also promotes the secretion of procoagulant and antifibrinolytic agents and dyslipidemia. These factors have shown a positive correlation with cardiovascular events[67–69] and apparently play an important role in the development and progression of atherosclerosis.

NAFLD is associated with derangements of the lipoprotein metabolism resembling atherogenic dyslipidemia seen in insulin-resistance states, such as obesity and diabetes.[70] Atherogenic dyslipidemia, a strong independent risk factor for cardiovascular events, is characterized by (1) an increased number of large very-low-density lipoprotein particles; (2) an increased number of small, dense, low-density lipoprotein particles; and (3) by low levels of high-density lipoprotein cholesterol.[71] The link between low levels of high-density lipoprotein cholesterol and CVD is well established. The precise mechanism of low high-density lipoprotein cholesterol levels in NAFLD reflects a formation and maturation defect and, thus, seems not solely linked to insulin resistance (Fuchs and colleagues, unpublished data, 2012). The hypothesis that high-density lipoprotein function, rather than the absolute concentration of this lipoprotein, is key for developing CVD is gaining strength. Given the substantial heterogeneity in the particle size, charge, and protein composition of high-density lipoproteins, it may not be surprising that high-density lipoprotein cholesterol levels are poor functional surrogates for this lipoprotein. Cholesterol efflux capacity of high-density lipoprotein particles defined as the capacity of high-density lipoproteins to uptake lipids

Table 2
Longitudinal studies linking CVD as the leading cause of death in biopsy-proven NAFLD

Authors	Study Population	NAFLD Participants	Follow-Up Duration (y)	Outcomes	Major Findings
Adams et al,[64] 2005	420 patients in Olmsted County, Minnesota	65 diagnosed by imaging and biopsy, 5 by biopsy alone, and 348 by imaging alone	7.6	Death from any cause	Deaths mainly from malignancy, followed by ischemic heart disease and liver-related causes among patients with NAFLD
Sanyal et al,[65] 2006	152 adult patients with NASH and cirrhosis seen at Virginia Commonwealth University Medical Center	152 with cirrhosis caused by NASH and 150 controls with cirrhosis caused by HCV	10.0	Death from any cause	Deaths mainly from infection in both patients with NASH and HCV cirrhosis, followed by heart disease in patients with NASH and cirrhosis; Higher mortality from heart disease in patients with NASH and cirrhosis than patients with HCV and cirrhosis
Ekstedt et al,[24] 2006	212 patients in Sweden with persistently elevated serum aminotransferases or alkaline phosphatase	129 NAFLD at baseline (71 with NASH)	13.7	Death from any cause	Deaths mainly from CAD, followed by extrahepatic malignancy and liver-related causes among patients with NASH
Rafiq et al,[26] 2009	173 patients (131 from Cleveland Clinic Foundation and 42 from Clinic for Liver Diseases cohort)	173 NAFLD (101 with non-NASH and 72 with NASH)	18.5	Death from any cause	Deaths mainly from CAD, followed by extrahepatic malignancy and liver-related causes among patients with NAFLD
Soderberg et al,[25] 2010	256 patients in Sweden with persistently elevated serum aminotransferases	118 NAFLD (67 with bland steatosis and 51 with NASH)	21.0	Death from any cause	Deaths mainly from CVD, followed by extrahepatic malignancy and liver-related causes among patients with NAFLD

Abbreviations: CAD, coronary artery disease; HCV, hepatitis C virus.

from macrophages for biliary removal as part of the reverse cholesterol pathway has been shown to be independent of high-density lipoprotein cholesterol levels and inversely associated with carotid intima-media thickness and angiographically confirmed coronary artery disease.[72] Interestingly and not anticipated, patients with NASH had a cholesterol efflux capacity that was not impaired compared with controls (Fuchs and colleagues, unpublished data). This finding suggests that antioxidant or antiinflammatory properties of the high-density lipoprotein particles are linked to the increased CVD in NAFLD. This observation may become of great clinical importance because the farnesoid X receptor agonist obeticholic acid (INT-747), a promising new treatment approach for NAFLD,[73] is lowering high-density lipoprotein cholesterol levels likely via hepatic upregulation of the scavenger receptor B1 or the inhibition of apoA1 synthesis.[74,75] It is mandatory to prove that obeticholic acid, despite its high-density lipoprotein cholesterol lowering effect, will not increase the cardiovascular risk associated with NAFLD.

SUMMARY AND CLINICAL PERSPECTIVE

A growing body of evidence supports the association of NAFLD and in particular its necroinflammatory state, NASH, with the future incidence of cardiovascular events independent of traditional risk factors and features of the metabolic syndrome. It is accepted that CVD is the leading cause of morbidity and mortality in patients with NAFLD long before the development of clinically significant liver disease.

Awareness and prompt recognition of NAFLD is a first but critical step to initiate screening for the early detection of subclinical atherosclerosis in patients with NAFLD. Once identified at increased risk for adverse cardiac events, patients can be offered appropriate preventive therapy and education for behavioral change. Thus, the risk stratification of asymptomatic patients and identification of high-risk patients are critical initial steps in preventing future adverse cardiac events such as myocardial infarction and sudden cardiac death. The Framingham risk score is a traditional risk factor inventory-based scoring system that uses readily available variables, such as gender, age, total cholesterol, high-density lipoprotein cholesterol, systolic blood pressure, and cigarette use, to calculate the 10-year risk for cardiovascular events. Albeit suboptimal in cardiovascular risk stratification, it is recommended as a first step in coronary risk assessment.[76]

The use of ultrasonography to identify the intima-media thickness of the carotid artery and computed tomography for coronary artery calcifications evaluation can provide incremental prognostic information over the Framingham risk score.[76] Guidelines by the American College of Cardiology Foundation and American Heart Association recommend screening for carotid artery intima-media thickness in intermediate-risk asymptomatic individuals and for coronary artery calcifications in patients with diabetes who are aged 40 years and older and low- to intermediate-risk asymptomatic individuals.[77] Because NAFLD severity is associated with higher carotid artery intima-media thickness and coronary artery calcifications,[34,78] it seems reasonable to consider screening patients with NAFLD, especially those with NASH, with one or the other of these imaging modalities. Although coronary artery calcifications may have a superior prognostic value in predicting future coronary heart disease than intima-media thickness of the carotid artery,[79] cost and radiation exposure are major concerns. Therefore, ultrasonography may be the initial screening test of choice.

Abundant data from the past several decades indicate that inflammation plays an important role in the pathobiology of atherosclerosis, and NAFLD itself may independently contribute to low-grade systemic inflammation. C-reactive protein as a biomarker of inflammation offers only modest predictive value of coronary heart disease risk.[80] However, C-reactive protein correlates with the histologic severity of NAFLD[81] and, therefore, the measurement of serum C-reactive protein may be useful in the primary prevention of CVD in patients with NAFLD. GGT, a surrogate marker of NAFLD, may be a promising prognostic marker in cardiovascular risk stratification because epidemiologic studies have corroborated its strong independent association with incident CVD.[50–53,82] Further studies are needed to evaluate GGT's overall importance independent from C-reactive protein and other presently accepted biomarkers and relative to the traditional risk factors used for predicting CVD in patients with NAFLD.

Once a diagnosis of NAFLD is established, either in the presence or in the absence of features of the metabolic syndrome, the evaluation of global CVD risk must be sought. A multidisciplinary team approach is necessary, and the timely referral by primary care physicians to appropriate specialists is important not only for early intervention for their liver disease but also for aggressive treatment aimed at modifying cardiovascular risk factors. Lifestyle change with weight loss and exercise is the initial management among patients with NAFLD, whereas pharmacotherapy may be reserved in those with poor compliance or NASH.[83] Finally, appropriate-designed, large, randomized trials in patients with histologically proven NASH are needed to validate the prognostic value of NASH for future cardiovascular events and to elucidate whether ameliorating NASH will ultimately prevent or slow the development and progression of CVD.

REFERENCES

1. Angulo P. Nonalcoholic fatty liver disease. N Engl J Med 2002;346:1221–31.
2. Farrell GC, Larter CZ. Nonalcoholic fatty liver disease: from steatosis to cirrhosis. Hepatology 2006;43:S99–112.
3. Lazo M, Clark JM. The epidemiology of nonalcoholic fatty liver disease: a global perspective. Semin Liver Dis 2008;28:339–50.
4. Clark JM, Diehl AM. Nonalcoholic fatty liver disease: an underrecognized cause of cryptogenic cirrhosis. JAMA 2003;289:3000–4.
5. Neuschwander-Tetri BA, Caldwell SH. Nonalcoholic steatohepatitis: summary of an AASLD Single Topic Conference. Hepatology 2003;37:1202–19.
6. Browning JD, Szczepaniak LS, Dobbins R, et al. Prevalence of hepatic steatosis in an urban population in the United States: impact of ethnicity. Hepatology 2004; 40:1387–95.
7. Edmison J, McCullough AJ. Pathogenesis of non-alcoholic steatohepatitis: human data. Clin Liver Dis 2007;11:75–104.
8. Clark JM. The epidemiology of nonalcoholic fatty liver disease in adults. J Clin Gastroenterol 2006;40(Suppl 1):S5–10.
9. Dunn W, Schwimmer JB. The obesity epidemic and nonalcoholic fatty liver disease in children. Curr Gastroenterol Rep 2008;10:67–72.
10. Marchesini G, Brizi M, Bianchi G, et al. Nonalcoholic fatty liver disease: a feature of the metabolic syndrome. Diabetes 2001;50:1844–50.
11. Kotronen A, Yki-Järvinen H. Fatty liver: a novel component of the metabolic syndrome. Arterioscler Thromb Vasc Biol 2008;28:27–38.
12. Marchesini G, Bugianesi E, Forlani G, et al. Nonalcoholic fatty liver, steatohepatitis, and the metabolic syndrome. Hepatology 2003;37:917–23.
13. Marchesini G, Marzocchi R, Agostini F, et al. Nonalcoholic fatty liver disease and the metabolic syndrome. Curr Opin Lipidol 2005;16:421–7.

14. Mensah GA, Mokdad AH, Ford E, et al. Obesity, metabolic syndrome, and type 2 diabetes: emerging epidemics and their cardiovascular implications. Cardiol Clin 2004;22:485–504.

15. Yusuf S, Hawken S, Ounpuu S, et al. Effect of potentially modifiable risk factors associated with myocardial infarction in 52 countries (the INTERHEART study): case-control study. Lancet 2004;364:937–52.

16. Lorenzo C, Williams K, Hunt KJ, et al. The National Cholesterol Education Program - Adult Treatment Panel III, International Diabetes Federation, and World Health Organization definitions of the metabolic syndrome as predictors of incident cardiovascular disease and diabetes. Diabetes Care 2007;30:8–13.

17. Mottillo S, Filion KB, Genest J, et al. The metabolic syndrome and cardiovascular risk a systematic review and meta-analysis. J Am Coll Cardiol 2010;56:1113–32.

18. Targher G, Day CP, Bonora E. Risk of cardiovascular disease in patients with nonalcoholic fatty liver disease. N Engl J Med 2010;363:1341–50.

19. Targher G, Bertolini L, Padovani R, et al. Prevalence of nonalcoholic fatty liver disease and its association with cardiovascular disease among type 2 diabetic patients. Diabetes Care 2007;30:1212–8.

20. Targher G, Bertolini L, Padovani R, et al. Prevalence of non-alcoholic fatty liver disease and its association with cardiovascular disease in patients with type 1 diabetes. J Hepatol 2010;53:713–8.

21. Picardi A, Vespasiani-Gentilucci U. Association between non-alcoholic fatty liver disease and cardiovascular disease: a first message should pass. Am J Gastroenterol 2008;103:3036–8.

22. Ong JP, Pitts A, Younossi ZM. Increased overall mortality and liver-related mortality in non-alcoholic fatty liver disease. J Hepatol 2008;49:608–12.

23. Dunn W, Xu R, Wingard DL, et al. Suspected nonalcoholic fatty liver disease and mortality risk in a population-based cohort study. Am J Gastroenterol 2008;103:2263–71.

24. Ekstedt M, Franzén LE, Mathiesen UL, et al. Long-term follow-up of patients with NAFLD and elevated liver enzymes. Hepatology 2006;44:865–73.

25. Söderberg C, Stål P, Askling J, et al. Decreased survival of subjects with elevated liver function tests during a 28-year follow-up. Hepatology 2010;51:595–602.

26. Rafiq N, Bai C, Fang Y, et al. Long-term follow-up of patients with nonalcoholic fatty liver. Clin Gastroenterol Hepatol 2009;7:234–8.

27. Lazo M, Hernaez R, Bonekamp S, et al. Non-alcoholic fatty liver disease and mortality among US adults: prospective cohort study. BMJ 2011;343:d6891.

28. Simon A, Chironi G, Levenson J. Comparative performance of subclinical atherosclerosis tests in predicting coronary heart disease in asymptomatic individuals. Eur Heart J 2007;28:2967–71.

29. Lorenz MW, Markus HS, Bots ML, et al. Prediction of clinical cardiovascular events with carotid intima-media thickness: a systematic review and meta-analysis. Circulation 2007;115:459–67.

30. Cao JJ, Arnold AM, Manolio TA, et al. Association of carotid artery intima-media thickness, plaques, and C-reactive protein with future cardiovascular disease and all-cause mortality: the Cardiovascular Health study. Circulation 2007;116:32–8.

31. Simon A, Megnien JL, Chironi G. The value of carotid intima-media thickness for predicting cardiovascular risk. Arterioscler Thromb Vasc Biol 2010;30:182–5.

32. McKimmie RL, Daniel KR, Carr JJ, et al. Hepatic steatosis and subclinical cardiovascular disease in a cohort enriched for type 2 diabetes: the Diabetes Heart Study. Am J Gastroenterol 2008;103:3029–35.

33. Manco M, Bedogni G, Monti L, et al. Intima-media thickness and liver histology in obese children and adolescents with non-alcoholic fatty liver disease. Atherosclerosis 2010;209:463–8.
34. Targher G, Bertolini L, Padovani R, et al. Relations between carotid artery wall thickness and liver histology in subjects with nonalcoholic fatty liver disease. Diabetes Care 2006;29:1325–30.
35. Sookoian S, Pirola CJ. Non-alcoholic fatty liver disease is strongly associated with carotid atherosclerosis: a systematic review. J Hepatol 2008;49:600–7.
36. Johnsen SH, Mathiesen EB, Joakimsen O, et al. Carotid atherosclerosis is a stronger predictor of myocardial infarction in women than in men: a 6-year follow-up study of 6226 persons: the Tromsø study. Stroke 2007;38:2873–80.
37. Plichart M, Celermajer DS, Zureik M, et al. Carotid intima-media thickness in plaque-free site, carotid plaques and coronary heart disease risk prediction in older adults. The Three-City study. Atherosclerosis 2011;219:917–24.
38. Jain A, McClelland RL, Polak JF, et al. Cardiovascular imaging for assessing cardiovascular risk in asymptomatic men versus women: the multi-ethnic study of atherosclerosis (MESA). Circ Cardiovasc Imaging 2011;4:8–15.
39. Chen CH, Nien CK, Yang CC, et al. Association between nonalcoholic fatty liver disease and coronary artery calcification. Dig Dis Sci 2010;55:1752–60.
40. Assy N, Djibre A, Farah R, et al. Presence of coronary plaques in patients with nonalcoholic fatty liver disease. Radiology 2010;254:393–400.
41. Jung DH, Lee YJ, Ahn HY, et al. Relationship of hepatic steatosis and alanine aminotransferase with coronary calcification. Clin Chem Lab Med 2010;48:1829–34.
42. Arad Y, Goodman KJ, Roth M, et al. Coronary calcification, coronary disease risk factors, C-reactive protein, and atherosclerotic cardiovascular disease events: the St. Francis Heart study. J Am Coll Cardiol 2005;46:158–65.
43. Villanova N, Moscatiello S, Ramilli S, et al. Endothelial dysfunction and cardiovascular risk profile in nonalcoholic fatty liver disease. Hepatology 2005;42:473–80.
44. Yeboah J, Folsom AR, Burke GL, et al. Predictive value of brachial flow-mediated dilation for incident cardiovascular events in a population-based study: the multi-ethnic study of atherosclerosis. Circulation 2009;120:502–9.
45. Laurent S, Cockcroft J, Van Bortel L, et al. Expert consensus document on arterial stiffness: methodological issues and clinical applications. Eur Heart J 2006;27:2588–605.
46. Mattace-Raso FU, van der Cammen TJ, Hofman A, et al. Arterial stiffness and risk of coronary heart disease and stroke: the Rotterdam study. Circulation 2006;113:657–63.
47. Sutton-Tyrrell K, Najjar SS, Boudreau RM, et al. Elevated aortic pulse wave velocity, a marker of arterial stiffness, predicts cardiovascular events in well-functioning older adults. Circulation 2005;111:3384–90.
48. Salvi P, Ruffini R, Agnoletti D, et al. Increased arterial stiffness in nonalcoholic fatty liver disease: the Cardio-GOOSE study. J Hypertens 2010;28:1699–707.
49. Vlachopoulos C, Manesis E, Baou K, et al. Increased arterial stiffness and impaired endothelial function in nonalcoholic Fatty liver disease: a pilot study. Am J Hypertens 2010;23:1183–9.
50. Ruttmann E, Brant LJ, Concin H, et al. Gamma-glutamyl transferase as a risk factor for cardiovascular disease mortality: an epidemiological investigation in a cohort of 163,944 Austrian adults. Circulation 2005;112:2130–7.
51. Strasak AM, Kelleher CC, Klenk J, et al. Longitudinal change in serum gamma-glutamyl transferase and cardiovascular disease mortality: a prospective

population-based study in 76,113 Austrian adults. Arterioscler Thromb Vasc Biol 2008;28:1857–65.

52. Fraser A, Harris R, Sattar N, et al. Gamma-glutamyl transferase is associated with incident vascular events independently of alcohol intake: analysis of the British Women's Heart and Health Study and Meta-Analysis. Arterioscler Thromb Vasc Biol 2007;27:2729–35.

53. Wannamethee SG, Lennon L, Shaper AG. The value of gamma-glutamyl transferase in cardiovascular risk prediction in men without diagnosed cardiovascular disease or diabetes. Atherosclerosis 2008;201:168–75.

54. Schindhelm RK, Dekker JM, Nijpels G, et al. Alanine aminotransferase predicts coronary heart disease events: a 10-year follow-up of the Hoorn study. Atherosclerosis 2007;191:391–6.

55. Ioannou GN, Weiss NS, Boyko EJ, et al. Elevated serum alanine aminotransferase activity and calculated risk of coronary heart disease in the United States. Hepatology 2006;43:1145–51.

56. Goessling W, Massaro JM, Vasan RS, et al. Aminotransferase levels and 20-year risk of metabolic syndrome, diabetes, and cardiovascular disease. Gastroenterology 2008;135:1935–44.

57. Olynyk JK, Knuiman MW, Divitini ML, et al. Serum alanine aminotransferase, metabolic syndrome, and cardiovascular disease in an Australian population. Am J Gastroenterol 2009;104:1715–22.

58. Emdin M, Pompella A, Paolicchi A. Gamma-glutamyl transferase, atherosclerosis, and cardiovascular disease: triggering oxidative stress within the plaque. Circulation 2005;112:2078–80.

59. Targher G, Bertolini L, Poli F, et al. Nonalcoholic fatty liver disease and risk of future cardiovascular events among type 2 diabetic patients. Diabetes 2005; 54:3541–6.

60. Targher G, Bertolini L, Rodella S, et al. Nonalcoholic fatty liver disease is independently associated with an increased incidence of cardiovascular events in type 2 diabetic patients. Diabetes Care 2007;30:2119–21.

61. Hamaguchi M, Kojima T, Takeda N, et al. Nonalcoholic fatty liver disease is a novel predictor of cardiovascular disease. World J Gastroenterol 2007;13:1579–84.

62. Haring R, Wallaschofski H, Nauck M, et al. Ultrasonographic hepatic steatosis increases prediction of mortality risk from elevated serum gamma-glutamyl transpeptidase levels. Hepatology 2009;50:1403–11.

63. Saadeh S, Younossi ZM, Remer EM, et al. The utility of radiological imaging in nonalcoholic fatty liver disease. Gastroenterology 2002;123:745–50.

64. Adams LA, Lymp JF, St Sauver J, et al. The natural history of nonalcoholic fatty liver disease: a population-based cohort study. Gastroenterology 2005;129:113–21.

65. Sanyal AJ, Banas C, Sargeant C, et al. Similarities and differences in outcomes of cirrhosis due to nonalcoholic steatohepatitis and hepatitis C. Hepatology 2006; 43:682–9.

66. Fuchs M, Sanyal AJ. Non-alcoholic fatty liver disease: a pathophysiological perspective. In: Arias IM, Alter HJ, Boyer JL, et al, editors. The liver: biology and pathobiology. 5th edition. Chichester (UK): John Wiley & Sons; 2009. p. 719–41.

67. Ridker PM, Rifai N, Rose L, et al. Comparison of C-reactive protein and low-density lipoprotein cholesterol levels in the prediction of first cardiovascular events. N Engl J Med 2002;347:1557–65.

68. Cesari M, Penninx BW, Newman AB, et al. Inflammatory markers and onset of cardiovascular events: results from the Health ABC study. Circulation 2003;108: 2317–22.

69. Thögersen AM, Jansson JH, Boman K, et al. High plasminogen activator inhibitor and tissue plasminogen activator levels in plasma precede a first acute myocardial infarction in both men and women: evidence for the fibrinolytic system as an independent primary risk factor. Circulation 1998;98:2241–7.
70. Adiels M, Taskinen MR, Borén J. Fatty liver, insulin resistance, and dyslipidemia. Curr Diab Rep 2008;8:60–4.
71. Bamba V, Rader DJ. Obesity and atherogenic dyslipidemia. Gastroenterology 2007;132:2181–90.
72. Khera AV, Cuchel M, de la Llera-Moya M, et al. Cholesterol efflux capacity, high-density lipoprotein function, and atherosclerosis. N Engl J Med 2011;364:127–35.
73. Sanyal AJ, Mudaliar S, Henry RR, et al. A new therapy for nonalcoholic fatty liver disease and diabetes? INT-747–the first FXR hepatic therapeutic study. Hepatology 2009;50:389A.
74. Claudel T, Sturm E, Duez H, et al. Bile acid-activated nuclear receptor FXR suppresses apolipoprotein A-I transcription via a negative FXR response element. J Clin Invest 2002;109:961–71.
75. Evans MJ, Mahaney PE, Borges-Marcucci L, et al. A synthetic farnesoid X receptor (FXR) agonist promotes cholesterol lowering in models of dyslipidemia. Am J Physiol Gastrointest Liver Physiol 2009;296:G543–52.
76. Shah PK. Screening asymptomatic subjects for subclinical atherosclerosis: can we, does it matter, and should we? J Am Coll Cardiol 2010;56:98–105.
77. Greenland P, Alpert JS, Beller GA, et al. 2010 ACCF/AHA guideline for assessment of cardiovascular risk in asymptomatic adults: a report of the American College of Cardiology Foundation/American Heart Association Task Force on Practice Guidelines. J Am Coll Cardiol 2010;56:e50–103.
78. Lee YH, Wu YJ, Liu CC, et al. The severity of Fatty liver disease relating to metabolic abnormalities independently predicts coronary calcification. Radiol Res Pract 2011;2011:8. DOI: 10.1155/2011/586785 Article ID 586785.
79. Folsom AR, Kronmal RA, Detrano RC, et al. Coronary artery calcification compared with carotid intima-media thickness in the prediction of cardiovascular disease incidence: the Multi-Ethnic Study of Atherosclerosis (MESA). Arch Intern Med 2008;168:1333–9.
80. Danesh J, Wheeler JG, Hirschfield GM, et al. C-reactive protein and other circulating markers of inflammation in the prediction of coronary heart disease. N Engl J Med 2004;350:1387–97.
81. Yoneda M, Mawatari H, Fujita K, et al. High-sensitivity C-reactive protein is an independent clinical feature of nonalcoholic steatohepatitis (NASH) and also of the severity of fibrosis in NASH. J Gastroenterol 2007;42:573–82.
82. Lee DS, Evans JC, Robins SJ, et al. Gamma glutamyl transferase and metabolic syndrome, cardiovascular disease, and mortality risk: the Framingham Heart Study. Arterioscler Thromb Vasc Biol 2007;27:127–33 [Epub 2006 Nov 9].
83. Adams LA, Angulo P. Treatment of non-alcoholic fatty liver disease. Postgrad Med J 2006;82:315–22.

Psychological and Psychiatric Aspects of Treatment of Obesity and Nonalcoholic Fatty Liver Disease

Karen E. Stewart, PhD*, James L. Levenson, MD

KEYWORDS

- Psychiatric care • Psychological care • Nonalcoholic fatty liver disease • Obesity

KEY POINTS

- Chronic illnesses incur a tremendous cost to American lives in both dollars and quality of life.
- Multiple psychiatric conditions are associated with increased risk of obesity and these conditions can interfere with efforts at weight loss.
- The major relevant clinical issues regarding the use of psychiatric drugs in patients with nonalcoholic steatohepatitis include the effects of liver disease on pharmacokinetics; the potential adverse effects of hepatotoxicity, weight gain, glucose intolerance, and hyperlipidemia; and potential drug interactions with statins and other hypolipidemic drugs.
- Optimal management of comorbid mental health and chronic illness problems requires a multidisciplinary approach and a shift in our current treatment paradigm.

Chronic illnesses incur a tremendous cost to American lives in both dollars and quality of life. Outcomes in these illnesses are often affected by psychological, behavioral, and pharmacologic issues related to mental illness and psychological symptoms. This article focuses on psychological and psychiatric issues related to the treatment of obesity and NAFLD, including available weight-loss interventions, the complex relationship between psychiatric disorders and obesity, and special considerations in the use of psychiatric drugs in patients with or at risk for NAFLD and obesity. Recommendations for collaborative care of individuals with comorbid NAFLD and psychological disorders/symptoms are discussed.

The authors have no conflicts of interest to report.
Department of Psychiatry, Virginia Commonwealth University, 1200 East Broad Street, PO Box 980268, Richmond, VA 23298-0268, USA
* Corresponding author.
E-mail address: kstewart2@mcvh-vcu.edu

Clin Liver Dis 16 (2012) 615–629
doi:10.1016/j.cld.2012.05.007
1089-3261/12/$ – see front matter © 2012 Elsevier Inc. All rights reserved.

OBESITY AND NAFLD

NAFLD affects an estimated 20% to 30% of adults living in Western countries, with up to 80% of obese individuals being affected.[1] Prospective studies have documented that among individuals initially free of NAFLD, persons who developed NAFLD over the course of a 7-year follow-up had higher baseline body mass index (BMI; calculated as weight in kilograms divided by height in meters squared, ie, kg/m^2) and gained more weight than those who did not.[2] In persons with documented NAFLD, weight gain is associated with progression of liver fibrosis over long-term (13.8 ± 1.2 years) follow-up,[3] and weight loss, whether achieved through lifestyle change or medication, is associated with improvements in liver histopathology. Specifically, weight losses of 7% and more are associated with improved NAFLD Activity Score (NAS; a scoring system comprising 14 histologic features) whereas losses of 5% and greater are associated with improvement in steatosis only.[4] Thus, weight management is a critical component of care for the patient with NAFLD.

Obesity is a complex condition that calls for a multidisciplinary approach. Many disciplines (eg, genetics, neuroscience, endocrinology, psychology, public health) have identified factors that contribute to the risk of developing obesity; however, considerable work remains in determining its optimal prevention and treatment. Available treatment options for obesity include bariatric surgery, medications, and behaviorally based lifestyle interventions. Each of these options presents unique benefits and drawbacks, and each carries a risk of long-term weight regain, emphasizing the need for further research in promotion of long-term weight management.

WEIGHT-LOSS INTERVENTIONS

Weight-loss medications serve to reduce body weight by reducing appetite, increasing satiety, reducing absorption of nutrients, or increasing energy expenditure. On average, these medications can produce statistically significant, albeit modest weight loss (generally 2–7.9 kg compared with placebo); however, the lost weight most often is regained after the medication is discontinued. No weight-loss medication has been demonstrated to be safe, effective, and well-tolerated for long-term use. Many of these medications have suffered unfavorable risk-benefit profiles or serious adverse events over long-term use, and have ultimately been removed from the market (eg, fenfluramines, rimonabant, dinitrophenol, aminorex, and sibutramine). Several medications have been prescribed off-label for weight loss (fluoxetine, buproprion, topiramate), but randomized clinical trial data are lacking. At present, diethylpropion (an amphetamine-like analogue) and phentermine (a 5-hydroxytryptamine agonist) are approved by the Food and Drug Administration (FDA) for short-term use (up to 12 weeks), and only orlistat (a lipase inhibitor) is approved for long-term use. Unfortunately, weight loss with orlistat is relatively modest, and is not well tolerated because of unpleasant gastrointestinal side effects.[5] In comparing patients with nonalcoholic steatohepatitis (NASH) receiving diet and vitamin E therapy with or without the addition of orlistat, the orlistat group lost slightly more weight than the comparison group (8.3% vs 6.0% of initial body weight); however, this difference was not significant nor did the groups differ in their improvement in serum aminotransferases, steatosis, necroinflammation, ballooning, or NAS scores.[6]

Bariatric surgery is a treatment for high-risk individuals with clinically severe obesity. Current standards remain consistent with the 1991 recommendations delivered by the National Institutes of Health Consensus Development Conference Panel.[7] These guidelines recommend that to be a surgical candidate, a patient should have a BMI of 40 or greater, or a BMI of at least 35 if the individual has serious weight-related comorbidities (eg, severe obstructive sleep apnea, type 2 diabetes mellitus, or obesity-related cardiomyopathy). Weight loss after bariatric surgery varies according to type of surgery, and ranges from 48% of excess body weight (gastric banding) to 70% of excess body weight (bypass procedures).[8] Pooling across surgery types, approximately 92% of patients demonstrate improvement or resolution of steatosis following surgery, with 82% experiencing resolution or improvement of NASH and 66% experiencing improvement in fibrosis.[9]

Behaviorally based weight-management interventions commonly include weekly group or individual sessions for 6 months to a year. These programs focus on energy balance by increasing physical activity and reducing calorie intake, and teach specific behavioral skills for achieving these goals. Specifically, these interventions combine nutritional education with behavioral interventions including self-monitoring, changing environmental cues for overeating and inactivity, problem solving, goal setting, planning, restructuring maladaptive thinking patterns, and relapse prevention. Self-monitoring (ie, writing down one's daily food intake and physical activity, and tracking one's weight) is a central component of these interventions and appears to be an important predictor of long-term maintenance of weight loss.[10] Weight loss in such programs averages 9 kg or approximately 10% of initial body weight.[11] Weight regain commonly occurs when the intervention ends; however, extended contact with the provider can help sustain lifelong adherence to healthy eating and physical activity behaviors. Thus, obesity must be considered a chronic health problem, and some level of ongoing support is likely necessary to maintain treatment effects in the long term.[12] These interventions can be translated into Internet-based delivery systems and are capable of producing meaningful weight loss, although the average weight loss in such programs appears to be modest (4–7 kg) compared with traditional in-person behavioral programs.[13] Internet and mobile technologies nonetheless represent a ripe area for wide dissemination of such interventions. Another important priority in behavioral weight-management research is on improving outcomes by tailoring interventions to individual patient need.

SUBOPTIMAL WEIGHT LOSS AND WEIGHT REGAIN IN WEIGHT-LOSS PROGRAMS

In each of these types of weight-loss programs, a significant proportion of individuals either fail to achieve significant weight loss or regain weight following the initial stages of treatment. For example, fewer than 50% of individuals in 2 randomized clinical behavioral weight-loss trials in NAFLD achieved the 7% weight loss associated with improved outcomes.[14,15] Weight loss following bariatric surgery is maximal at 1 year, at which point progressive weight regain commonly begins (eg, 38% ± 7% of initial body weight following gastric bypass at 1 year becomes 25% ± 11% net loss at 10 years after gastric bypass). A deterioration in some of the specific health benefits of weight loss seems to accompany this weight regain, although an overall reduced risk of mortality is seen in bariatric samples compared with matched individuals receiving usual care of obesity.[16,17] These findings highlight the need for a greater understanding of the psychosocial forces that contribute to suboptimal weight loss and weight regain.

RELATION BETWEEN PSYCHIATRIC DISORDERS AND OBESITY

Weight-loss intervention trials typically exclude individuals with severe psychopathology (defined, eg, by Lazo and colleagues[15] as hospitalization for depression within the past 6 months and current diagnosis of psychotic or bipolar disorder; and by Promrat and colleagues[14] as psychiatric problems significant enough to prevent participation). Less severe psychiatric problems and eating disorders are often not tracked or reported in these trials, and the presence of these conditions may partially account for weight-loss outcomes. The following sections review the relation between different psychiatric conditions and obesity and the impact of these conditions on outcomes in weight-management programs.

Mood/Anxiety Disorders

Relation to obesity

Mood disorders are associated with a greater risk of obesity after controlling for the use of psychotropic medications that can cause weight gain.[18] Unipolar depression and obesity demonstrate a bidirectional relationship; that is, the presence of either condition at baseline confers a greater risk of developing the other condition in prospective analyses.[19,20] Increased prevalence of overweight has been noted in an Italian sample of drug-naïve patients with bipolar disorder (40.8% compared with the national rate estimated to be ~16% during the time of data collection).[21]

A past-year diagnosis with an anxiety disorder is also associated with increased risk of obesity.[18] A large population-based sample recently demonstrated that a past-year diagnosis of posttraumatic stress disorder (PTSD) is associated with increased risk of obesity compared with individuals with no lifetime history of PTSD after adjusting for psychotropic medication use, sociodemographic factors, and depression.[22] Obesity was associated with a past-year history of panic attacks in men participating in a large Canadian nationally representative survey. For women participating in this survey, obesity was associated with a past-year history of social phobia or lifetime history of agoraphobia without panic disorder.[23]

Impact on outcomes in weight-loss interventions

Depression is relatively common in individuals seeking behavioral weight-management services, and depressed individuals have poorer weight-loss outcomes when participating in these interventions. In one clinic-based program, 17% of treatment-seeking obese individuals were diagnosed with major depression. Only 16% of depressed individuals met the program goal of losing 7% or more of initial body weight, compared with 38% of nondepressed participants meeting this goal. Depressed individuals may be more likely to drop out of a weight-loss program,[24] and depressive symptoms are a risk factor for weight regain.[10] Fortunately, it appears that depressed individuals experience a significant reduction in depressive symptoms when participating in a behavioral weight-management program. Exercise-only interventions also appear to have a slightly more modest, but significant positive impact on depressive symptoms.[25]

Eating Disorders

Relation to obesity

Binge-eating disorder (BED) and night-eating syndrome (NES) are commonly associated with increased BMI. BED is not a formal diagnosis in the American Psychiatric Association *Diagnostic and Statistical Manual of Mental Disorders* (Fourth Edition, Text Revised) (DSM-IV), but is included as a diagnosis for further study.[26] BED, a condition characterized by binge eating without the use of compensatory strategies (eg, vomiting, laxative use, over-exercising) has been recommended by the Eating Disorders Workgroup for inclusion in the forthcoming DSM-V.[27] BED is estimated to occur in 2% of the general population, and in from 10% to 20% of patients in obesity clinics. Rates of BED in patients seeking bariatric surgery have been variable (6%–47%).[28] This variability likely is due to inconsistencies in assessment methods and diagnostic criteria, and these rates are much lower when gold-standard assessment tools and strict diagnostic criteria are used (eg, 4.2%–6.6% in a rigorously assessed bariatric sample).[29] Although obesity is not required for a diagnosis of BED, the two are closely related, with 42.4% of individuals with BED qualifying as obese (BMI ≥30) in a national comorbidity study.[30]

NES is a condition not currently included in the DSM-IV. The core feature of this condition is excessive nighttime eating defined as at least 25% of food intake occurring after the evening meal and/or waking during the night to eat. This condition is frequently accompanied by morning anorexia, sleep difficulties, and worsening mood during evening hours.[31] NES is estimated to occur in 1.5% of the general population, in 9% to 14% of treatment-seeking obese individuals, and in 9% to 42% of bariatric surgery candidates.[28] As with BED, rates of NES are typically lower in samples where strict diagnostic criteria and rigorous assessment methods are used (eg, 1.9%–8.9% in a bariatric sample).[29] Although rates of NES are elevated in samples of persons with weight problems, the prevalence of obesity in those with NES remains equivocal, partly because of variability in defining this condition.[32]

Impact on outcomes in weight-management interventions

The presence of BED is associated with poorer weight-loss outcomes in weight-loss studies.[24] However, individuals with BED have reported rather unstable recent weight histories on enrolling in treatment cohorts. For example, participants reported gaining an average of 4.3 kg (range −18.1 kg to +28.1 kg) in the year before initiating therapy. Thus, maintaining a stable weight or losing a modest amount of weight might represent a significant improvement for individuals with BED as they gain control over their eating patterns.[33] CBT for BED is superior to behavioral weight management in achieving abstinence from binge eating; however, weight-loss outcomes in CBT are poorer than those seen in weight-management interventions.[34] A recent study compared CBT with behavioral weight loss and a sequenced CBT followed by behavioral weight-loss intervention. As expected, CBT was superior for abstinence from binge eating, behavioral weight loss was superior for weight loss, and the sequenced program did not improve results on either outcome. Thus, patients will likely benefit most from either CBT or behavioral weight loss, and treatment selection may best be determined by the patient's preferred treatment goal.

Other Psychiatric Disorders

Relation to obesity

Whether schizophrenia contributes to risk of obesity independent of the effect of the use of psychotropic medication remains uncertain. One study has documented increased BMI, visceral fat, and plasma cortisol in drug-naïve and drug-free schizophrenics compared with age-matched healthy controls. This sample was small (n = 15 schizophrenics, 7 were drug naïve and 8 were drug free), however, and drug free was defined as no oral neuroleptics for 6 weeks and no intramuscular treatments for 6 months,[35] so the generalizability of these findings is limited.

Attention-deficit/hyperactivity disorder (ADHD) has also been demonstrated to be associated with greater likelihood of being overweight or obese in a nationally representative sample, and the relationship between ADHD and obesity appears to be partially accounted for by associated BED.[36]

Impact on outcomes in weight-management interventions

Individuals with schizophrenia are often not included in standard weight-management programs, although several studies have evaluated medications to prevent/treat antipsychotic medication-related weight gain. Metformin has shown the greatest weight-loss potential (mean −2.94 kg) compared with placebo in these patients.[37] Some of these studies have combined lifestyle intervention with medication treatment, and this combination appears to improve outcomes more than medication therapy alone.[38]

POTENTIAL MECHANISMS LINKING MENTAL HEALTH AND OBESITY

In addition to weight gain associated with psychotropic medications, several common factors may contribute to the risk of both obesity and psychiatric disorders, including habitual inactivity, neuroinflammation, insufficient access to health care, alterations in neurometabolism, and oxidative stress.[39] Psychiatric illnesses also alter behavioral patterns in ways that could increase the risk of obesity. A large study using United States national representative data found that the link between major depression and obesity in women may be accounted for by shifts in food intake and physical activity levels.[40] Analysis of the 1999 Large Health Survey of Veterans (N = 501,161) revealed that compared with their healthy peers, veterans with schizophrenia, PTSD, or bipolar disorder were at elevated risk of reporting a pattern of poor health behaviors, defined as the co-occurrence of obesity, inactivity, and current smoking.[41]

PSYCHOTHERAPIES

The evidence base for cognitive-behavioral therapies (CBT) for mood, anxiety, and eating disorders is quite strong (see Ref.[42] for a review of meta-analyses). CBT emphasizes the links between thoughts, feelings, and behaviors, and seeks to guide patients to bring about improvements in mood and psychosocial functioning through altering maladaptive patterns of thought and behavior. One meta-analysis of direct comparisons of CBT against psychiatric medications for the treatment of anxiety and depression concluded that these 2 treatment modalities appear to have roughly comparable short-term outcomes, with an advantage for CBT in the treatment of panic disorder and a small nonsignificant advantage for edication in the treatment of social anxiety.[43] Other types of efficacious psychotherapies include interpersonal psychotherapy, problem-solving therapy, nondirective supportive therapy, behavioral activation therapy,[44] social skills training, and psychodynamic therapies.[45]

THE USE OF PSYCHIATRIC DRUGS IN PATIENTS WITH NASH

The major relevant clinical issues regarding the use of psychiatric drugs in patients with NASH include the effects of liver disease on pharmacokinetics; the potential adverse effects of hepatotoxicity, weight gain, glucose intolerance, and hyperlipidemia; and potential drug interactions with statins and other hypolipidemic drugs.

Effects of Liver Disease on Pharmacokinetics

Most psychiatric drugs are eliminated via metabolism by the liver and/or excretion by the kidney. There are 2 phases of hepatic metabolism: phase I metabolism consists of oxidation (ie, cytochrome P450 system), reduction, or hydrolysis, and phase II metabolism consists of conjugation (glucuronidation, acetylation, and sulfation). Clearance of drugs may be limited by either the rate of delivery (ie, hepatic blood flow) of the drug to the liver or the capacity of hepatic enzymes to metabolize the drug. Clinically significant decreases in hepatic blood flow occur only in severe cirrhosis, whereby portosystemic shunting reduces metabolic capacity.

Early fatty liver disease (steatosis) usually does not require dose alteration of psychiatrics, but steatohepatitis may require dosage adjustment depending on the severity of liver dysfunction. In patients whose disease has progressed to cirrhosis, drug dosing will require significant modification. All plasma proteins are synthesized in the liver, so protein binding is altered in liver disease. The main clinical significance of this is that in chronic severe liver disease, blood levels of psychiatrics that bind to plasma proteins (eg, tricyclic antidepressants and α1-acid glycoprotein) must be interpreted while taking into account the reduction in protein binding. When prescribing hepatically metabolized psychiatric drugs to patients with impaired liver function, it is advisable to reduce the initial dose and titrate more slowly. For more detailed reviews of these principles, see Ferrando and colleagues,[46] Crone and colleagues,[47] and Owen.[48]

Antidepressants

Antidepressant drugs are used to treat mood, anxiety, eating, and some somatoform disorders as well as insomnia, enuresis, incontinence, headaches, and chronic pain. All antidepressants rarely can cause idiosyncratic hepatotoxicity. Because severe hepatotoxicity appeared to be more common with nefazodone, it was removed from the market in many countries (it is still available generically in the United States), and it should not be used in patients with preexisting liver disease.[49] Reports of duloxetine-associated hepatotoxicity in 1% of patients prompted product warnings, but a subsequent review suggests hepatotoxicity is no more common with duloxetine than with other antidepressants.[50]

Weight gain is a relatively common problem during both acute and chronic treatment with antidepressants. Tricyclic antidepressants (TCAs) and mirtazapine most commonly cause weight gain, which is less common with serotonin reuptake inhibitors (SSRIs), and even less so with serotonin-norepinephrine reuptake inhibitors (SNRIs). Bupropion is the only antidepressant that appears to never cause weight gain.[51]

In the absence of weight gain, antidepressants do not cause glucose intolerance, but there is reason to think that SSRIs might (slightly) improve glucose metabolism. However, in diabetic patients with neuropathic pain, TCAs or SNRIs are preferred for their analgesic effects.

Several antidepressants, including mirtazapine, paroxetine, and sertraline, have been reported to increase low-density lipoprotein (LDL) cholesterol, but this effect appears to be linked to weight gain.[52,53]

All antidepressants are extensively metabolized by the liver, resulting in decreased clearance and prolonged half-life in patients with significant hepatic dysfunction. In such patients the starting dose should be reduced 50% and maintenance doses should also be reduced. Fluoxetine has an especially long half-life (because of the long half-life of its pharmacologically active metabolite norfluoxetine), and may require dosing less often than daily. Anticholinergic TCAs may precipitate or aggravate hepatic encephalopathy in patients with cirrhosis through anticholinergic central nervous system effects and through slowing gastrointestinal transit.

Lithium

Lithium is used to treat bipolar disorder, and in treatment-resistant depression to augment antidepressant response. Lithium does not have any hepatotoxicity. Weight gain is the second most common reason cited by patients for lithium noncompliance.[54] Increased thirst and polyuria are nearly universal side effects caused by lithium's blockade of antidiuretic hormone in the kidney, and some of the weight gain in patients taking lithium has been attributed to increased consumption of high-calorie fluids in response to thirst.[55] Another possible contribution to weight gain with chronic lithium treatment is overt (8%–10%) or subclinical hypothyroidism (20%). In the absence of weight gain and hypothyroidism, lithium does not cause glucose intolerance or hyperlipidemia.

Although lithium is excreted entirely by the kidney, its use may be difficult in patients with advanced cirrhosis because of fluid shifts due to ascites, diuretics, secondary hyperaldosteronism, and gastrointestinal bleeding, as well as other changes in renal function.

Anticonvulsant Mood Stabilizers

Anticonvulsant mood stabilizers (not all anticonvulsants) are used to treat bipolar disorders as well as chronic pain. Valproate, carbamazepine, and oxcarbazepine are the most commonly used anticonvulsant mood stabilizers for the treatment of mania, and lamotrigine for bipolar depression. Anticonvulsants commonly cause transient elevations in liver enzymes.[56] Significant changes in liver function are usually reversible with dosage reduction or discontinuation, but fatal hepatotoxicity has been reported with valproate and carbamazepine. The risk of hepatic failure may be increased by combination therapy and/or the presence of chronic liver disease.[57]

Weight gain is a common cause of noncompliance, especially with valproate. Carbamazepine less commonly causes weight gain, lamotrigine has little effect on weight, and topiramate causes a small weight loss.[58–60] In the absence of weight gain, anticonvulsants appear to have little effect on glucose or lipid metabolism.

Most anticonvulsants are extensively metabolized by the liver, resulting in decreased clearance and prolonged half-life in patients with significant hepatic dysfunction. Lower starting and maintenance doses are advisable. Oxcarbazepine requires less dose reduction than carbamazepine. Gabapentin and pregabalin are renally excreted, and dose adjustment is not necessary unless renal function is impaired.

Antipsychotics

Antipsychotics are used to treat schizophrenia, bipolar disorder, treatment-resistant depression and anxiety disorders, delirium, and psychosis in patients with dementia. Liver enzyme elevations during antipsychotic therapy have long been reported but seldom require drug discontinuation. If present, mild to moderate elevations in hepatic aminotransferases and alkaline phosphatase usually occur early in treatment and are unlikely to result in hepatic dysfunction. Cholestatic jaundice is a rare idiosyncratic reaction reported with phenothiazines.

Almost all antipsychotics can cause weight gain, to varying degrees. Among the older typical antipsychotics, the greatest risk of weight gain is with low-potency agents such as thioridazine and chlorpromazine. Molindone appeared to be the only typical antipsychotic that did not cause weight gain, but this agent is no longer available in the United States. With some of the newer atypical antipsychotics, substantial weight gain has been a serious clinical problem. The greatest to least likelihood of weight gain is: clozapine > olanzapine >> quetiapine > risperidone = paliperidone > aripiprazole > ziprasidone.[61]

The atypical antipsychotics have been reported to cause hyperglycemia, new-onset type 2 diabetes, and occasionally ketoacidosis. These effects are not solely explained by weight gain. Patients may also be at risk because schizophrenia and bipolar disorder are themselves associated with increased risk for type 2 diabetes. Similar to the risk for weight gain, the relative risk for causing or aggravating glucose intolerance is: clozapine = olanzapine > quetiapine > risperidone.[62] It is not clear that ziprasidone and aripiprazole cause hyperglycemia, but the FDA warning has been applied to the entire class of atypical antipsychotics.

Phenothiazines (eg, chlorpromazine), but not butyrophenones (eg, haloperidol) have long been known to elevate serum levels of cholesterol and triglycerides. The risk of hyperlipidemia among atypical antipsychotics is highest with clozapine, olanzapine, and quetiapine, and lowest with risperidone, ziprasidone, and aripiprazole.[63] Thus, in a patient with NASH the preferred antipsychotics would be those least likely to cause weight gain, glucose intolerance, and hyperlipidemia, for example, ziprasidone and aripiprazole among the atypical antipsychotics, and haloperidol and fluphenazine among the typical antipsychotics. Guidelines for the use of atypical antipsychotics jointly developed by the American Diabetes Association and the American Psychiatric Association[64] require regular monitoring of weight, waist circumference, blood pressure, fasting glucose, and lipid profile.

All antipsychotics are extensively metabolized by the liver, resulting in decreased clearance and prolonged half-life in patients with significant hepatic dysfunction. Lower starting and maintenance doses are advisable with all antipsychotics.

Benzodiazepines and Nonbenzodiazepine Sedatives

Benzodiazepines are used to treat anxiety disorders, sleep disorders, and alcohol withdrawal. Nonbenzodiazepine sedatives (eszopiclone, zopiclone, zolpidem, zaleplon) are prescribed for insomnia. Neither is associated with hepatotoxicity, weight gain, glucose intolerance, or hyperlipidemia. However, in patients with cirrhosis, benzodiazepines and nonbenzodiazepine sedatives (including barbiturates) can precipitate hepatic encephalopathy. Most benzodiazepines and nonbenzodiazepine sedatives are extensively metabolized by the liver. The exceptions are lorazepam, temazepam, and oxazepam, because they are metabolized predominantly by phase II conjugation, which is relatively preserved in chronic liver disease, making them the preferred sedatives in patients with impaired liver function.

Buspirone

Buspirone is used to treat generalized anxiety disorder, and has no significant effects on hepatic function, weight, glucose, or lipid metabolism. Buspirone is extensively metabolized by the liver, so lower starting and maintenance doses are advisable in patients with impaired liver function.

Psychostimulants

Psychostimulants are used in the treatment of ADHD, narcolepsy, treatment-resistant depression, apathy, and analgesia augmentation in severe pain. The commonly prescribed psychostimulant medications include methylphenidate, various amphetamines, atomoxetine, modafinil, and armodafinil. Pemoline has been withdrawn in many countries including the United States because of its potentially fatal hepatotoxicity. Although psychostimulants may cause appetite suppression and weight loss, this is uncommon at therapeutic doses. Psychostimulants at therapeutic doses have no appreciable effects on hepatic function, glucose, or lipid metabolism. All psychostimulants are extensively metabolized by the liver, requiring dose reduction in patients with significant hepatic dysfunction. The exception is methylphenidate, which appears to be predominantly metabolized in the bloodstream.

Cholinesterase Inhibitors and Memantine

Tacrine is now rarely prescribed because of frequent reversible hepatotoxicity.[65] Other cholinesterase inhibitors and memantine are well tolerated, with no appreciable effects on hepatic function, weight, glucose, or lipid metabolism. While all of the cholinesterase inhibitors require hepatic metabolism, donepezil requires less dose adjustment than galantamine and rivastigmine. Memantine is primarily eliminated by the kidney and does not require dose adjustment in patients with liver disease.

Drug Interactions Between Hypolipidemic and Psychiatric Drugs

The statins are all substrates for CYP 3A4. Nefazodone and carbamazepine are potent 3A4 inhibitors and can raise statin levels significantly. Less strong inhibition of 3A4 occurs with norfluoxetine (primary metabolite of fluoxetine) and oxcarbazepine. Lovastatin, simvastatin, atorvastatin, and fenofibrate are inhibitors of P-glycoprotein, and can increase absorption of buspirone by a factor of 5 to 10.[48,49] A summary of the potential hepatotoxicity, weight gain, glucose intolerance, hyperlipidemia, and metabolism/excretion with psychiatric medication is given in **Table 1**.

RECOMMENDATIONS FOR CLINICAL DECISION MAKING

NAFLD is a serious obesity-related condition, and bariatric surgery should be considered for patients with NAFLD and BMI of 35 or greater, as this treatment currently offers the greatest long-term potential for weight loss. Patients with a BMI less than 35 or who prefer nonsurgical weight loss should be referred for behavioral weight-management services. Group interventions or individual therapy with a behaviorally trained mental health professional with experience in health behavior change can be effective in promoting and maintaining weight loss. Although individuals with depression and/or BED may have poorer weight-loss outcomes than others, they can lose weight and they may benefit both psychologically and physically by participating in a weight-management program. Interventions that sequence treatment to focus first on BED and then weight loss do not appear to enhance either weight loss or abstinence from binge-eating outcomes, thus patients should be referred for either BED treatment or weight-management–focused treatment according to their preference. Individuals with severe mental illness (eg, suicidal ideation, avolition, psychotic symptoms, severe anxiety) should, of course, be referred for psychological/psychiatric evaluation and treatment. Medications for weight loss are not recommended, as no existing options have been demonstrated to be both safe and effective for long-term use.

Optimal management of comorbid mental health and chronic illness problems requires a shift in our current treatment paradigm. Models that integrate medical and mental health care in the clinic setting have received growing interest in recent years and have been demonstrated to provide superior outcomes compared with usual care. Collaborative care models vary in their specific structure, but a program implemented at the University of Washington serves as an excellent example. In their intervention group, nurses, primary care physicians, a psychiatrist, and a psychologist collaborated in providing structured visits with patients with diabetes, coronary heart disease, or both conditions, and comorbid depression. Compared with usual care, the patients receiving collaborative care showed greater improvement in all 4 disease-outcome measures (glycated hemoglobin, systolic blood pressure, LDL cholesterol, and depressive symptoms). Collaborative care patients were also more satisfied

Table 1
Psychiatric drugs in patients with NASH

Drug	Potential Hepatotoxicity	Weight Gain	Glucose Intolerance	Hyperlipidemia	Metabolism/ Excretion
Antidepressants					
Tricyclics	Rare	++	–	–	Hepatic
SSRIs, SNRIs	Rare	+	–	–	Hepatic
Bupropion	Rare	–	–	–	Hepatic
Mirtazapine	Rare	++	–	–	Hepatic
Trazodone	Rare	++	–	–	Hepatic
Mood Stabilizers					
Lithium	–	++	–	–	Renal
Valproate	+	++	–	–	Hepatic
Carbamazepine	+	+	–	–	Hepatic
Oxcarbazepine	Rare	+	–	–	Hepatic
Lamotrigine	Rare	–	–	–	Hepatic
Antipsychotics					
Chlorpromazine	+	++	–	–	Hepatic
Haloperidol	Rare	+	–	–	Hepatic
Clozapine	+	+++	++	++	Hepatic
Olanzapine	Rare	+++	++	++	Hepatic
Quetiapine	Rare	++	+	+	Hepatic
Risperidone	Rare	+	±	±	Hepatic
Aripiprazole	Rare	rare	–	–	Hepatic
Ziprasidone	Rare	–	–	–	Hepatic
Sedative-Hypnotics					
Lorazepam, temazepam, oxazepam	Hepatic encephalopathy in cirrhosis	–	–	–	Hepatic phase II conjugation
Other benzodiazepines	Hepatic encephalopathy in cirrhosis	–	–	–	Hepatic phase I and II
Eszopiclone, zopiclone, zolpidem, zaleplon	Hepatic encephalopathy in cirrhosis	–	–	–	Hepatic
Buspirone	Rare	–	–	–	Hepatic
Stimulants					
Methylphenidate	–	–	–	–	Bloodstream
Amphetamines	–	–	–	–	Hepatic

with their care,[66] and satisfaction has been previously linked to better self-care behaviors and better outcomes.[67]

REFERENCES

1. Ruhl C, Everhart J. Epidemiology of nonalcoholic fatty liver. Clin Liver Dis 2004;8: 501–19, vii.

2. Zelber Sagi S, Lotan R, Shlomai A, et al. Predictors for incidence and remission of NAFLD in the general population during a seven-year prospective follow-up. J Hepatol 2012;56(5):1145–51.

3. Ekstedt M, Franzn L, Mathiesen U, et al. Long-term follow-up of patients with NAFLD and elevated liver enzymes. Hepatology 2006;44:865–73.

4. Musso G, Cassader M, Rosina F, et al. Impact of current treatments on liver disease, glucose metabolism and cardiovascular risk in non-alcoholic fatty liver disease (NAFLD): a systematic review and meta-analysis of randomised trials. Diabetologia 2012;55(4):885–904.

5. Ioannides Demos L, Piccenna L, McNeil J. Pharmacotherapies for obesity: past, current, and future therapies. J Obes 2011;2011:179674.

6. Harrison S, Fecht W, Brunt E, et al. Orlistat for overweight subjects with nonalcoholic steatohepatitis: a randomized, prospective trial. Hepatology 2009;49:80–6.

7. Gastrointestinal surgery for severe obesity: National Institutes of Health Consensus Development Conference Statement. Am J Clin Nutr 1992;55: 615S–9S.

8. Buchwald H, Avidor Y, Braunwald E, et al. Bariatric surgery: a systematic review and meta-analysis. JAMA 2004;292:1724–37.

9. Mummadi R, Kasturi K, Chennareddygari S, et al. Effect of bariatric surgery on nonalcoholic fatty liver disease: systematic review and meta-analysis. Clin Gastroenterol Hepatol 2008;6:1396–402.

10. Wing R, Phelan S. Long-term weight loss maintenance. Am J Clin Nutr 2005;82: 222S–5S.

11. Wing RR. Behavioral weight control. In: Wadden TA, Stunkard AJ, editors. Handbook of obesity treatment. New York: The Guilford Press; 2002. p. 301–16.

12. Perri MG, Corsica JA. Improving the maintenance of weight lost in behavioral treatment of obesity. In: Wadden TA, Stunkard AJ, editors. Handbook of obesity treatment. New York: The Guilford Press; 2002. p. 357–82.

13. Tate D. A series of studies examining Internet treatment of obesity to inform Internet interventions for substance use and misuse. Subst Use Misuse 2011; 46:57–65.

14. Promrat K, Kleiner D, Niemeier H, et al. Randomized controlled trial testing the effects of weight loss on nonalcoholic steatohepatitis. Hepatology 2010;51: 121–9.

15. Lazo M, Solga S, Horska A, et al. Effect of a 12-month intensive lifestyle intervention on hepatic steatosis in adults with type 2 diabetes. Diabetes Care 2010;33: 2156–63.

16. Sjstrm L, Lindroos A, Peltonen M, et al. Lifestyle, diabetes, and cardiovascular risk factors 10 years after bariatric surgery. N Engl J Med 2004;351:2683–93.

17. Sjstrm L, Narbro K, Sjstrm CD, et al. Effects of bariatric surgery on mortality in Swedish obese subjects. N Engl J Med 2007;357:741–52.

18. Bodenlos J, Lemon S, Schneider K, et al. Associations of mood and anxiety disorders with obesity: comparisons by ethnicity. J Psychosom Res 2011;71: 319–24.

19. Luppino F, de Wit L, Bouvy P, et al. Overweight, obesity, and depression: a systematic review and meta-analysis of longitudinal studies. Arch Gen Psychiatry 2010;67:220–9.

20. Blaine B. Does depression cause obesity?: a meta-analysis of longitudinal studies of depression and weight control. J Health Psychol 2008;13:1190–7.

21. Maina G, Salvi V, Vitalucci A, et al. Prevalence and correlates of overweight in drug-naïve patients with bipolar disorder. J Affect Disord 2008;110:149–55.

22. Pagoto S, Schneider K, Bodenlos J, et al. Association of post-traumatic stress disorder and obesity in a nationally representative sample. Obesity (Silver Spring) 2012;20:200–5.

23. Mather A, Cox B, Enns M, et al. Associations of obesity with psychiatric disorders and suicidal behaviors in a nationally representative sample. J Psychosom Res 2009;66:277–85.

24. Pagoto S, Bodenlos J, Kantor L, et al. Association of major depression and binge eating disorder with weight loss in a clinical setting. Obesity (Silver Spring) 2007; 15:2557–9.

25. Fabricatore AN, Wadden TA, Higginbotham AJ, et al. Intentional weight loss and changes in symptoms of depression: a systematic review and meta-analysis. Int J Obes 2011;35:1363–76.

26. AMA. Diagnostics and statistics manual of mental disorders. Text Revision. 4th edition. Washington, DC: American Psychiatric Association; 2000.

27. American Psychiatric Association: DSM 5 development. Available at: http://www.dsm5.org/ProposedRevision/Pages/FeedingandEatingDisorders.aspx. Accessed February 27, 2012.

28. Allison K, Crow S, Reeves R, et al. Binge eating disorder and night eating syndrome in adults with type 2 diabetes. Obesity (Silver Spring) 2007;15:1287–93.

29. Allison K, Wadden T, Sarwer D, et al. Night eating syndrome and binge eating disorder among persons seeking bariatric surgery: prevalence and related features. Obesity (Silver Spring) 2006;14(Suppl 2):77S–82S.

30. Hudson J, Hiripi E, Pope H, et al. The prevalence and correlates of eating disorders in the National Comorbidity Survey Replication. Biol Psychiatry 2007;61:348–58.

31. Allison K, Lundgren J, O'Reardon J, et al. Proposed diagnostic criteria for night eating syndrome. Int J Eat Disord 2010;43:241–7.

32. Gallant AR, Lundgren J, Drapeau V. The night-eating syndrome and obesity. Obes Rev 2012;13(6):528–36.

33. Barnes R, Blomquist K, Grilo C. Exploring pretreatment weight trajectories in obese patients with binge eating disorder. Compr Psychiatry 2011;52:312–8.

34. Masheb R, Grilo C, Rolls B. A randomized controlled trial for obesity and binge eating disorder: low-energy-density dietary counseling and cognitive-behavioral therapy. Behav Res Ther 2011;49:821–9.

35. Thakore JH, Mann JN, Vlahos I, et al. Increased visceral fat distribution in drug-naive and drug-free patients with schizophrenia. Int J Obes 2002;26:137–41.

36. Pagoto S, Curtin C, Lemon S, et al. Association between adult attention deficit/hyperactivity disorder and obesity in the US population. Obesity (Silver Spring) 2009;17:539–44.

37. Maayan L, Vakhrusheva J, Correll C. Effectiveness of medications used to attenuate antipsychotic-related weight gain and metabolic abnormalities: a systematic review and meta-analysis. Neuropsychopharmacology 2010;35:1520–30.

38. Wu R, Zhao J, Jin H, et al. Lifestyle intervention and metformin for treatment of antipsychotic-induced weight gain: a randomized controlled trial. JAMA 2008; 299:185–93.

39. McIntyre R, Alsuwaidan M, Goldstein B, et al. The Canadian Network for Mood and Anxiety Treatments (CANMAT) task force recommendations for the management of patients with mood disorders and comorbid metabolic disorders. Ann Clin Psychiatry 2012;24:69–81.

40. Dave D, Tennant J, Colman G. Isolating the effect of major depression on obesity: role of selection bias. J Ment Health Policy Econ 2011;14:165–86.

41. Chwastiak L, Rosenheck R, Kazis L. Association of psychiatric illness and obesity, physical inactivity, and smoking among a national sample of veterans. Psychosomatics 2011;52:230–6.

42. Butler A, Chapman J, Forman E, et al. The empirical status of cognitive-behavioral therapy: a review of meta-analyses. Clin Psychol Rev 2006;26:17–31.

43. Roshanaei Moghaddam B, Pauly M, Atkins D, et al. Relative effects of CBT and pharmacotherapy in depression versus anxiety: is medication somewhat better for depression, and CBT somewhat better for anxiety? Depress Anxiety 2011; 28:560–7.

44. Cuijpers P, Andersson G, Donker T, et al. Psychological treatment of depression: results of a series of meta-analyses. Nord J Psychiatry 2011;65:354–64.

45. Cuijpers P, van Straten A, Andersson G, et al. Psychotherapy for depression in adults: a meta-analysis of comparative outcome studies. J Consult Clin Psychol 2008;76:909–22.

46. Ferrando SJ, Owen JA, Levenson JL, editors. Clinical manual of psychopharmacology in the medically ill. Washington, DC: American Psychiatric Publishing, Inc; 2010.

47. Crone CC, Dobbelstein CR. Gastrointestinal disorders. In: Levenson JL, editor. American Psychiatric Publishing textbook of psychosomatic medicine. second edition. Washington, DC: American Psychiatric Publishing, Inc; 2011. p. 463–90.

48. Owen JA. Psychopharmacology. In: Levenson JL, editor. American Psychiatric Publishing textbook of psychosomatic medicine. 2nd edition. Washington, DC: American Psychiatric Publishing, Inc; 2011. p. 957–1020.

49. Stewart DE. Hepatic adverse reactions associated with nefazodone. Can J Psychiatry 2002;47:375–7.

50. McIntyre RS, Panjwani ZD, Nguyen HT, et al. The hepatic safety profile of duloxetine: a review. Expert Opin Drug Metab Toxicol 2008;4:281–5.

51. Papakostas GI. Tolerability of modern antidepressants. J Clin Psychiatry 2008; 69(Suppl E1):8–13.

52. Le Melledo JM, Pilar Castillo AM, Newman S, et al. The effects of newer antidepressants on low-density lipoprotein cholesterol levels. J Clin Psychiatry 2004;65: 1017–8.

53. McIntyre RS, Soczynska JK, Konarski JZ, et al. The effect of antidepressants on lipid homeostasis: a cardiac safety concern? Expert Opin Drug Saf 2006;5: 523–37.

54. Gitlin MJ, Cochran SD, Jamison KR. Maintenance lithium treatment: side effects and compliance. J Clin Psychiatry 1989;50:127–31.

55. McEvoy GE. American Hospital Formulary Service (AHFS) drug information 2008. Bethesda (MD): American Society of Health-System Pharmacists Inc; 2008.

56. Bjornsson E. Hepatotoxicity associated with antiepileptic drugs. Acta Neurol Scand 2008;118:281–90.

57. Konig SA, Schenk M, Sick C, et al. Fatal liver failure associated with valproate therapy in a patient with Friedreich's disease: review of valproate hepatotoxicity in adults. Epilepsia 1999;40:1036–40.

58. Mendlewicz J, Souery D, Rivelli SK. Short-term and long-term treatment for bipolar patients: beyond the guidelines. J Affect Disord 1999;55:79–85.

59. Chengappa KN, Chalasani L, Brar JS, et al. Changes in body weight and body mass index among psychiatric patients receiving lithium, valproate, or topiramate: an open-label, nonrandomized chart review. Clin Ther 2002;24:1576–84.

60. Biton V, Mirza W, Montouris G, et al. Weight change associated with valproate and lamotrigine monotherapy in patients with epilepsy. Neurology 2001;56:172–7.

61. Haddad P. Weight change with atypical antipsychotics in the treatment of schizophrenia. J Psychopharmacol 2005;19:16–27.
62. Miller EA, Leslie DL, Rosenheck RA. Incidence of new-onset diabetes mellitus among patients receiving atypical neuroleptics in the treatment of mental illness: evidence from a privately insured population. J Nerv Ment Dis 2005;193:387–95.
63. Meyer JM, Koro CE. The effects of antipsychotic therapy on serum lipids: a comprehensive review. Schizophr Res 2004;70:1–17.
64. American Diabetes Association, American Psychiatric Association, American Association of Clincial Endocrinologists. Consensus development conference on antipsychotic drugs and obesity and diabetes. Diabetes Care 2004;27: 596–601.
65. Watkins PB, Zimmerman HJ, Knapp MJ, et al. Hepatotoxic effects of tacrine administration in patients with Alzheimer's disease. JAMA 1994;271:992–8.
66. Katon W, Lin EH, Von Korff M, et al. Collaborative care for patients with depression and chronic illnesses. N Engl J Med 2010;363:2611–20.
67. Sherbourne C. Antecedents of adherence to medical recommendations: results from the Medical Outcomes Study. J Behav Med 1992;15:447–68.

Management of Nonalcoholic Steatohepatitis

An Evidence-Based Approach

Suzanne E. Mahady, MD[a,b], Jacob George, MD, PhD[a],*

KEYWORDS

- Nonalcoholic steatohepatitis • Fatty liver • Therapy • Exercise • Diet

KEY POINTS

- This review of the current evidence base for the management of nonalcoholic steatohepatitis highlights the paucity of data relative to the high prevalence of the disease. In hepatology, this is all the more apparent given the major advances in the treatment of other liver disorders such as viral hepatitis and hepatocellular carcinoma.
- Current practice comprises a mixture of lifestyle modification with nutraceutical and potential pharmacologic treatments, without a high level of evidence that any of these approaches improves liver-related outcomes.
- Better designed and adequately powered studies of current approaches and novel treatments, with clinical end points, are urgently required.

INTRODUCTION

Nonalcoholic fatty liver disease (NAFLD) and its progressive form, nonalcoholic steatohepatitis (NASH), are an increasingly common cause of chronic liver disease in the developed world, with NASH projected to be the leading cause of liver transplantation in the United States by 2020.[1] The aim of treatment in NASH is to reduce progression to advanced fibrosis, cirrhosis, and its sequelae. However, the optimal treatment remains uncertain because of the perceived futility of lifestyle modification, adverse effects of drug therapies, and the narrow selection criteria, suboptimal availability, and costs of bariatric surgery. Effective therapies for NASH are a research priority not only to reduce the projected burden of liver disease but also because of emerging evidence that NASH is associated with incident cardiovascular disease independent of traditional risk factors.[2]

Disclosures: None.
[a] Storr Liver Unit, Westmead Millennium Institute, University of Sydney and Department of Gastroenterology and Hepatology, Westmead Hospital, Hawkesbury Road, Westmead, New South Wales 2145, Australia; [b] Sydney School of Public Health, University of Sydney, Camperdown, New South Wales 2006, Australia
* Corresponding author.
E-mail address: jacob.george@sydney.edu.au

Clin Liver Dis 16 (2012) 631–645
doi:10.1016/j.cld.2012.05.003
1089-3261/12/$ – see front matter © 2012 Elsevier Inc. All rights reserved.

liver.theclinics.com

This review addresses current data from the perspective of levels of evidence[3] for the various therapeutic options in NASH, including lifestyle modification, drug therapies, and bariatric surgery. Such an approach has not previously been taken, including in the published guidelines by the American Association for the Study of Liver Diseases,[4] the European Association for the Study of the Liver,[5] and the Asian Pacific Association for the Study of the Liver,[6] and is therefore timely. In particular, behavioral therapies to assist patients in adopting lifestyle changes are highlighted and a research agenda for future NASH management is presented.

LIFESTYLE MODIFICATION

Lifestyle modification remains the standard of care for patients with NASH. By definition, it is a tripartite and holistic approach incorporating dietary, exercise, and behavioral changes. However, there is little robust evidence to support these recommendations, with minimal trial-based data and the relevant observational studies at high risk of multiple biases. The lack of adequate methodology led to the publication of a position paper that addresses desirable aspects of study design for trials in NASH,[7] in particular the use of histologic end points as the preferred outcome measure.

Despite these limitations, lifestyle modification should be promoted because it offers a range of associated health benefits. It reduces progression to diabetes in susceptible patients,[8–10] which is sustained[11] and reproducible across ethnicities.[12] Lifestyle modification improves associated cardiovascular risk factors including hypertension[13] and all-cause mortality,[14,15] and is not associated with significant side effects.

What Evidence is Available from Controlled Trials of Lifestyle Modification in People with NASH?

To date, there are few randomized controlled trials of lifestyle modification in NASH with liver histology as the primary outcome. At present, the best evidence comes from a trial by Promrat and colleagues.[16] This trial in 31 patients used portion-controlled meals, exercise (200 minutes per week), and behavioral strategies with a weight loss aim of 7% to 10% from baseline. Change in NASH histologic score at 48 weeks was the primary outcome measure. The investigators found a significant improvement in steatohepatitis in patients in the intensive treatment arm, proportional to weight loss; however, an improvement in fibrosis was not observed (possibly due to short trial duration). A second trial of 60 patients with histologically confirmed NASH[17] treated with a low-fat diet and exercise (200 minutes per week), and with 30 participants additionally randomized to an antioxidant supplement, also found significant improvements in necroinflammation. These studies provide good evidence that rigorous lifestyle modification translates to histologic benefit, but the generalizability of these results to average clinic patients outside intensively supported trial conditions is unclear. Furthermore, long-term outcomes including sustainability of change remain unstudied in NASH. For patients across the spectrum of NAFLD, several other trials using hepatic steatosis or measures of insulin resistance as their outcome measure also show a benefit from lifestyle intervention.[18–20]

What Evidence is Provided by Observational Studies of Lifestyle Modification in People with NASH?

Observational studies of lifestyle modification are affected by a range of factors conferring a high likelihood of bias, and it is difficult to glean additional information over that provided by trials. The patient populations are heterogeneous, with variable definitions of NAFLD or NASH including abnormal transaminases or imaging with undefined increases in liver fat. This inconsistent case definition is likely to result in a substantial degree of misclassification bias. A recent systematic review of lifestyle modification in NASH found poor recording of alcohol intake and steatogenic drugs, likely further contributing to bias.[21] Other methodological concerns with observational studies include invalid and/or inaccurate measurement of study factors such as exercise. Self-reported questionnaires are often used instead of objective, validated tools, with some exceptions.[22] Choice and measurement of outcomes is lacking, with use of surrogate markers such as liver function tests or biochemical measures of insulin resistance, which are neither specific nor sensitive for histologic change associated with NASH. Therefore, well-conducted cohort studies with better defined study exposures and end points are needed to provide information applicable to patients who are atypical of trial populations.

Dietary Recommendations: What Evidence Exists to Support General Dietary Advice for People with NASH?

In both trials and observational studies, caloric restriction as a therapy for NASH has been used in several different formats including fat-restricted diets, carbohydrate-restricted diets, low-carbohydrate ketogenic diets, and high-protein diets. To date, they have not been directly compared in people with NASH, and it is unclear whether one diet is superior to another, with previous expert opinion supporting low-fat diets with a normal amount of carbohydrate (60%) and protein (>15%).[23] A recent, large-scale trial in overweight adults addressed this question with respect to efficacy in producing weight loss, comparing 4 different diets in more than 800 subjects over 2 years.[24] The investigators found that any caloric restriction resulted in a similar degree of weight loss irrespective of the macronutrient composition. However, sustainability of weight loss was not seen, as many participants regained weight at 12 months. At the other end of the spectrum, rapid weight loss (as may occur with ketogenic diets) may worsen steatohepatitis and should be avoided.[25–27] Therefore, patient-related factors such as personal preference may be the most important factor when choosing a diet type, but focusing on change in macronutrient composition and foods to avoid, rather than a calorically restricted diet, may prove more sustainable over the long term.

Dietary Recommendations on Specific Macronutrients: Omega-3 and the Mediterranean Diet

Certain macronutrients may offer additional benefit, and limited data suggest that changing macronutrient composition alone can be beneficial. Supplementation with polyunsaturated fatty acids has been of increasing interest after research indicated beneficial effects on hepatic lipogenesis and steatosis.[28] To support this hypothesis, people with NAFLD have lower dietary intake of polyunsaturated fatty acids,[29] a higher ratio of omega-6/omega-3 polyunsaturated fatty acids,[30] with the ratio in Western diets currently estimated at 1:16 compared with 1:1 in traditional diets,[31] and lower fish intake.[32] Increasing consumption of omega-3 polyunsaturated fatty acids improves hepatic lipid metabolism[33] and hepatic steatosis in cohort studies,[34,35] with limited trial-based data.[36,37] The lack of significant side effects[38] makes this an attractive therapeutic addition, and randomized controlled diets in humans to clarify the degree of benefit, timing, and dose are needed.

The Mediterranean diet has been used in the treatment of NAFLD. A small but well-conducted crossover trial[39] looked a 12 patients with NAFLD defined by magnetic resonance spectroscopy. Half of the patients were randomized to a Mediterranean diet and the others to a low-fat diet consistent with recommendations of the National Heart Foundation,[40] with a crossover at 6 weeks. Patients on the Mediterranean diet showed significant improvements in insulin sensitivity and reduction in liver fat of 39% in the absence of weight loss. Other trial-based data support significant improvements in insulin sensitivity in obese subjects.[41] It is likely that the principles of a Mediterranean diet will be beneficial for patients with NAFLD; however, the cost may be prohibitive for some.

Dietary Recommendations: Fructose and High-Fructose Corn Syrup

High levels of dietary fructose may be an independent risk factor for NAFLD.[42] Recent data have highlighted the differential hepatic metabolism of fructose compared with other sugars such as glucose, which may contribute to the development of the metabolic syndrome. In brief, glucose ingestion stimulates insulin secretion from the pancreas, causing leptin secretion and consequent satiety, whereas fructose does not.[43] Fructose also results in high rates of de novo lipogenesis, an effect not seen with glucose.[43] In animal models, high fructose consumption induces insulin resistance and impaired glucose tolerance.[44,45] These data, though not definitive, suggest a pathogenic role for fructose, and it seems reasonable to recommend that high dietary consumption of fructose should be avoided, although modest amounts of naturally occurring sources such as fruit are permissible.

A particular form of fructose, high-fructose corn syrup, is best avoided altogether. High-fructose corn syrup is produced by an industrial process involving the enzymatic isomerization of dextrose to fructose,[46] and was virtually absent from Western diets before 1970. Since then, the intake has steadily increased because of its inclusion in a wide range of soft drinks and processed foods, paralleling the increase in the metabolic syndrome in epidemiologic studies.[47] High-fructose corn syrup is detrimental for several reasons including its dense caloric content, impairment of normal satiety,[48,49] and its consumption often occurring in association with foods high in saturated fat.

Exercise Recommendations

Exercise provides metabolic benefits independent of weight loss in patients with NAFLD or NASH. A trial in obese patients with hepatic steatosis found that 4 weeks of cycling produced significant improvements in hepatic triglyceride, visceral adipose tissue, and free fatty acids, although weight was not significantly altered.[50] Further trial-based data in NAFLD supports a benefit of aerobic training without weight loss[20,22] with the benefit proportional to exercise intensity[22]; the benefits were reproducible in an older age group (mean >70 years).[51] Furthermore, trial evidence clearly indicates that exercise reduces associated cardiovascular risk factors. The totality of evidence for the numerous benefits of exercise should be highlighted to patients. Indeed, an increase in exercise alone may be the primary therapeutic focus in patients consistently unable to lose weight with caloric restriction, and who lose motivation for lifestyle changes because of this.

Exercise may not be a panacea for all, however, as mitochondrial biogenesis may be reduced in patients with NAFLD,[52] thereby reducing their response to this form of therapy. Moderate levels of mitochondrial dysfunction may be heritable in people with insulin resistance.[53] Furthermore, exercise may be precluded by cardiovascular comorbidities and osteoarthritis,[54] and a meta-analysis of counseling by primary care physicians indicated that intensive efforts did not necessarily increase physical activity.[55]

Behavioral Therapy

Clinicians who treat patients with NASH need to know not only the evidence for and rationale behind various recommendations but also how to counsel patients to improve adherence. Therefore, it is important to understand the principles of behavioral therapy, which is not part of the traditional domain of hepatologists but a critical part of managing those with NASH. Behavioral therapies are well studied in the diabetic literature, with good evidence for their efficacy. For example, both the Finnish Diabetes Prevention Study[8] and the US Diabetes Prevention Program[9] have shown that behavior change–based therapy is much more effective than usual care or metformin treatment in the prevention of diabetes in obese adults with impaired glucose tolerance.

Behavioral therapy is broadly defined as the use of psychological techniques to modify maladaptive behaviors, and differs on a theoretical basis from cognitive-behavioral therapy (CBT). Nevertheless, the application is similar in the management of obesity-related conditions[56] and CBT itself is likely to be effective in people with NAFLD.[57] In general, clinicians should adopt an "engaging counseling style"[58] that uses empathy, works with the patient to identify barriers to change, avoids stigmatization of the obese individual, and supports an individual's self efficacy, as empowerment is considered a key factor in success.[58] One should initially engage patients by discussing the benefits of lifestyle change and identifying barriers. For instance, lack of confidence and fear of falling have been independently associated with reluctance to exercise in a NAFLD cohort.[59] As an example, acknowledgment of the difficulty of losing weight (empathy) could be used, but followed by encouragement of uptake of self-proposed strategies (empowerment). Specific tools could be suggested, including self monitoring with food diaries, exercise logs, or pedometers. Previously fit patients should find encouragement in data suggesting that those with high cardiovascular fitness previously tend to gain fitness at a faster rate than those who were never fit.[60] Dietary modification should be instituted in small steps and reiterated at visits with other providers such as primary care physicians. Finally, a multidisciplinary approach with dietitians or psychologists delivering education in a group setting is helpful in patients with the metabolic syndrome,[8] and should be offered where available.

What Information Should be Offered Regarding Weight Loss?

Although the aforementioned data suggest that benefits in NAFLD can occur with change in macronutrient composition and exercise independent of weight loss, some patients may be highly motivated to lose weight, and clinicians should be cognizant of the amount that may be beneficial. Weight-loss aims have previously been recommended at 10% of body weight, based on historical data showing improvement in liver enzymes in overweight patients.[61] More recently, position statements from international associations recommend 7%.[5] In counseling patients on weight loss, it is important to highlight that even small amounts of weight loss may contribute significantly to reduction in intrahepatic fat, despite minimal change in total body weight, and reduction in hepatic fat is highly predictive of associated metabolic improvements.[62]

PHARMACOLOGIC THERAPIES FOR NASH

While lifestyle modification should remain the initial therapeutic approach for people with NASH, it will not be successful in a significant proportion and thus may not be sufficient to control disease progression. However, there is no consensus on the indications for pharmacologic treatment in NASH and when to initiate it, the clinical outcomes that should be achieved, and when treatment can be safely stopped. Current therapeutic options include insulin sensitizers, antioxidants, and a range of hepatoprotective agents.

Insulin Sensitizers

Insulin resistance is almost universal in NASH,[63,64] and amelioration of this with insulin sensitizers such as thiazolidinediones has been the subject of intense interest.

Thiazolidinediones improve insulin sensitivity via their action on peroxisome proliferator–activated receptor γ,[65] have anti-inflammatory[66] and antiatherosclerotic effects,[67] and increase circulating adiponectin.[68] Several well-conducted trials have been undertaken,[69–73] all with histologic end points, and generally show an improvement in steatosis and necroinflammation that occurs early.[74] A subsequent meta-analysis showed a small but significant improvement in fibrosis, with a number needed to treat to improve fibrosis of 1 in 13.[75]

However, the side effects of thiazolidinediones are clinically challenging and render these drugs unsuitable for routine use. On average, patients gain around 4 kg,[75] which is often unacceptable to patients who are overweight to begin with. Other side effects include cardiovascular morbidity with rosiglitazone[76] (not currently shown for pioglitazone[77]), bone loss and fracture risk[78,79] and, possibly, an increased risk of bladder cancer.[80] The risk-benefit ratio of thiazolidinediones is likely to be most favorable in older patients with advanced fibrosis who are unable to adopt lifestyle changes and have continuing risk factors for disease progression.[81] As an aside, patients with impaired glucose tolerance may gain additional benefit from thiazolidinediones, owing to their ability to prevent development of diabetes.[82,83]

Vitamin E

Vitamin E inhibits profibrotic activity in the liver,[84,85] and is inexpensive and well tolerated. Despite initial small, negative trials,[86,87] a large, well-conducted study of high-dose vitamin E in nondiabetic patients with biopsy-proven NASH (PIVENS[72]) showed a reduction in hepatic inflammation but not fibrosis. Vitamin E was not associated with any significant adverse effects in this trial; however, a meta-analysis of more than 135,000 patients taking vitamin E supplements found an increase in all-cause mortality (an additional 39 deaths per 10,000 people) for those on high-dose (400 IU) vitamin E.[88] This increase was dose dependent and began at 150 IU/d, clearly much less than the 800 IU/d trialed in PIVENS. These results should be borne in mind when using vitamin E, although the applicability is unclear because most patients in the meta-analysis had chronic health conditions that may have confounded the results.

Other Pharmacologic Therapies Trialed in NASH

Multiple other pharmacologic therapies have been trialed in NASH patients. Orlistat, an inhibitor of fat absorption, has been tested in a small but well-conducted trial,[89] where patients commenced on caloric restriction and vitamin E were randomized to receive orlistat or placebo. Histologic improvement was the primary end point at 36 weeks. Orlistat was not associated with statistically significant levels of weight loss or histologic improvement, but in patients who did lose weight, histologic improvement was proportional to the amount of weight lost. Other trials have also failed to show significant weight loss with orlistat,[90] therefore it cannot currently be recommended for people with NASH. Other drugs tested in trial-based settings include metformin,[73,87,91] ursodeoxycholic acid,[92–94] statins,[95] gemfibrozil,[96] probucol,[97] vitamin C,[98] betaine,[99] and N-acetylcysteine,[100] but convincing or consistent evidence for a benefit from any of these agents is lacking.

BARIATRIC SURGERY FOR NASH

Surgical treatment of obesity is attractive because of its ability to achieve a more sustained weight loss compared with medical therapy, but the selection criteria are narrow.[101] Bariatric surgery includes restrictive procedures (laparoscopic adjustable gastric banding [LAGB]) and malabsorptive procedures (Roux-en-Y gastric bypass, biliopancreatic diversion), and is indicated for morbid obesity (body mass index >40 or >35 kg/m^2) if associated with comorbidities such as insulin resistance, obstructive sleep apnea, and hypertension.[102] NASH alone is currently not an indication for bariatric surgery, and there are no controlled trials of bariatric surgery in NASH patients. Thus, data on changes in liver histology after surgery is mainly retrospective and heavily influenced by selection bias, and this should be borne in mind when applying the data to patients in the clinic.

In the context of selection bias, bariatric surgery results in impressive and sustained weight loss, and widespread improvement in metabolic abnormalities and liver histology. LAGB in 36 highly selected obese patients resulted in a mean weight loss of 34 kg and improvements in all histologic parameters including fibrosis.[103] Other case series have shown regression in fibrosis,[104] but this has not been seen in all studies.[105] A prospective cohort study shows that improvement in histology parallels that in insulin resistance.[106] A meta-analysis of the effect of bariatric surgery on NASH histology with 766 paired liver biopsies concluded that there were large and significant benefits in most parameters (66% of patients had improved fibrosis and 70% had complete resolution of NASH), but methodological flaws such as pooling in the presence of heterogeneity and likely publication bias make the quantitative results unreliable.[107] Whether one form of bariatric surgery is superior with respect to liver histology is unclear, but efficacy in causing weight loss is similar with both procedures.[108] The choice of bariatric surgery is usually determined by local regulatory and insurance factors, with gastric bypass commonly performed in the United States and LAGB the commonest procedure in countries such as Australia.[109]

Overall, the benefit of bariatric surgery for NASH remains controversial. Although there is good evidence that bariatric surgery improves aspects of the metabolic syndrome such as resolution of type 2 diabetes,[110] some experts question whether bariatric surgery is as effective in treating NASH,[111] particularly as fibrosis may continue to progress despite weight loss.[106] Of concern to hepatologists is the potential worsening of steatohepatitis with rapid weight loss induced by malabsorption, and the risk of hepatic decompensation in those with preexisting liver disease.[112] The side-effect profile is appreciable, although mortality has markedly improved since the advent of bariatric surgery in the 1950s; morbidity is currently estimated at 0.05% for LAGB and 0% to 5% for bypass procedures. Other side effects with LAGB include stomach prolapse, tube breakage, and erosions.[109]

NASH MANAGEMENT: A FUTURE RESEARCH AGENDA

A summary of the various treatment approaches for people with NASH, along with the associated level of evidence, is presented in **Table 1**. From this table it is clear that several areas remain a research priority if patients with NASH are to be treated effectively. Patient-related outcomes have not been well studied, and preferences for different treatment approaches in NASH are unknown. This information is needed to improve adherence to treatment, and to this end quality-of-life data should be included as an outcome in clinical trials of NASH, currently available for only one trial.[72] Trials of lifestyle modification should include well-defined diet and exercise interventions with histologic and clinical end points. For policy makers, cost-effectiveness data on treatment options and screening for metabolic comorbidities would be informative. Finally, there is increasing interest in a "parallel hits" hypothesis to account for the pathophysiology of NASH,[113] including the role of gut microbiota in the promotion of hepatic inflammation,[114] implying that therapeutic targets beyond insulin resistance may be the focus of future clinical trials.

Table 1
Levels of evidence[3] and methodological aspects of therapeutic studies in NASH

Therapeutic Option	Level of Evidence[a]	Histologic End Points	Liver-Related Clinical Outcomes Studied?	Patient-Oriented Outcomes (eg, QoL) Studied?	Cost-Efficacy Data Available?	Comments
Lifestyle modification (tripartite)	Low	Yes	No	No	No	
Exercise alone	Low	No	No	No	No	Trial data on NAFLD, not NASH patients
Thiazolidinediones	Moderate	Yes	No	Yes	No	
Vitamin E	Moderate	Yes	No	Yes	No	
Bariatric surgery	Very low	Yes	No	No	No	High risk of selection bias

Abbreviation: QoL, quality of life.

[a] Levels of evidence as per GRADE[3]: Moderate = further research is likely to have an important impact on our confidence in the estimate of effect and may change the estimate; Low = further research is very likely to have an important impact on our confidence in the estimate of effect and is likely to change the estimate; Very low = any estimate of effect is very uncertain.

SUMMARY

This review of the current evidence base for NASH management highlights the paucity of data relative to the high prevalence of the disease. In hepatology, this is all the more apparent given the major advances in the treatment of other liver disorders such as viral hepatitis and hepatocellular carcinoma. Current practice comprises a mixture of lifestyle modification with nutraceutical and potential pharmacologic treatments, without a high level of evidence that any of these approaches improves liver-related outcomes. Better designed and adequately powered studies of both current approaches and novel treatments, with clinical end points, are urgently required.

REFERENCES

1. Charlton MR, Burns JM, Pedersen RA, et al. Frequency and outcomes of liver transplantation for nonalcoholic steatohepatitis in the United States. Gastroenterology 2011;141:1249–53.
2. Targher G, Day CP, Bonora E. Risk of cardiovascular disease in patients with nonalcoholic fatty liver disease. N Engl J Med 2010;363:1341–50.
3. Atkins D, Best D, Briss PA, et al. Grading quality of evidence and strength of recommendations. BMJ 2004;328:1490.
4. Sanyal AJ. AGA technical review on nonalcoholic fatty liver disease. Gastroenterology 2002;123:1705–25.
5. Ratziu V, Bellentani S, Cortez-Pinto H, et al. A position statement on NAFLD/NASH based on the EASL 2009 special conference. J Hepatol 2010;53:372–84.
6. Farrell GC, Chitturi S, Lau GK, et al. Guidelines for the assessment and management of non-alcoholic fatty liver disease in the Asia-Pacific region: executive summary. J Gastroenterol Hepatol 2007;22:775–7.
7. Sanyal AJ, Brunt EM, Kleiner DE, et al. Endpoints and clinical trial design for nonalcoholic steatohepatitis. Hepatology 2011;54:344–53.
8. Tuomilehto J, Lindstrom J, Eriksson JG, et al. Prevention of type 2 diabetes mellitus by changes in lifestyle among subjects with impaired glucose tolerance. N Engl J Med 2001;344:1343–50.
9. Knowler WC, Barrett-Connor E, Fowler SE, et al. Reduction in the incidence of type 2 diabetes with lifestyle intervention or metformin. N Engl J Med 2002;346:393–403.
10. Ramachandran A, Snehalatha C, Mary S, et al. The Indian Diabetes Prevention Programme shows that lifestyle modification and metformin prevent type 2 diabetes in Asian Indian subjects with impaired glucose tolerance (IDPP-1). Diabetologia 2006;49:289–97.
11. Lindstrom J, Ilanne-Parikka P, Peltonen M, et al. Sustained reduction in the incidence of type 2 diabetes by lifestyle intervention: follow-up of the Finnish Diabetes Prevention Study. Lancet 2006;368:1673–9.
12. Kosaka K, Noda M, Kuzuya T. Prevention of type 2 diabetes by lifestyle intervention: a Japanese trial in IGT males. Diabetes Res Clin Pract 2005;67:152–62.
13. Laaksonen DE, Lindstrom J, Lakka TA, et al. Physical activity in the prevention of type 2 diabetes: the Finnish diabetes prevention study. Diabetes 2005;54:158–65.
14. Sesso HD, Paffenbarger RS Jr, Lee IM. Physical activity and coronary heart disease in men: the Harvard Alumni Health Study. Circulation 2000;102:975–80.
15. Wei M, Kampert JB, Barlow CE, et al. Relationship between low cardiorespiratory fitness and mortality in normal-weight, overweight, and obese men. JAMA 1999;282:1547–53.

16. Promrat K, Kleiner DE, Niemeier HM, et al. Randomized controlled trial testing the effects of weight loss on nonalcoholic steatohepatitis. Hepatology 2010; 51:121–9.

17. Vilar Gomez E, Rodriguez De Miranda A, Gra Oramas B, et al. Clinical trial: a nutritional supplement Viusid, in combination with diet and exercise, in patients with nonalcoholic fatty liver disease. Aliment Pharmacol Ther 2009;30:999–1009.

18. Lazo M, Solga SF, Horska A, et al. Effect of a 12-month intensive lifestyle intervention on hepatic steatosis in adults with type 2 diabetes. Diabetes Care 2010; 33:2156–63.

19. St George A, Bauman A, Johnston A, et al. Effect of a lifestyle intervention in patients with abnormal liver enzymes and metabolic risk factors. J Gastroenterol Hepatol 2009;24:399–407.

20. Sreenivasa Baba C, Alexander G, Kalyani B, et al. Effect of exercise and dietary modification on serum aminotransferase levels in patients with nonalcoholic steatohepatitis. J Gastroenterol Hepatol 2006;21:191–8.

21. Thoma C, Day CP, Trenell MI. Lifestyle interventions for the treatment of nonalcoholic fatty liver disease in adults: a systematic review. J Hepatol 2012; 56(1):255–66. DOI: 10.1016/j.jhep.2011.06.010 [Epub 2011 Jul 1].

22. St George A, Bauman A, Johnston A, et al. Independent effects of physical activity in patients with nonalcoholic fatty liver disease. Hepatology 2009;50: 68–76.

23. Zivkovic AM, German JB, Sanyal AJ. Comparative review of diets for the metabolic syndrome: implications for nonalcoholic fatty liver disease. Am J Clin Nutr 2007;86:285–300.

24. Sacks FM, Bray GA, Carey VJ, et al. Comparison of weight-loss diets with different compositions of fat, protein, and carbohydrates. N Engl J Med 2009; 360:859–73.

25. Andersen T, Gluud C, Franzmann MB, et al. Hepatic effects of dietary weight loss in morbidly obese subjects. J Hepatol 1991;12:224–9.

26. Rozental P, Biava C, Spencer H, et al. Liver morphology and function tests in obesity and during total starvation. Am J Dig Dis 1967;12:198–208.

27. Capron JP, Delamarre J, Dupas JL, et al. Fasting in obesity: another cause of liver injury with alcoholic hyaline? Dig Dis Sci 1982;27:265–8.

28. Xu J, Cho H, O'Malley S, et al. Dietary polyunsaturated fats regulate rat liver sterol regulatory element binding proteins-1 and -2 in three distinct stages and by different mechanisms. J Nutr 2002;132:3333–9.

29. Musso G, Gambino R, De Michieli F, et al. Dietary habits and their relations to insulin resistance and postprandial lipemia in nonalcoholic steatohepatitis. Hepatology 2003;37:909–16.

30. Cortez-Pinto H, Jesus L, Barros H, et al. How different is the dietary pattern in non-alcoholic steatohepatitis patients? Clin Nutr 2006;25:816–23.

31. Simopoulos AP. The importance of the ratio of omega-6/omega-3 essential fatty acids. Biomed Pharmacother 2002;56:365–79.

32. Zelber-Sagi S, Nitzan-Kaluski D, Goldsmith R, et al. Long term nutritional intake and the risk for non-alcoholic fatty liver disease (NAFLD): a population based study. J Hepatol 2007;47:711–7.

33. Levy JR, Clore JN, Stevens W. Dietary n-3 polyunsaturated fatty acids decrease hepatic triglycerides in Fischer 344 rats. Hepatology 2004;39:608–16.

34. Sekiya M, Yahagi N, Matsuzaka T, et al. Polyunsaturated fatty acids ameliorate hepatic steatosis in obese mice by SREBP-1 suppression. Hepatology 2003;38: 1529–39.

35. Capanni M, Calella F, Biagini MR, et al. Prolonged n-3 polyunsaturated fatty acid supplementation ameliorates hepatic steatosis in patients with non-alcoholic fatty liver disease: a pilot study. Aliment Pharmacol Ther 2006;23: 1143–51.

36. Zhu FS, Liu S, Chen XM, et al. Effects of n-3 polyunsaturated fatty acids from seal oils on nonalcoholic fatty liver disease associated with hyperlipidemia. World J Gastroenterol 2008;14:6395–400.

37. Spadaro L, Magliocco O, Spampinato D, et al. Effects of n-3 polyunsaturated fatty acids in subjects with nonalcoholic fatty liver disease. Dig Liver Dis 2008;40:194–9.

38. Parker HM, Johnson NA, Burdon CA, et al. Omega-3 supplementation and non-alcoholic fatty liver disease: a systematic review and meta analysis. J Hepatol 2011. DOI: 10.1016/j.jhep.2011.08.018.

39. Ryan MC, Itsiopoulos C, Ward G, et al. The Mediterranean diet: improvement in hepatic steatosis and insulin sensitivity in individuals with NAFLD. Hepatology 2011;54(Suppl 4):212A.

40. Canberra: National Health and Medical Research Council. Department of Health; 2005. Available at: http://www.nhmrc.gov.au/_files_nhmrc/publications/attachments/n31.pdf. Accessed February, 2012.

41. Shai I, Schwarzfuchs D, Henkin Y, et al. Weight loss with a low-carbohydrate, Mediterranean, or low-fat diet. N Engl J Med 2008;359:229–41.

42. Ouyang X, Cirillo P, Sautin Y, et al. Fructose consumption as a risk factor for non-alcoholic fatty liver disease. J Hepatol 2008;48:993–9.

43. Elliott SS, Keim NL, Stern JS, et al. Fructose, weight gain, and the insulin resistance syndrome. Am J Clin Nutr 2002;76:911–22.

44. Fields M, Lewis CG, Lure MD. Responses of insulin to oral glucose and fructose loads in marginally copper-deficient rats fed starch or fructose. Nutrition 1996; 12:524–8.

45. Martinez FJ, Rizza RA, Romero JC. High-fructose feeding elicits insulin resistance, hyperinsulinism, and hypertension in normal mongrel dogs. Hypertension 1994;23:456–63.

46. Bhosale SH, Rao MB, Deshpande VV. Molecular and industrial aspects of glucose isomerase. Microbiol Rev 1996;60:280–300.

47. Bray GA, Nielsen SJ, Popkin BM. Consumption of high-fructose corn syrup in beverages may play a role in the epidemic of obesity. Am J Clin Nutr 2004; 79:537–43.

48. Teff KL, Elliott SS, Tschop M, et al. Dietary fructose reduces circulating insulin and leptin, attenuates postprandial suppression of ghrelin, and increases triglycerides in women. J Clin Endocrinol Metab 2004;89:2963–72.

49. Shapiro A, Mu W, Roncal C, et al. Fructose-induced leptin resistance exacerbates weight gain in response to subsequent high-fat feeding. Am J Physiol Regul Integr Comp Physiol 2008;295:R1370–5.

50. Johnson NA, Sachinwalla T, Walton DW, et al. Aerobic exercise training reduces hepatic and visceral lipids in obese individuals without weight loss. Hepatology 2009;50:1105–12.

51. Finucane FM, Sharp SJ, Purslow LR, et al. The effects of aerobic exercise on metabolic risk, insulin sensitivity and intrahepatic lipid in healthy older people from the Hertfordshire Cohort Study: a randomised controlled trial. Diabetologia 2010;53:624–31.

52. Pessayre D. Role of mitochondria in non-alcoholic fatty liver disease. J Gastroenterol Hepatol 2007;22(Suppl 1):S20–7.

53. Petersen KF, Dufour S, Befroy D, et al. Impaired mitochondrial activity in the insulin-resistant offspring of patients with type 2 diabetes. N Engl J Med 2004;350:664–71.
54. Skarfors ET, Wegener TA, Lithell H, et al. Physical training as treatment for type 2 (non-insulin-dependent) diabetes in elderly men. A feasibility study over 2 years. Diabetologia 1987;30:930–3.
55. Eden KB, Orleans CT, Mulrow CD, et al. Does counseling by clinicians improve physical activity? a summary of the evidence for the U.S. Preventive Services Task Force. Ann Intern Med 2002;137:208–15.
56. Fabricatore AN. Behavior therapy and cognitive-behavioral therapy of obesity: is there a difference? J Am Diet Assoc 2007;107:92–9.
57. Moscatiello S, Di Luzio R, Bugianesi E, et al. Cognitive-behavioral treatment of nonalcoholic fatty liver disease: a propensity score-adjusted observational study. Obesity 2011;19:763–70.
58. Bellentani S, Dalle Grave R, Suppini A, et al. Behavior therapy for nonalcoholic fatty liver disease: the need for a multidisciplinary approach. Hepatology 2008; 47:746–54.
59. Frith J, Day CP, Robinson L, et al. Potential strategies to improve uptake of exercise interventions in non-alcoholic fatty liver disease. J Hepatol 2010;52:112–6.
60. Kantartzis K, Thamer C, Peter A, et al. High cardiorespiratory fitness is an independent predictor of the reduction in liver fat during a lifestyle intervention in non-alcoholic fatty liver disease. Gut 2009;58:1281–8.
61. Palmer M, Schaffner F. Effect of weight reduction on hepatic abnormalities in overweight patients. Gastroenterology 1990;99:1408–13.
62. Albu JB, Heilbronn LK, Kelley DE, et al. Metabolic changes following a 1-year diet and exercise intervention in patients with type 2 diabetes. Diabetes 2010; 59:627–33.
63. Marchesini G, Brizi M, Morselli-Labate AM, et al. Association of nonalcoholic fatty liver disease with insulin resistance. Am J Med 1999;107:450–5.
64. Chitturi S, Abeygunasekera S, Farrell GC, et al. NASH and insulin resistance: Insulin hypersecretion and specific association with the insulin resistance syndrome. Hepatology 2002;35:373–9.
65. Yki-Jarvinen H. Thiazolidinediones. N Engl J Med 2004;351:1106–18.
66. Ialenti A, Grassia G, Di Meglio P, et al. Mechanism of the anti-inflammatory effect of thiazolidinediones: relationship with the glucocorticoid pathway. Mol Pharmacol 2005;67:1620–8.
67. Sidhu JS, Kaposzta Z, Markus HS, et al. Effect of rosiglitazone on common carotid intima-media thickness progression in coronary artery disease patients without diabetes mellitus. Arterioscler Thromb Vasc Biol 2004;24:930–4.
68. Tonelli J, Li W, Kishore P, et al. Mechanisms of early insulin-sensitizing effects of thiazolidinediones in type 2 diabetes. Diabetes 2004;53:1621–9.
69. Belfort R, Harrison SA, Brown K, et al. A placebo-controlled trial of pioglitazone in subjects with nonalcoholic steatohepatitis. N Engl J Med 2006;355: 2297–307.
70. Ratziu V, Giral P, Jacqueminet S, et al. Rosiglitazone for nonalcoholic steatohepatitis: one-year results of the randomized placebo-controlled Fatty Liver Improvement with Rosiglitazone Therapy (FLIRT) Trial. Gastroenterology 2008; 135:100–10.
71. Aithal GP, Thomas JA, Kaye PV, et al. Randomized, placebo-controlled trial of pioglitazone in nondiabetic subjects with nonalcoholic steatohepatitis. Gastroenterology 2008;135:1176–84.

72. Sanyal AJ, Chalasani N, Kowdley KV, et al. Pioglitazone, vitamin E, or placebo for nonalcoholic steatohepatitis. N Engl J Med 2010;362:1675–85.

73. Idilman R, Mizrak D, Corapcioglu D, et al. Clinical trial: insulin-sensitizing agents may reduce consequences of insulin resistance in individuals with non-alcoholic steatohepatitis. Aliment Pharmacol Ther 2008;28:200–8.

74. Ratziu V, Charlotte F, Bernhardt C, et al. Long-term efficacy of rosiglitazone in nonalcoholic steatohepatitis: results of the Fatty Liver Improvement by Rosiglitazone Therapy (FLIRT 2) extension trial. Hepatology 2010;51: 445–53.

75. Mahady SE, Walker S, Sanyal A, et al. The role of thiazolidinediones in non-alcoholic steatohepatitis—a systematic review and meta analysis. J Hepatol 2011;55:1383–90.

76. Singh S, Loke YK, Furberg CD. Long-term risk of cardiovascular events with rosiglitazone: a meta-analysis. JAMA 2007;298:1189–95.

77. Lincoff AM, Wolski K, Nicholls SJ, et al. Pioglitazone and risk of cardiovascular events in patients with type 2 diabetes mellitus: a meta-analysis of randomized trials. JAMA 2007;298:1180–8.

78. Murphy CE, Rodgers PT. Effects of thiazolidinediones on bone loss and fracture. Ann Pharmacother 2007;41:2014–8.

79. Schwartz AV, Sellmeyer DE, Vittinghoff E, et al. Thiazolidinedione use and bone loss in older diabetic adults. J Clin Endocrinol Metab 2006;91: 3349–54.

80. Lewis JD, Ferrara A, Peng T, et al. Risk of bladder cancer among diabetic patients treated with pioglitazone: interim report of a longitudinal cohort study. Diabetes Care 2011;34:916–22.

81. Pagadala M, Zein CO. Predictors of steatohepatitis and advanced fibrosis in non-alcoholic fatty liver disease. Clin Liver Dis 2009;13:591–606.

82. Durbin RJ. Thiazolidinedione therapy in the prevention/delay of type 2 diabetes in patients with impaired glucose tolerance and insulin resistance. Diabetes Obes Metab 2004;6:280–5.

83. Gerstein HC, Yusuf S, Bosch J, et al. Effect of rosiglitazone on the frequency of diabetes in patients with impaired glucose tolerance or impaired fasting glucose: a randomised controlled trial. Lancet 2006;368:1096–105.

84. Parola M, Muraca R, Dianzani I, et al. Vitamin E dietary supplementation inhibits transforming growth factor beta 1 gene expression in the rat liver. FEBS Lett 1992;308:267–70.

85. Houglum K, Venkataramani A, Lyche K, et al. A pilot study of the effects of d-alpha-tocopherol on hepatic stellate cell activation in chronic hepatitis C. Gastroenterology 1997;113:1069–73.

86. Nobili V, Manco M, Devito R, et al. Lifestyle intervention and antioxidant therapy in children with nonalcoholic fatty liver disease: a randomized, controlled trial. Hepatology 2008;48:119–28.

87. Bugianesi E, Gentilcore E, Manini R, et al. A randomized controlled trial of metformin versus vitamin E or prescriptive diet in nonalcoholic fatty liver disease. Am J Gastroenterol 2005;100:1082–90.

88. Miller ER 3rd, Pastor-Barriuso R, Dalal D, et al. Meta-analysis: high-dosage vitamin E supplementation may increase all-cause mortality. Ann Intern Med 2005;142:37–46.

89. Harrison SA, Fecht W, Brunt EM, et al. Orlistat for overweight subjects with nonalcoholic steatohepatitis: a randomized, prospective trial. Hepatology 2009;49:80–6.

90. Zelber-Sagi S, Kessler A, Brazowsky E, et al. A double-blind randomized placebo-controlled trial of orlistat for the treatment of nonalcoholic fatty liver disease. Clin Gastroenterol Hepatol 2006;4:639–44.

91. Omer Z, Cetinkalp S, Akyildiz M, et al. Efficacy of insulin sensitizing agents in nonalcoholic fatty liver disease. Eur J Gastroenterol Hepatol 2010;22:18–23.

92. Lindor KD, Kowdley KV, Heathcote EJ, et al. Ursodeoxycholic acid for treatment of nonalcoholic steatohepatitis: results of a randomized trial. Hepatology 2004; 39:770–8.

93. Dufour JF, Oneta CM, Gonvers JJ, et al. Randomized placebo-controlled trial of ursodeoxycholic acid with vitamin E in nonalcoholic steatohepatitis. Clin Gastroenterol Hepatol 2006;4:1537–43.

94. Santos VN, Lanzoni VP, Szejnfeld J, et al. A randomized double-blind study of the short-time treatment of obese patients with nonalcoholic fatty liver disease with ursodeoxycholic acid. Braz J Med Biol Res 2003;36:723–9.

95. Nelson A, Torres DM, Morgan AE, et al. A pilot study using simvastatin in the treatment of nonalcoholic steatohepatitis: a randomized placebo-controlled trial. J Clin Gastroenterol 2009;43:990–4.

96. Basaranoglu M, Acbay O, Sonsuz A. A controlled trial of gemfibrozil in the treatment of patients with nonalcoholic steatohepatitis. J Hepatol 1999;31:384.

97. Merat S, Malekzadeh R, Sohrabi MR, et al. Probucol in the treatment of nonalcoholic steatohepatitis: a double-blind randomized controlled study. J Hepatol 2003;38:414–8.

98. Harrison SA, Torgerson S, Hayashi P, et al. Vitamin E and vitamin C treatment improves fibrosis in patients with nonalcoholic steatohepatitis. Am J Gastroenterol 2003;98:2485–90.

99. Abdelmalek MF, Sanderson SO, Angulo P, et al. Betaine for nonalcoholic fatty liver disease: results of a randomized placebo-controlled trial. Hepatology 2009;50:1818–26.

100. Pamuk GE, Sonsuz A. N-acetylcysteine in the treatment of non-alcoholic steatohepatitis. J Gastroenterol Hepatol 2003;18:1220–1.

101. Livingston EH. Procedure incidence and in-hospital complication rates of bariatric surgery in the United States. Am J Surg 2004;188:105–10.

102. NIH conference. Gastrointestinal surgery for severe obesity. Consensus development conference panel. Ann Intern Med 1991;115:956–61.

103. Dixon JB, Bhathal PS, Hughes NR, et al. Nonalcoholic fatty liver disease: Improvement in liver histological analysis with weight loss. Hepatology 2004; 39:1647–54.

104. Kral JG, Thung SN, Biron S, et al. Effects of surgical treatment of the metabolic syndrome on liver fibrosis and cirrhosis. Surgery 2004;135:48–58.

105. Klein S, Mittendorfer B, Eagon JC, et al. Gastric bypass surgery improves metabolic and hepatic abnormalities associated with nonalcoholic fatty liver disease. Gastroenterology 2006;130:1564–72.

106. Mathurin P, Hollebecque A, Arnalsteen L, et al. Prospective study of the long-term effects of bariatric surgery on liver injury in patients without advanced disease. Gastroenterology 2009;137:532–40.

107. Mummadi RR, Kasturi KS, Chennareddygari S, et al. Effect of bariatric surgery on nonalcoholic fatty liver disease: systematic review and meta-analysis. Clin Gastroenterol Hepatol 2008;6:1396–402.

108. O'Brien PE, Dixon JB, Brown W. Obesity is a surgical disease: overview of obesity and bariatric surgery. ANZ J Surg 2004;74:200–4.

109. O'Brien PE, Brown WA, Dixon JB. Obesity, weight loss and bariatric surgery. Med J Aust 2005;183:310–4.
110. Buchwald H, Avidor Y, Braunwald E, et al. Bariatric surgery: a systematic review and meta-analysis. JAMA 2004;292:1724–37.
111. Angulo P. NAFLD, obesity, and bariatric surgery. Gastroenterology 2006;130: 1848–52.
112. Cotler SJ, Vitello JM, Guzman G, et al. Hepatic decompensation after gastric bypass surgery for severe obesity. Dig Dis Sci 2004;49:1563–8.
113. Tilg H, Moschen AR. Evolution of inflammation in nonalcoholic fatty liver disease: the multiple parallel hits hypothesis. Hepatology 2010;52:1836–46.
114. Musso G, Gambino R, Cassader M. Obesity, diabetes, and gut microbiota: the hygiene hypothesis expanded? Diabetes Care 2010;33:2277–84.

Index

Note: Page numbers of article titles are in **boldface** type.

A

Abetalipoproteinemia
  NASH and, 537
Acquired errors of metabolism
  NASH and, 536–537
Amiodarone
  steatohepatitis due to, 527
Anticonvulsant mood stabilizers
  in NASH patients, 622
Antidepressant(s)
  in NASH patients, 621
Antipsychotic agents
  in NASH patients, 622–623
Antiretroviral therapy
  steatohepatitis due to, 530–531
Apoptosis
  as Hh signaling amplifier, 552–553
  markers of
    in noninvasive diagnosis of NASH, 570
Autocrine signaling, 551

B

Bacterial overgrowth
  NASH due to, 534–535
Ballooning
  in NASH prognosis, 492
Bariatric surgery
  in NASH management, 636–637
Behavioral therapy
  in NASH management, 634–635
Benzodiazepine sedatives
  in NASH patients, 623
Brachial artery
  flow-mediated vasodilation of
    NAFLD and, 601–602
Buspirone
  in NASH patients, 623

Clin Liver Dis 16 (2012) 647–657
doi:10.1016/S1089-3261(12)00072-4
1089-3261/12/$ – see front matter © 2012 Elsevier Inc. All rights reserved.

liver.theclinics.com

C

Cannabis
  steatohepatitis due to, 531–532
Canonical signaling, 550–551
Cardiovascular disease (CVD)
  NAFLD and
    biologic mechanisms in, 606–608
    incidence of, 602–606
    mortality associated with, 606
Cardiovascular disease (CVD) markers
  subclinical
    NAFLD and, 600–602
Cardiovascular system
  NAFLD and, **599–613**. *See also* Nonalcoholic fatty liver disease (NAFLD), cardiovascular
    link to
Carotid artery
  ultrasound of, 600–601
Celiac disease
  NASH and, 536
Chemotherapy-associated steatohepatitis, 530
Children
  NAFLD in
    vs. adults, **587–598**. *See also* Nonalcoholic fatty liver disease (NAFLD), in children *vs.*
      adults
Cholinesterase inhibitors
  in NASH patients, 624
Cirrhosis, 557
Computed tomography (CT)
  of coronary artery calcifications
    NAFLD and, 601
  in fibrosis assessment in NASH, 580
CT. *See* Computed tomography (CT)
CVD. *See* Cardiovascular disease (CVD)

D

DEAEH. *See* 4,4'-Diethylaminoethoxyhexestrol (DEAEH)
Diet
  in NASH management, 633–634
Dietary factors
  in hepatic steatosis, 515–517
4,4'-Diethylaminoethoxyhexestrol (DEAEH)
  steatohepatitis due to, 527–529
Drug-induced steatohepatitis, 526–532
  amiodarone, 527
  antiretroviral therapy, 530–531
  cannabis, 531–532
  chemotherapies, 530
  glucocorticoids, 530
  methotrexate, 529–530

perhexiline maleate and DEAEH, 527–529
prevalence of, 526
tamoxifen, 529

E

Eating disorders
    obesity and, 618–619
Elastography
    magnetic resonance
        in fibrosis assessment in NASH, 579–580
    transient
        in fibrosis assessment in NASH, 578–579
Enzyme(s)
    liver
        as surrogate marker in NAFLD diagnosis, 602–603
Epigenetics
    in NAFLD, 482–483
Exercise
    in NASH management, 634

F

Familial hypobetalipoproteinemia
    NASH and, 537
Fatty liver disease
    gut microbiota and, 518–519
Fibrosis. *See* Liver fibrosis

G

Gene(s)
    in NAFLD, 480–481
Genetic(s)
    in hepatic steatosis, 514–515
    in NAFLD, 589–590
Genetic diseases
    metabolic diseases and, 536–537
Glucocorticoids
    steatohepatitis due to, 530
Glucose homeostasis
    in hepatic steatosis
        micro-RNA regulation of, 517–518
Growth hormone deficiency
    NASH and, 532–533
Gut microbiota
    fatty liver disease due to, 518–519

H

HCC. *See* Hepatocellular carcinoma (HCC)
HDL. *See* High-density lipoprotein (HDL)
Hedgehog (Hh) ligands, 551

Hedgehog (Hh) signaling pathway
    amplifiers of
        apoptosis and inflammation, 552–553
    canonical signaling, 550–551
    in HCC
        dysregulation of, 557–558
    in injured liver
        activation of, 552
    noncanonical signaling, 551
    overview of, 550–551
    in repair and regeneration, 553–556
        extracellular matrix, 556
        fibrogenesis and fibrogenic repair, 555
        growth of progenitor population of cells and epithelial-to-mesenchymal transition
            response, 554–555
        OPN and fibrogenesis, 556
        vascular remodeling, 556
Hepatic steatosis
    dietary factors in, 515–517
    genetics in, 514–515
    glucose homeostasis in
        micro-RNA regulation of, 517–518
    gut microbiota and, 518–519
    inflammatory factors in, 507–514
    insulin signaling in
        micro-RNA regulation of, 517–518
    mechanisms of, **505–526**
    metabolic factors in, 506–514
    transcriptional factors in, 507–514
Hepatocellular carcinoma (HCC)
    Hh signaling in
        dysregulation of, 557–558
    in NASH
        risk factors for, 549–550
Hh signaling pathway. *See* Hedgehog (Hh) signaling pathway
High-density lipoprotein (HDL)
    in CVD link to NAFLD, 606–608
Histologic scoring systems
    in prediction of clinically meaningful outcomes in NASH, 488–490
Hypobetalipoproteinemia
    familial
        NASH and, 537
Hypothyroidism
    NASH and, 533–534
Hypoxia
    in NAFLD pathogenesis, 471–476

    I

IBD. *See* Inflammatory bowel disease (IBD)
Inborn errors of metabolism
    NASH and, 536–537

Inflammation
    as Hh signaling amplifier, 552–553
Inflammatory bowel disease (IBD)
    NASH and, 535–536
Inflammatory factors
    in hepatic stenosis, 507–514
Insulin sensitizers
    in NASH management, 635–636
Insulin signaling
    in hepatic steatosis
        micro-RNA regulation of, 517–518
Intestinal factors
    NASH associated with, 534–536

L

Lifestyle modification
    in NASH management, 632–635
        behavioral therapy, 634–635
        dietary recommendations, 633–634
        evidence from controlled trials, 632
        evidence from observational studies, 632–633
        exercise, 634
        weight loss, 635
Ligand(s)
    Hh, 551
Lipodystrophy(ies)
    NASH and, 537
Lipoprotein
    high-density
        in CVD link to NAFLD, 606–608
Lithium
    in NASH patients, 621–622
Liver biopsy
    in NASH diagnosis and staging, 568
        limitations of, 499–500, 568–569
Liver disease(s). *See also specific diseases*
    pharmacokinetic effects of, 620–621
Liver enzymes
    as surrogate marker in NAFLD diagnosis, 602–603
Liver "fat remodeling" hypothesis
    PNPLA3 and, 469–470
Liver fibrosis
    in NASH
        imaging assessment of, 578–580
            CT in, 580
            MRE in, 579–580
            MRI in, 580
            transient elastography in, 578–579
        prognostic indicators, 490–491
        risk factors for, 549–550

Liver (*continued*)
      serum markers of, 572–577
         direct markers, 576
         proprietary predictive panels, 576–577
         simple laboratory tests, 572–573
            with clinical markers, 573–576
    stellate cell and, 557
    2-hit model of, 550
Liver histology
    in NASH
        in predicting clinically meaningful outcomes, **487–504**. *See also* Nonalcoholic
            steatohepatitis (NASH), clinically meaningful outcomes in, liver histology in
            prediction of

M

Magnetic resonance elastography (MRE)
    in fibrosis assessment in NASH, 579–580
Magnetic resonance imaging (MRI)
    in fibrosis assessment in NASH, 580
Mallory-Denk bodies (MDBs)
    in NASH prognosis, 491–492
MDBs. *See* Mallory-Denk bodies (MDBs)
Memantine
    in NASH patients, 624
Mental health
    obesity and
        mechanisms linking, 620
Metabolic diseases
    NASH and, 536–537
Metabolic factors
    in hepatic stenosis, 506–514
Methotrexate
    steatohepatitis due to, 529–530
Micro-RNA regulation
    in hepatic steatosis
        in insulin signaling and glucose homeostasis, 517–518
Microbiota
    gut
        fatty liver disease due to, 518–519
Mood/anxiety disorders
    obesity and, 618
MRE. *See* Magnetic resonance elastography (MRE)
MRI. *See* Magnetic resonance imaging (MRI)

N

NAFLD. *See* Nonalcoholic fatty liver disease (NAFLD)
NASH. *See* Nonalcoholic steatohepatitis (NASH)
Nonalcoholic fatty liver disease (NAFLD)
    cardiovascular link to, **599–613**
        biologic mechanisms in, 606–608
        clinical perspective on, 608–609

HDL in, 606–608
incidence of, 602–606
mortality-related, 606
subclinical CVD
   brachial artery flow-mediated vasodilation in, 601–602
   coronary artery calcifications in
     CT of, 601
   marker for, 600–602
   pulse-wave velocity in, 602
   ultrasound of carotid artery in, 600–601
in children *vs.* adults, **587–598**
   diagnosis, 591–593
   genetics, 589–590
   histology, 591–593
   management, 593–595
   natural history, 590–591
   pathophysiology of, 589
   quality of life, 590–591
described, 587–589
diagnosis of
   in children *vs.* adults, 591–593
   liver enzymes as surrogate marker in, 602–603
   ultrasound as surrogate marker in, 603–606
epidemiology of
   genetic, **467–485**. *See also* Nonalcoholic fatty liver disease (NAFLD), genetic
     epidemiology of
epigenetics in, 482–483
gene(s) in, 480–481
genetic architecture of, 476–480
genetic epidemiology of, **467–485**
   beyond DNA sequence variation, 482–483
   described, 467–469
   future challenges related to, 480–481
   joining effects of genetic variants from multiple pathways, 470–471
   next-generation sequencing techniques
     potential advance generated by, 481–482
   PNPLA3 in, 469–470
   prioritization based on previous reported loci, 471–476
   systems biology approaches, 470–471
genetic susceptibility to, 470–471
histology of
   in children *vs.* adults, 591–593
mortality due to
   CVD and, 606
natural history of
   in children *vs.* adults, 590–591
obesity and, 616. *See also* Obesity
pathogenesis of
   molecular mediators of, 471–476
pathophysiology of
   in children *vs.* adults, 589

Nonalcoholic (*continued*)
    prevalence of, 505, 599–600
    quality of life with
        in children *vs.* adults, 590–591
    sexual dimorphism of
        RS738409 variant and, 470
    treatment of
        in children *vs.* adults, 593–595
        psychiatric drugs in, **615–629**
            recommendations for clinical decision making,
                624–625
Nonalcoholic steatohepatitis (NASH)
    background of, 567–568
    bacterial overgrowth and, 534–535
    celiac disease and, 536
    clinically meaningful outcomes in
        liver histology in prediction of, **487–504**
            histologic features in prognostication, 490–492, 498–500
                ballooning, 490–491
                fibrosis, 492
                MDBs, 491–492
            histologic scoring systems, 488–490
            limitations of, 499–500
            variability in diagnosing individual pathologic lesions, 499
    definition of
        lack of consensus for, 499
    described, 488, 525–526, 631–632
    diagnosis of
        liver biopsy in, 568
            limitations of, 568–569
        noninvasive, **567–585**
            apoptosis markers in, 570
            clinical and laboratory variables in, 570
            routine imaging studies in, 570–571
    disease progression in
        fibrosis and stellate cell, 557
        mechanisms of, **549–565**. *See also specific mechanisms and* Hedgehog (Hh)
            signaling pathway
            future directions in, 558–559
        repair gone awry, 557–558
    fibrosis in
        imaging assessment of, 578–580. *See also* Liver fibrosis, in NASH, imaging
            assessment of
        risk factors for, 549–550
        serum markers of, 572–577. *See also* Liver fibrosis, in NASH, serum markers of
    genetic diseases and, 536–537
    growth hormone deficiency and, 532–533
    HCC in
        risk factors for, 549–550
    histologic progression of, 488
    hypothyroidism and, 533–534

IBD and, 535–536
intestinal factors in, 534–536
lipodystrophies and, 537
metabolic diseases and, 536–537
mortality associated with, 493–498
   all-cause related, 493–496
   cardiovascular-related, 496–497
   liver-related, 497
   posttransplant-related, 498
nutritional factors in, 534
pathways to, **525–548**
pharmacokinetic effects of, 620–621
prevalence of, 488, 505
staging of
   liver biopsy in, 568
treatment of, **631–645**
   bariatric surgery in, 636–637
   future research agenda in, 637
   lifestyle modification in, 632–635. *See also* Lifestyle modification, in NASH
      management
   pharmacologic, 635–636
      psychiatric drugs in
         anticonvulsant mood stabilizers, 622
         antidepressants, 621
         antipsychotics, 622–623
         benzodiazepine sedatives, 623
         buspirone, 623
         cholinesterase inhibitors, 624
         interactions between hypolipidemic and psychiatric drugs, 624
         lithium, 621–622
         memantine, 624
         nonbenzodiazepine sedatives, 623
         pharmacokinetic effects, 620–624
         psychostimulants, 623
      psychological, **615–629**
in twenty-first century, 549–550
Noncanonical signaling, 551
Nuclear receptors
in NAFLD pathogenesis, 471–476
Nutritional factors
NASH associated with, 534

O

Obesity
mental health and
   mechanisms linking, 620
NAFLD and, 616
psychiatric disorders and, 617–620. *See also specific disorders*
   eating disorders, 618–619
   mood/anxiety disorders, 618

Obesity (*continued*)
    relationship between, 617–620
    schizophrenia, 619–620
  psychological and psychiatric management of, **615–629**
  weight-loss interventions for, 616–617
  weight-loss programs for
    suboptimal weight loss and weight regain in, 617
Occupational steatohepatitis, 532
OPN
  fibrogenesis and, 556
Orlistat
  in NASH management, 636

P

Paracrine signaling, 551
Perhexiline maleate
  steatohepatitis due to, 527–529
PNPLA3 gene
  liver "fat remodeling" hypothesis and, 469–470
  NAFLD and, 469–470
  sex interaction and, 470
Psychiatric disorders
  obesity and, 617–620. *See also specific disorders and* Obesity, psychiatric disorders
    and
Psychostimulants
  in NASH patients, 623
Pulse-wave velocity
  NAFLD and, 602

Q

Quality of life
  NAFLD effects on
    in children *vs.* adults, 590–591

R

RS738409 variant
  in sexual dimorphism of NAFLD, 470

S

Sex interaction
  gene by
    PNPLA3 and, 470
Steatohepatitis
  chemotherapy-associated, 530
  drug-induced, 526–532. *See also* Drug-induced steatohepatitis
  nonalcoholic. *See* Nonalcoholic steatohepatitis (NASH)
  occupational, 532

Steatosis
    diagnosis of
        noninvasive, 569
            clinical and laboratory variables in, 569
    hepatic
        mechanisms of, **505–526**. *See also* Hepatic steatosis
Stellate cells
    liver fibrosis and, 557

T

Tamoxifen
    steatohepatitis due to, 529
Transcriptional factors
    in hepatic stenosis, 507–514
Transient elastography
    in fibrosis assessment in NASH, 578–579

U

Ultrasound
    of carotid artery, 600–601
    as surrogate marker in NAFLD diagnosis, 603–606

V

Vasodilation
    flow-mediated
        of brachial artery
            NAFLD and, 601–602
Vitamin E
    in NASH management, 636

W

Weber-Christian disease
    NASH and, 537
Weight loss
    interventions for, 616–617
    in NASH management, 635
    suboptimal
        in weight-loss programs, 617
Weight-loss programs
    suboptimal weight loss and weight regain in, 617
Weight regain
    in weight-loss programs, 617
Wilson disease
    NASH and, 536

Moving?

Make sure your subscription moves with you!

To notify us of your new address, find your **Clinics Account Number** (located on your mailing label above your name), and contact customer service at:

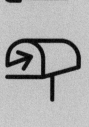

Email: journalscustomerservice-usa@elsevier.com

800-654-2452 (subscribers in the U.S. & Canada)
314-447-8871 (subscribers outside of the U.S. & Canada)

Fax number: 314-447-8029

Elsevier Health Sciences Division
Subscription Customer Service
3251 Riverport Lane
Maryland Heights, MO 63043

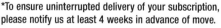